Clinical and Educational Child Psychology

Clinical and Educational Child Psychology

An Ecological-Transactional Approach to Understanding Child Problems and Interventions

Linda Wilmshurst

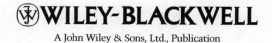

WILEY-BLACKWELL

A John Wiley & Sons, Ltd., Publication

Wiley-Blackwell is an imprint of John Wiley & Sons, formed by the merger of Wiley's global Scientific, Technical and Medical business with Blackwell Publishing.

Registered Office
John Wiley & Sons Ltd, The Atrium, Southern Gate, Chichester, West Sussex, PO19 8SQ, UK

Editorial Offices
350 Main Street, Malden, MA 02148-5020, USA
9600 Garsington Road, Oxford, OX4 2DQ, UK
The Atrium, Southern Gate, Chichester, West Sussex, PO19 8SQ, UK

For details of our global editorial offices, for customer services, and for information about how to apply for permission to reuse the copyright material in this book please see our website at www.wiley.com/wiley-blackwell.

Library of Congress Cataloging-in-Publication Data

Wilmshurst, Linda.
  Clinical and educational child psychology : an ecological-transactional approach to understanding child problems and interventions / Linda Wilmshurst.
    p. cm.
  Includes index.
  ISBN 978-1-119-95226-8 (cloth) – ISBN 978-1-119-95225-1 (pbk.)   1. Developmental psychology.   2. Child psychology.   3. Clinical child psychology.   I. Title.
  BF713.W55 2013
  618.92'89–dc23

                                                                           2012029604

A catalogue record for this book is available from the British Library.

Cover image: Photo © Cathy Yeutet / 123RF
Cover design by www.cyandesign.co.uk

1   2013

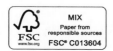

Contents

Part One
The Foundations

1
Child and Adolescent Development: Normal and Atypical Variations

Introduction

What is normal behavior and when does deviation from the norm become serious enough to warrant a label of "abnormal" behavior? Can behavior be considered normal in one context and abnormal in another? Can behavior be considered "normal" at one age and "abnormal" or atypical at another age? These are some of the questions that will be addressed throughout this book and in the case study in this chapter.

A case in practice

As you read the case study in the sidebar, ask yourself the question: *"How serious is Pat's problem?"* Pat is experiencing problems in a number of different areas, including social, emotional, and educational. If you were a clinical or educational/school psychologist, and Pat's mother or teacher asked if you thought Pat was in need of intervention, how would you determine the severity of Pat's problems and what important information would you need to know? *What is the first question you should ask?* The first question should be: *How old is Pat?* Because children are growing and

Case study of Pat: an introduction

Pat is experiencing problems in school. Pat never seems to finish assignments on time and takes forever to get started on a task. Yesterday, Pat sat for 15 minutes staring into space, before putting pencil to paper.

When Pat enters the classroom, you can tell immediately if it is going to be a good day or a bad day. One day, Pat can be moody, irritable, and very hard to get along with, and o___ another day, Pat can be happy and almost giddy with excitement. However, on these occasions, it is very easy for Pat to escalate out of control.

Because of the mood swings, Pat is not popular with peers, and basically has no friends, at school. As a result, Pat is often on the sidelines watching as others socialize and have fun.

Fortunately, Pat is a member of the community soccer team, which affords an opportunity to engage in activities with peers on the weekend.

changing, it is imperative to know what the expectations are for Pat, given the age level. If Pat were a preschooler, the mood swings would likely be due to immaturity in emotional control and emotion regulation which is in the process of being

Clinical and Educational Child Psychology, First Edition. Linda Wilmshurst.
© 2013 John Wiley & Sons, Ltd. Published 2013 by John Wiley & Sons, Ltd.

Table 1.1 Guideposts to the study of child development

1. Development unfolds in a *predictable* pattern.
2. Patterns of behavior and skills (thoughts, emotions, motor skills) *build upon previously acquired skills* and progress *towards increasingly complex variants* of these behaviors throughout childhood and adolescence.
3. Although children pass through similar stages or sequences of development, the *rate of mastery* of various milestones can vary widely due to *individual differences*.
4. Some factors that can *influence* a child's rate of skill acquisition, for better or worse, include: **child variables**, such as *heredity, temperament, cognitive ability, motor, affective, and social maturation*; and **environmental variables**, such as *parenting practices, socio-economic status, peers, quality of schooling, culture*, as well as *availability of and access to community resources*. As a result, development is the outcome of the on-going **transactions** between the child and his or her environment.
5. In the **transactional model** (Sameroff & Chandler, 1975), child and parent outcomes are seen to be the result of the on-going interplay of child and environmental factors that influence, respond to, and adapt to changes on several **ecological** levels (Bronfenbrenner, 1979). The application of these models as an over-arching framework for understanding child development across biological, psychological, and social domains has resulted in a complex and comprehensive perspective: the **ecological transactional model** (Cicchetti & Lynch, 1993).

stabilized during this period. However, if Pat is an eight- or 10-year-old child, then our expectation would be for significantly more maturity in areas of emotional control and self-regulation. Additionally, the age of the child would determine which assessment instruments should be used and the type of pre-assessment information that might be useful. Initially, regardless of the focus of concern, understanding the problem requires a fundamental understanding of the nature and course of development.

The nature and course of development

The study of human **development** in the formative years focuses on **predictable** "age-related changes that are *orderly, cumulative and directional*" (DeHart, Sroufe, & Cooper, 2004, p. 4). Knowledge of normal development is a prerequisite to understanding the extent and nature of any deviations from the norm that may exist in social, emotional, or behavioral functioning. In normal development, skills and competencies build on previous foundations, becoming increasingly refined and complex. It is from this predictable framework that deviations in the acquisition of developmental milestones (*physical, cognitive, behavioral, emotional, social*) can be assessed using normal developmental expectations as the guide.

There are several guiding principles from the study of **normal development** that have significant implications for understanding deviations in child development from a clinical and educational perspective. Some of the salient features are presented in Table 1.1.

Transactional processes

The term "transactional" is used to refer to the "interrelations among dynamic biological, psychological and social systems" that provide the necessary framework for the "ongoing and multiple transactions among environmental forces, caregiver characteristics and child characteristics as dynamic, reciprocal contributions" that increase or decrease the likelihood of well-being or psychopathology (Cicchetti & Toth, 1998, p. 226).

The nature of developmental change

Historically, developmental change has been conceptualized as following either a **discontinuous** or **continuous** course, while the major contributing forces have been attributed to the influences of **nature** (*heredity*) or **nurture** (*environment*). Within this framework, outcomes in the form of milestones or benchmarks assist in making comparisons between levels of achievements mastered relative to predicted developmental expectations. The following discussion looks at how theorists have conceptualized the nature of developmental change over time.

Discontinuous versus continuous change

Discontinuous change   Theorists who propose a **discontinuous** pathway conceptualize development as a series of steps or stages which involve the mastery of levels that are distinctively different at each stage. Theoretical models that share this framework include, but are not limited to: Piaget's stages of cognitive development, Freud's psychosexual stage theory, and Erikson's stages of psychosocial development. Within this framework, theorists view change as *quantitative* and *universal* with a consistent set of sequences and a fixed order of progression, regardless of cultural or global context.

Continuous change   Other theorists believe that developmental change progresses in a smooth and **continuous** manner. For example, *information processing theorists* would be interested in studying how a child's memory strategies evolve over time, as the child adds new strategies and skills to his or her repertoire. Memory strategies adopted later in development would be *qualitatively* different from earlier methods used and would build on earlier skill sets. Within this framework, *behavioral theorists* would also consider the development of behavioral patterns as a continuous process of increasingly complex skills that build upon earlier patterns.

Nature versus nurture: historical beginnings   One of the most controversial themes surrounding child development that has sparked endless debate is the relative contribution of **nature** (heredity) versus **nurture** (environment).

Nature   On one side of the historical debate, the eighteenth-century French philosopher Jean-Jacques Rousseau challenged assumptions regarding the importance of the environment for one's development and argued that nature was the supreme influence over the course of development. According to Rousseau, if parents were to adopt a **laissez-faire** approach (leaving the child alone and not interfering), the child would unfold naturally and blossom like a flower. For Rousseau, development was best represented as a series of stages (infancy, childhood, late childhood, and adolescence) that were programmed to unfold in a predictable pattern (discontinuous process).

Nurture   On the other side of the debate, proponents supported the views of the seventeenth-century English philosopher John Locke, who argued for the importance of "nurturance" in child rearing. According to Locke, children begin their existence as a **tabula rasa**, or blank slate, and are dependent on those around them to nurture their existence by filling their slates with knowledge. Locke would have been supportive of change as a continuous process, evident in the increasingly complex changes that result under the tutelage of adult mentors.

Nature's child   Just prior to 1800, a 12-year-old **feral** child was discovered in a forest in Aveyron, France that would put the nature/nurture debate to the test. A medical student, Jean Itard, took the *wild boy of Aveyron* into his home and devoted years to an attempt to civilize the boy whom he named Victor. However, after many years of instruction, Victor made minimal progress in improving his language and social skills. Victor's late discovery and subsequent failure to acquire language not only stressed the importance of **nurture** (early environment) on development, but also suggested the existence of critical or **sensitive periods** for the acquisition of certain skill sets.

Feral children today

Dramatic evidence of the importance of nurture continues to come forth in the occasional reports of "feral" children (children raised in isolation or by animals) who are discovered living in the wild or in severe isolation (cases of severe confinement and abuse). Support for the importance of early environmental stimulation is apparent, since the feral children often demonstrate significant and irreversible developmental delays.

Nature and nurture: contemporary trends   Today, theorists focus on the dynamic *interaction* between nature and nurture. While it was once thought that the direction of influence was primarily unilateral, from the parent to the child (parent → child), social cognitive and social learning theorists such as Albert Bandura (1986) expanded this notion to emphasize the **bidirectional** nature of the process, where the parent influences the child but the child is also instrumental in influencing responses from the parent (parent ←→ child). Furthermore, influences were seen to be evident in three important contexts, including the environment (persons and situational events), personal/cognitive factors (temperament, affect, biological factors), and behavior (see Figure 1.1).

In Bandura's social learning model, **reciprocal determinism** represents the dynamic interchange between the person, the behavior, and the environment. This model of **triadic reciprocity** encompasses an on-going process where individuals adapt and adjust behavioral responses to changes in environmental demands by adjusting their cognition, affect, and beliefs in responses to feedback. A scenario that follows Bandura's model would include, for example, parents (*environmental*) who attempt to improve a child's weak social skills (*personal/cognitive factor*) by enrolling the child in a social group experience to improve social behaviors (*behavior*), or a teacher who provides remedial academic support (*environment*), for a student whose academic self-esteem is low (*personal factor*) in order to improve on-task behavior and academic

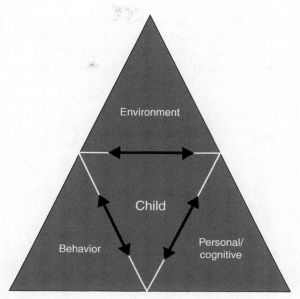

Figure 1.1 Reciprocal determinism.

According to Bandura's (1986) theory of reciprocal determinism, the contexts that can influence a child's behavior include: the *environment* and potential reinforcers (people, situations, physical surroundings), *personal/cognitive factors* (temperament, response style, cognitive-developmental level, which influence beliefs, expectations, and future responses), and *behavior* (responses that may or may not have been reinforced in the past. It is important to note that the arrows are bidirectional, in that a response in one area will impact responses in another and vice versa.

success (*behavior*). Although Bandura's model increased our understanding of the reciprocal and triadic nature of influences, the model did not address how biological or maturational factors might impact this process. More recently, theorists have focused on the **transactional nature** of the process (i.e., *influences of change are themselves changed in the process*) and have attempted to incorporate this model into a developmental framework (Cicchetti & Lynch, 1993).

Transactional processes in action: a case example

After careful deliberation, Jane decides to attend a university in Paris despite the fact that the majority of her friends will remain in London and she is not completely fluent in French. Her choice represents the starting point for a number of experiences and changes that will be very different from what she would have encountered had she remained in London. Furthermore, the resulting changes (attitudes, behaviors, her manner of dress and language) will also exert their influence on how she responds to her environment and how those in her environment respond to her. Jane's case is an example of the transactional process in action.

As will be discussed in *Chapter 2*, the first few years of life represent a time when the developing brain is highly vulnerable to environmental stimulation, as new neural connections are being created, and old, under-stimulated pathways are being discarded. Research has informed us that the quality of early stimulation, both mentally and emotionally, can have a profound and often prolonged influence on later development. There is also evidence to suggest that early emotional trauma may cause profound changes in one's future ability to respond to stressful situations. For example, elevated levels of the neurotransmitter **norepinephrine** and the hormone **cortisol** may, over time, alter the ability of the **hippocampus** (the portion of the brain that regulates stress hormones) to adapt to stressful circumstances (Bremner, 1999).

The high cost of living in an orphanage

O'Connor et al. (2000) studied severely deprived children from Romanian orphanages who were subsequently adopted into homes in the United Kingdom. The study compared outcomes for children who were adopted in the first six months with those that had remained in the orphanage for up to two years. Results indicated that although all the children demonstrated significant improvement, those who had been at the orphanage longest (for two years' duration) continued to experience significant cognitive impairment four to six years post adoption.

In a discussion of the impact of environmental and biological influences on development, Bronfenbrenner (2001) discusses the results of a study conducted in the Dutch city of Nijmegen, by a developmental psychologist (Riksen-Walraven, as cited in Bronfenbrenner, 2001). In this study involving 100 nine-month-old infants, parents were given a "Workbook for Parents" designed to reflect one of three conditions: a stimulation group, a responsiveness group, and a combined group. In the stimulation group, parents were advised that stimulation was the key to positive growth and their workbook contained a number of activities for parents to direct and promote engaged learning. Parents in the responsiveness group were instructed, much as Rousseau would have advised, to let the children "blossom" on their own, not to interfere or direct, but to provide opportunities for self-discovery. Workbooks for the third group of parents contained a mix of the two approaches.

Results revealed that children in the responsiveness group demonstrated the most significant gains on tasks of exploration and learning, followed next by the stimulation group, and lastly, the combined group. Furthermore, long-term follow-up, at 7, 10, and 12 years of age, revealed lasting effects for the responsiveness group, with teachers rating these children as more "competent and skillful" than peers in the other two groups; however, this was true only for the girls, and not the boys. The authors reasoned that during the course of the experiment (which took place in the late 1970s and 1980s), parents' beliefs in the need for responsiveness strengthened their parenting practices by allowing females far more independence and exploration than would have taken place originally. The experiment was a testimony to the powerful effects that can occur in interactions between biology and the environment. In *Chapter 2*, the focus will be on the nature of theoretical models and how these different perspectives contribute to our understanding of child and adolescent development from a variety of different perspectives: biological, cognitive behavioral, psychodynamic, and parenting practices and family dynamics.

Milestones and periods of development

Milestones in development represent benchmarks for developmental change. Based on the assumption that development proceeds through a predictable set of skills that are acquired, on average, at certain age levels, it is possible to chart an individual child's progress relative to "normal" peer development in several areas, including: social, emotional, cognitive, and behavioral expectations.

Periods of development and expectations for change

Investigators have charted the course of normal development, highlighting milestones (benchmarks) that are predicted to occur within a given range of age-related expectations. Given a child's age and stage of development, it is possible to compare a child's progress relative to normal expectations concerning physical, cognitive, behavioral, emotional, and social development. The actual age ranges included in each stage of development can be arbitrary; however, most sources divide child and adolescent development into five stages:

- infant (0–12 months);
- toddler (12–30 months);
- early childhood or preschool-age (21/2–5 years);
- middle childhood or school-age (6–10/11 years);
- adolescence (11/12–19 years).

The topic of developmental milestones will be addressed at greater length in *Chapter 3* (which addresses milestones in early childhood and school-age children) and again in *Chapter 4* (adolescence).

Risk and protective factors

We know that there are several factors that can place children and youth at increased **risk** for difficulties, behavior problems, and school failure, such as: low birth weight, having a difficult temperament, living in an impoverished neighborhood, attending poor quality schools, adverse family conditions, and negative peer influences (Bates, Pettit, Dodge, & Ridge, 1998; Breslau, Paneth, & Lucia, 2004). However, we also know that there are **protective factors** that can help buffer an individual from harm, such as: above average intelligence, supportive parents, and social competence (Williams, Anderson, McGee, & Silva, 1990).

In our opening case study, *was Pat a boy or girl?* If you said that Pat was a boy, you have just placed Pat at increased risk for having a mental health problem, since being male is a risk factor (Rutter, 1989). However, the fact that Pat is involved in sports, and can share activities with peers, provides a protective buffer (Bearman & Moody, 2004). If, on the other hand, Pat is a girl, then she would be at increased risk for developing an eating disorder, depression, and suicidal ideation, since girls who feel isolated and friendless have twice the risk of suicide than their peers (Bearman & Moody, 2004). Throughout the text, risks and protective factors will be discussed, as they relate to the problems and challenges that children and youth face.

Determining the nature and severity of problems

The severity of a given problem or behavior can be evaluated by determining: the **frequency** of the behavior (e.g., *Does the behavior occur on a daily, weekly basis?*); the **duration** of the behavior (*Is the behavior recent versus on-going?*); and whether the behavior is **pervasive** across situations (*Is the behavior evident at home, school, or on the playground?*). Finding answers to these questions will provide an increased understanding of whether the problem represents an adjustment reaction or is a chronic response of a more serious and persistent nature.

Adjustment disorders are a temporary response to a *known* stressor, such as a relocation (e.g., a change of school). Most individuals with adjustment disorders recover within a relatively short period of time (six months), once they have developed the necessary skills to cope with the change. However, for some, the stress caused by the changes may be overwhelming and mark the beginning of a more serious and progressive decline in mental health. In this book, common stressors are identified in a number of different contexts, such as school (transitions), at home (parental or sibling conflict), or peer relationships. These stressful life events can place preschool and primary school-age children and adolescents at increased risk for more serious problems, if they are unable to develop successful strategies to cope with the stressors (*Chapter 6*). In adolescence, peer pressures are discussed that can place some youth at increased risk for opting out of a more traditional role, choosing a path that leads to identity formation as part of a street gang.

In the opening case study, readers were introduced to Pat. However, in the initial case presentation, there was little information given about Pat's age, gender, and family circumstances. Consider the additional information about Pat given in the box.

Case study of Pat: additional information

Pat is a 12-year-old male who lives with his mother who is a single parent. They live in an impoverished neighborhood, and his mother works long hours to make enough money to support them. Pat has no siblings, rarely sees his father, and has been struggling academically for the past two years. With all the physical and emotional changes taking place with the onset of puberty, Pat is having increased problems with regulating his emotions and is becoming increasingly moody. An increase in his academic workload has only added to his problems.

What is the next step? Given the severity of the problem, Pat's mother would be well advised to contact the school psychologist or a private clinician to pinpoint the nature of the problem and determine how significantly Pat's problems deviate from the norm. In addition to interviewing Pat's teachers and parent, there are a number of different assessment instruments available, including: psychometric assessment of intelligence, learning, cognitive, personality, and neuropsychological functioning; behavioral rating scales, projective tests, and tests of academic performance. The psychologist may also want to observe Pat and conduct a functional behavioral assessment to identify problem behaviors and the context in which they are occurring.

Results from the comprehensive psychological assessment reveal that Pat has a number of difficulties that are contributing to his problems. Pat has problems with inattention, concentration, sustaining attention for effortful tasks, disorganization, ease of distractibility, and follow-through to task completion. There are also mood fluctuations that range from irritability to giddy behaviors, evidence of grandiose beliefs, incessant talking, and racing thoughts. Socially, Pat feels isolated at school, although he is grateful that he can hang with his soccer buddies after the games. Although Pat does not admit to suicidal ideation, scores on the depression inventory are a cause for concern. Academically, Pat is scoring approximately two grades below level, despite intelligence in the high average range.

Diagnosis and classification

What is the benefit of a diagnosis?

At this point, we have confirmed that Pat has a number of significant problems. However, the specific nature of the problems, what is causing the problems (etiology), and how the problems can best be treated are not self-evident. As you read this book, the importance of a correct diagnosis will become increasingly apparent. Once a diagnosis is made, then an entire body of pre-existing knowledge becomes available to inform professionals about the nature and typical course of the disorder and the best empirically supported treatments available, clinically, or the best intervention plans that can be executed within the school setting.

Diagnosis from a clinical perspective There are two major systems of clinical classification for diagnostic purposes: the *Diagnostic and Statistical Manual of Mental Disorders* (DSM), published by the American Psychiatric Association (APA, 2000) and the *International Classification of Diseases* (ICD), published by the World Health Organization (WHO, 1992). The classification systems provide a list of symptoms and conditions that must be met in order to be given a specific diagnosis. These two systems are **categorical** systems (an either/or system or binary system) that the practitioner uses to decide whether conditions are met (does the client meet the criteria?) to warrant a diagnosis. While the DSM is used primarily in North America, the ICD is used widely throughout Europe.

Another method of classification that is not categorical and may be more conducive to describing child and adolescent problems is the **dimensional classification system**, which conceptualizes behavior along a continuum of severity. Information about behavior is obtained by having parents and teachers complete behavioral rating scales to indicate the extent to which a given behavior (e.g., playing alone) is evident (never, seldom, often, always). Once scored, these scales often generate a behavioral profile which compares the child's scores for each of the behavioral categories assessed (e.g., anxious/depressed; attention problems; social problems) with what is expected, given the child's age and gender. More information about each of the classification systems is available in *Chapter 5*.

Diagnosis from an educational perspective From an educational perspective, Pat's progress could be monitored and an observational assessment carried out to determine the factors within the classroom environment that exacerbate the difficulty he is experiencing. There may be a number of classroom- and curriculum-related factors that can be adapted to alleviate some of the pressure on Pat. Factors such as length of tasks, expectations, pace of work, type of lessons, and range of lessons can all be adjusted to accommodate his difficulties. In addition, there are many curriculum changes and methods of lesson delivery that can be altered to assist Pat with his learning problems and make his school experience more successful.

Diagnosis and mental health   Pat's symptoms possibly match criteria for a number of different disorders, primarily: attention deficit hyperactivity disorder (ADHD) (as it is called in the DSM) or hyperkinetic disorder of childhood (HDK) (as it is called in the ICD), bipolar disorder (BD), or depression. However, prescribing medication for ADHD/HDK could escalate symptoms of BD, causing violent aggressive outbursts, so it is very important to establish a differential diagnosis. In this case, family history could provide valuable information, since heritability is high in BD. Research has shown that if one parent is diagnosed with BD, there can be a 30–35% risk to the child of having the disorder (Chang, Steiner, & Ketter, 2000). According to Pat's mother, Pat's father was diagnosed with BD in his early twenties and the reason that their marriage broke up was due to his wild mood swings and his refusal to take medication to treat the disorder. Given the history of BD in the family, Pat is at increased risk for BD, a disorder that has alternating episodes of depression and mania. Tests of cognitive function also suggest a learning disability which explains why he has so much difficulty with written expression. Pat also demonstrates another common challenge in working with children and adolescents, which is the tendency for this population to exhibit **comorbidity** (more than one disorder concurrently).

One of the limitations of the current versions of the ICD and DSM classification systems is that they have relatively few diagnoses that are specifically for children, and while children may have some symptoms similar to adults, symptoms often can change relative to the child's developmental level. For example, *generalized anxiety disorder* (GAD) is a disorder characterized by high levels of worry that is "free floating," not attached to any specific cause, and unreasonable. However, while a child might be worried about not doing well at school, or not being liked by friends, an adult might worry that they may become ill, or get into a traffic accident. Depression is another example of how disorders may manifest differently in adults and children. While depression can often be evident in symptoms of sadness, self-blame, and fatigue in adults, it is often expressed as *irritability* in children.

Because of the emphasis on development in this book, the various disorders are presented and described as they would appear during different developmental levels and, rather than adhering to verbatim accounts of criteria from the DSM and ICD, characteristics will be described as they relate to how these problems manifest at different age levels. At the end of this chapter, readers can find an outline of the goals of the book and the presentation format.

Theoretical frameworks: questions of etiology and intervention

An investigation of developmental issues and concerns would not be complete without providing a foundation from which to examine how and why behaviors potentially develop and the nature of their deviation from the normal trajectory. With this goal in mind, *Chapter 2* provides an overview of the various theoretical frameworks that are available to increase our understanding of how and why a problem may have developed.

Returning to our case study of Pat as an example, let us imagine that Pat visits a number of therapists from different theoretical backgrounds who suggest different viewpoints as to the possible cause of and potential treatment for Pat's "depressive symptoms." A therapist from a *biological/neurological perspective* would likely view Pat's depressive symptoms as an indication of low levels of the neurotransmitter serotonin, and genetic vulnerability (Pat's father was diagnosed with BD). Treatment for BD would most likely involve medical management to restore levels to normal; in this case lithium, a mood stabilizer, might be prescribed. From a *behavioral perspective*, the therapist may surmise that Pat's depressive symptoms are being reinforced (rewarded) because every time there is a complaint or default on Pat's part, someone comes to the rescue. Or there is also the possibility that Pat may have learned the behavior by modeling or observing Pat's mother's low level of emotional responsiveness. (Pat's mother was recently also diagnosed with depression, which has been on-going, and undiagnosed, for years.) Developing a contingency plan for rewarding independent and positive behaviors would likely play a key role in the treatment program. A therapist from a *cognitive perspective* would evaluate maladaptive thinking patterns and may suggest that Pat has developed a negative thinking loop (negative triad) which is exaggerating the negative and minimizing the positive events in life. Treatment would involve reframing thought patterns to match more positive thinking models. Finally, a *psychodynamic* therapist might look at past history and discover that Pat has felt emotionally abandoned and has feelings of insecure attachment that influence Pat's ability to relate to others. Long-term psychodynamic therapy may be recommended, or if Pat were younger, play therapy might be a good alternative.

From the school perspective there are a number of initiatives that can be developed to assist Pat in becoming more successful in the classroom. Pat's lack of organizational skills may be a significant roadblock to completing written assignments as Pat seems to spend more time generating random thoughts than putting information down on paper in a logical and predictable sequence. Potential problems with learning, attention, and executive functions will be discussed in *Chapter 8*, along with suggestions for interventions and accommodations for these problems at home and at school.

A transactional ecological bio-psycho-social framework

The contribution that different theoretical models can add to our understanding of child problems is further enhanced when supported by Bronfenbrenner's (1979, 1989) ecological framework. More recently, Bronfenbrenner referred to his model as a bioecological model to emphasize the biological characteristics as fundamental to the dynamic interplay between the child and the environment (Bronfenbrenner & Morris, 1998). This framework assists in emphasizing the interaction between child characteristics (genetics, temperament) and environmental characteristics (immediate and more distal influences), in an on-going and **transactional nature**, such that changes beget changes and that influence is bidirectional in nature. Within this model, the child is in the center of a number of concentric circles that represent influences in the environment: the first wave is the **microsystem** that includes the immediate surroundings, including family, school, neighborhood, and peers; the next wave is the **exosystem** (extended family, economic conditions); and the final level of influence is the **macrosystem** (culture, laws). All of these factors influence and are in turn influenced by the child's individual characteristics (biological make-up, genetic vulnerabilities, intelligence). Interactions between the child and his or her environment ultimately will shape the nature and direction of the child's developmental trajectory as the child acquires the necessary skills for successful adaptation and communication. It is with a growing understanding of the on-going and transactional nature of the process that we have come to appreciate how changes within the child can result in transformations in the environment at all levels depicted above, and that, conversely, changes at all levels of influence can impact the growing individual child, for better or for worse. It is within this over-arching framework that development is presented and discussed as it unfolds in its normal and atypical variations.

Risks, protective factors, and the role of chaotic environments

There has been increased interest in the influence of chaos on human development, especially with respect to the impact of chaotic environments on children's lives. Bronfenbrenner (2001) discusses the rise in "developmental disarray" evident in the lives of children, adolescents, and families which he says permeates the primary life settings from peer groups, to schools, to health care systems. Wachs and Evans (2010) suggest an interesting framework for discussing chaotic environments, drawing upon Joachim Wohlwill's (1970) concept of environment stimulation and Urie Bronfenbrenner's bioecological model. Within this framework, the authors discuss a curvilinear model that addresses potential negative outcomes for over- and under-stimulation, within the contexts of Bronfenbrenner's model of proximal and more distal influences. Some of the environmental aspects influenced by chaos include: scarcity of resources at home or at school, lack of family routines, harsh parenting practices, instability in child care, noise levels in classrooms, and visually chaotic classrooms (Evans & Wachs, 2010). Throughout this book, the concept of chaos will be addressed, as it informs developmental influences in the broader vision of factors influencing development beyond that of a low socio-economic status environment.

Developmental deviations: clinical and educational perspectives

The role of clinical child psychologists and educational psychologists

As will become increasingly clear, clinical child psychologists and educational/school psychologists perform many of the same functions and use many of the same assessment techniques. However, differences may be evident in the specific language that these professions use (clinical versus educational terminology), the settings in which they work (hospitals, schools, mental health clinics), and the focus of their practice.

Clinical child psychologists The goal of the clinical child psychologist is to address the mental health needs of children and adolescents by reducing psychological distress and restoring psychological well-being. Clinical psychologists can be found as part of a multidisciplinary team, working alongside medical practitioners, social workers, and other health professionals, or they can work independently. Common areas of practice include the treatment of psychological disorders such as depression and anxiety, learning disabilities, or serious pathology, such as schizophrenia. The clinical child psychologist may work with the child or adolescent, individually or in a group, or within the context of the family (parents, caregivers). In the United Kingdom, clinical psychologists are most likely to be found "working in health and social care settings including hospitals, health centres, community mental health teams" (British Psychological Society (BPS); http://www.bps.org.uk/careers-education-training/how-become-psychologist/types-psychologists/becoming-educational-psycholo). In the United States, clinical child psychologists can also be found in similar settings (mental health clinics, residential treatment centers, and hospitals, and working within the juvenile justice or child welfare systems), although many clinicians work in private practice. More often than not, clinical psychologists will have a particular area of expertise, such as providing services to child and adolescent populations, rather than adult populations, or in specialized areas of practice, such as marital therapy, addictions, and eating disorders. They may provide on-going therapy to assist with transitions and emotional difficulties, and monitor progress through family contact. Some clinical psychologists teach, and/or are involved in research to investigate the etiology, course, and treatment of psychological disorders.

Historically, clinical child psychology as a discipline gained status in the mid-1980s when Sroufe and Rutter (1984) launched their journal *Development and Psychopathology*, giving the area of developmental psychopathology the unique recognition it deserved and setting it apart from adult clinical psychology.

Educational/school psychologists According to the BPS, "educational psychologists tackle the problems encountered by young people in education, which may involve learning difficulties and social or emotional problems" (www.BPS.org.uk). In the United States and Canada, the term **school psychologist** is used to refer to someone in this profession, and in spite of the difference in titles, the roles are quite similar in Canada, the United States, Western Europe, Australia, and New Zealand. Although educational psychologists also involve parents in gathering information and generally planning for the child, the primary context of intervention is within the school setting, primarily involving the child and his or her teachers, or related professionals (speech and language therapists, physical therapists, school counselors). The educational psychologist's concerns primarily relate to the child's learning needs and the child's ability to profit from his or her educational experiences, and to enable "teachers to become more aware of the social factors affecting teaching and learning" (BPS, http://www.bps.org.uk/careers-education-training/how-become-psychologist/types-psychologists/becoming-educational-psycholo).

Although within the United States the majority of school psychologists are primarily employed within the public school system, some may be employed in a liaison capacity with the public school system, in their employment within private practice, private schools, mental health facilities, learning centers, or hospitals. According to the BPS, the primary employer of educational psychologists in the United Kingdom is also the local education authorities, and as such educational psychologists are most likely to be found in "schools, colleges, nurseries and special units" and to "liaise with other professionals in education, health and social services." However, the BPS notes that there are growing numbers of educational psychologists who can be found working independently or as private consultants.

Historically, educational psychologists and school psychologists have faced similar challenges due to the enactment of educational policy in their respective locations.

The Education Acts of 1981 and 1993 in the United Kingdom placed emphasis on the identification of children with "special educational needs" (SEN) and clearly prioritized assessment as the primary function of educational psychologists (Fallon, Woods, & Rooney, 2010; Woods, 1994). In the United States, a similar movement was launched with the passing of the Education for All Handicapped Children Act (EHA, 1975) and its reauthorization as the Individuals with Disabilities Education Act (IDEA, 1990) which relegated school psychologists to a position as "gate keepers" to special education placements in their assessments to determine placements and on-going meetings to review placements (Dahl, Hoff, Peacock, & Ervin, 2011; Reschly & Ysseldyke, 1995). There is an increasing trend among these professionals, globally, to become more involved in research initiatives, providing input into educational policy, and to become more engaged in practices of training and professional development (Fallon, Woods, & Rooney, 2010; Nastasi & Varjas, 2011).

The intersection of clinical and educational psychology

In her article addressing critical issues children will face in the twenty-first century, Crockett (2004) lists issues including: poverty, violence, bullying and harassment, teen pregnancy/sexual behavior, alcohol and drug abuse, mental health issues and services, diversity and tolerance, and access to quality education and technology. Although this list of issues is based on statistics gathered concerning children in the United States, there is no question that these matters are of global concern in their overall impact on child development and well-being. Additionally, Crockett notes that although these issues represent challenges to all children, responding to these issues is even more challenging for children who experience these difficulties in conjunction with academic, behavioral, and emotional problems. Within this context, shifting roles and priorities, globally, have had an impact on professionals whose main goal is to work with children and adolescents facing these challenges with an increasing need to enhance their skills in all areas (professional training and collaboration). For example, in England, the training of educational psychologists "has moved from a one year Masters to a three year Doctoral programme" (Norwich, Richards, & Nash, 2010), while in the United States, greater numbers of school psychologists at the Master's level are returning to graduate school to upgrade to a Specialist or Doctoral level. Within the last 10 years, several universities in the United States have developed combined Doctoral programs that integrate clinical and school psychology.

Furthermore, policies such as Every Child Matters (DfES, 2004) in Europe and No Child Left Behind (US Department of Education, 2001) in the United States have impacted the further expansion of the role of educational psychologists into areas of consultation and intervention, further blurring the lines between these two "psychologies."

Clinical and educational psychology: international focus on psychology in the schools

According to the WHO (2005), between 5% and 20% of children and adolescents are in need of mental health services, globally. In their attempt to track and identify the mental health needs of children and adolescents, the WHO cites a number of difficulties encountered, including the fact that:

> Child mental health needs are often inter-sectoral or present in systems other than the health or mental health arena. Children with mental health problems are often first seen and first treated in the education, social service or juvenile justice systems. Since a great many problems of youth are identified in the education sector, these problems may or may not get recorded as mental health problems or needs.
>
> (WHO, 2005, p. 7)

In addition, shortage of services is a major roadblock to obtaining appropriate care for mental health issues for children and adolescents, with access rates ranging between 20% and 80%, globally. Scandinavian regions of Europe have the highest access rates, while those countries that have higher proportions of children have the least available services. In order to address growing concerns regarding availability of and access to mental health services for children and adolescents worldwide, the International School Psychology Association (ISPA) distributed a survey to 43 different countries to evaluate the roles, responsibilities, professional preparation, and challenges of school psychologists. The survey revealed that although these individuals shared common professional duties, such as *individual assessment* (of cognitive, social, emotional, and behavioral difficulties), *development of intervention plans*, and *consultation*, there was wide variation in their professional titles (school/educational psychologist, counselor, psychologist in schools/education, psychopedagogue) and the location where they delivered their services. While some professionals were located in the schools, others could be found in clinics, hospitals, and universities (Nastasi & Varjas, 2011). The survey revealed that school psychology services were best developed in the United States, Canada, Western Europe, Israel, Australia, and New Zealand (Jimerson, Oakland, & Farrell, 2007). In their chapter on international implications for school psychology, Nastasi and Varjas (2011, p. 815) emphasize the need to open the doors to more program focus on cultural and global concerns and the infusion of "culturally and contextually relevant (e.g., culturally constructed) programs, promotion of sustainability and institutionalizing, translation to other contexts and dissemination to facilitate international development of school psychology." In the spirit of addressing this need, this book provides an international focus on research, as well as emphasis on global concerns that will assist practitioners in their work with children and adolescents in clinical and educational settings across the world.

Goals and organizational format of this book

The goal of this book is to provide a comprehensive look at typical developmental patterns in childhood and adolescence (two to 18 years of age) and discuss how common challenges encountered during these key periods of development (stressors at home, at school, and in the environment) can influence the developmental trajectory for better or worse, depending on the child's ability to cope and master these challenges. The book will explain why children who encounter multiple stressors may not be successful in developing adequate abilities to control their emotions or regulate their behaviors relative to age-based expectations, and how these children, without important and necessary interventions, may become vulnerable to a host of clinical, educational, and mental health problems. The book is divided into two major parts:

Part One: The foundations;
Part Two: Child and adolescent problems and disorders.

Each part addresses key issues relevant to a better understanding of the extent and nature of child and adolescent problems.

Part One: The foundations

This introductory section consists of five chapters and provides the necessary theoretical background to assist readers in better understanding how children and adolescents develop their perceptions of their world, their feelings about themselves and others, and their responses to these perceptions and feelings.

In *Chapter 2*, readers are introduced to five theoretical models, including: the *biological model* (brain chemistry, anatomy, and function), the *cognitive behavioral model* (the development of thoughts about ourselves and others and how behaviors are learned), the *psychodynamic model* (unconscious motives and defenses, as well as issues in attachment), and *models of parenting practices and family dynamics* (parenting style and family systems theory). Ultimately, the chapter presents an over-arching framework, *a transactional, ecological bio-psycho-social framework* that integrates information from all the theoretical models and encompasses the total child.

In *Chapter 3* and *Chapter 4*, normal developmental milestones are discussed, to provide readers with the necessary benchmarks for development in early and middle childhood (*Chapter 3*) and adolescence (*Chapter 4*), as these changes relate to physical, neurological, cognitive, emotional, and social development. A thorough understanding of the expectations for development in these areas provides the foundation for evaluating the extent of deviation from the norm in later discussions of disordered behaviors. Each of these chapters concludes by presenting the latest contemporary research on the influences of attachment and parenting styles on child and adolescent development.

Chapter 5, the final chapter of Part One, provides an overview of the many ethical issues that are involved in working with children and adolescents, in research and clinical practice. The chapter provides clinical and educational perspectives on the nature of developmental deviations and how these may be assessed and evaluated. Discussion concerning issues of diagnosis and classification looks at some challenges in applying current systems to child and adolescent problems. Ethical issues and concerns facing practitioners working with children and adolescence are discussed as they relate to practice and research, internationally. Finally, international concerns of clinical and educational/school psychologists are discussed as they relate to contemporary child and adolescent issues and current challenges to practice.

Part Two: Child and adolescent problems and disorders

The first chapter of Part Two, *Chapter 6*, is devoted to adjustment problems that children and adolescents can face on a daily basis resulting from stressors in their school, family, and social environment. The discussion of adjustment problems is strategically placed at the beginning of the section because these are common stressors which can interfere with positive developmental outcomes on a temporary basis, but can evolve into more significant disorders if not recognized and addressed appropriately. In this way, these problems can be seen as a bridge between normal and disordered behaviors.

Sequencing of disorder presentation   Recent efforts to revise the *Diagnostic and Statistical Manual of Mental Disorders* (DSM) and *International Classification of Diseases* (ICD) have prompted discussions regarding how best to cluster or group disorders based on information available from recent research. With respect to the reclassification of childhood disorders, Andrews, Pine, Hobbs, Anderson, and Sutherland (2009) conducted a meta-analysis of childhood disorders that currently appear in the DSM (APA, 2000) in the category of "Disorders Usually First Diagnosed in Infancy, Childhood, or Adolescence" and the ICD categories of "Mental Retardation," "Disorders of Psychological Development," and "Behavioral and Emotional Disorders with Onset Usually Occurring in Childhood and Adolescence." As part of their review, Andrews et al. (2009) considered the validity of including different childhood disorders under the umbrella of neurodevelopmental disorders, including: conduct disorder (CD), separation anxiety disorder, attention deficit hyperactivity disorder (ADHD), mental retardation (intellectual disability), pervasive developmental disorders (autistic spectrum disorders), motor disorders, communication disorders, and learning disorders. However, while some disorders seemed to match a number of validating criteria, such as intellectual disability and pervasive developmental disorders, others, such as subtypes of ADHD, shared some features with neurodevelopmental and externalizing disorders, such as CD. Ultimately, Andrews et al. (2009) suggest the possibility of five disorders being clustered within the category of neurodevelopmental disorders, based on genetic etiology, symptom similarity, cognitive impairment, early onset, and persistence of course. The five disorders suggested are: mental retardation (intellectual disability), pervasive developmental disorders (autism spectrum disorders), motor disorders, communication disorders, and learning disorders.

For purposes of this book, *Chapter 7* includes three primary neurodevelopmental disorders (intellectual disability, autistic spectrum disorders, and communication disorders), as well as other disorders with early childhood onset (feeding disorders and selective mutism).

In *Chapter 8*, students are introduced to disorders that involve problems of learning (five types of specific learning disabilities) and attention disorders with or without hyperactivity and impulsivity and how these disorders impact academic performance, as well as social-emotional functioning. From a developmental perspective, these problems are most likely identified within the first two to three years of formal schooling. The chapter provides important information on etiology, identification, and intervention for these disorders.

In *Chapter 9*, the discussion evolves around a wide range of externalizing behaviors which are often the most frequent source of referrals for mental health services. A continuum of behavioral problems are introduced, ranging from mild forms of early aggression to bullying and victimization of peers, behaviors that challenge authority (oppositional defiant disorder), and behaviors that violate the rights of others (conduct disorder). The chapter also addresses recent emphasis on the callous and unemotional specifier for conduct disorder, and how the disorders are assessed and treated.

Internalizing disorders are the focus of *Chapter 10*. In this chapter, some of the most frequent disorders are discussed, including: anxiety disorders (phobias, separation anxiety disorder, generalized anxiety disorder, obsessive compulsive disorder, and panic disorder), mood disorders (major depression, dysthymia, and bipolar disorders), and somatization disorders and somatic concerns. The chapter addresses how these disorders manifest in children at different levels of development, as well as discussing assessment and treatment alternatives. Suicide, which increases greatly in adolescence, is also discussed in this chapter, as well as a very successful school-based suicide prevention program that is available.

There has been growing international concern about the increase in eating disorders and substance use and abuse among children and youth. In *Chapter 11*, these concerns are addressed by discussing the results of numerous surveys that have been conducted internationally to draw attention to the decreasing ages and increasing prevalence rates for eating disorders and substance use and abuse. Empirically supported treatment alternatives and prevention programs are presented.

In *Chapter 12*, the topic of child maltreatment is addressed from an international perspective, as it relates to physical, sexual, and emotional maltreatment, as well as child neglect and situations of multiple maltreatment. Self-injurious behaviors are also addressed in this chapter, because they are often triggered by perceived maltreatment. This chapter is strategically placed prior to discussions of child trauma and trauma disorders, since many children who are maltreated also develop post-traumatic stress disorder (PTSD).

Finally, in *Chapter 13*, the discussion will focus on child trauma and trauma-related disorders. Reactive attachment disorder and acute and post-traumatic stress disorder (PTSD) will be addressed, as well as how symptoms of these disorders manifest across the developmental spectrum. Discussion will focus on concerns regarding the identification of PTSD in preschool children.

Format of the presentation of the clinical disorders   Each of the chapters will be presented in a consistent format which includes a diagnostic description of the disorder, followed by a discussion of the nature and course of the disorder, etiology and prevalence rates, and assessment and treatment alternatives. The following is an overview of the types of information that will be presented in each of the sections outlined, as follows.

Nature and course   This section will provide a description of the disorder/problem. The intention is not to provide a verbatim account of diagnostic criteria as they appear in the DSM or ICD, since readers can access these manuals directly. What will be provided is general information about the disorder, such as symptoms and subtypes, as well as differential diagnostic considerations, and any disparities in how the disorders are conceptualized by the different classification systems.

The section will also provide a description of developmental characteristics, chart the course of the disorder, and present findings from research concerning how the disorder manifests across the different developmental levels.

Etiology and prevalence   Etiology will be discussed in relation to various theoretical frameworks (biological, cognitive-behavioral, psychodynamic (attachment) and parenting styles), and prevalence rates will be provided as they relate to current research in the field.

Assessment and treatment   There are many assessment instruments and checklists that can be used to provide general information about a child's personality, self-esteem, and behavioral profile. Depending on his or her age, questionnaires can be completed by the child/adolescent, or by an adult familiar with the child (parents, caregivers, teachers). In *Chapter 5*, many general assessment instruments are introduced as they relate to the evaluation of cognitive, academic, and psychological/behavioral functioning. This section will very briefly draw attention to symptom-specific instruments that are available to compare a child's or adolescent's level of responses in a particular area (e.g., anxiety, depression) relative to others in the same age range, and will serve to orient readers to other sources for more in-depth information on the instrument.

The importance of identifying empirically supported treatments has gained increasing emphasis, developmentally. The focus will be on providing developmentally appropriate methods of intervention that represent a wide variety of theoretical frameworks (cognitive-behavioral, family systems, play therapy, biomedical management, special education) and systems of delivery (individual, group, and family therapy).

References

American Psychiatric Association (APA). (2000). *Diagnostic and statistical manual of mental disorders* (4th ed., text revision). Washington, DC: Author.

Andrews, G., Pine, D. S., Hobbs, M. J., Anderson, T. M., & Sutherland, M. (2009). Neurodevelopmental disorders: Cluster 2 of the proposed meta-structure for DSM-V and ICD-11. *Psychological Medicine, 39,* 2013–2023.

Bandura, A. (1986). *Social foundations of thought and action: A social cognitive theory.* Englewood Cliffs, NJ: Prentice Hall.

Bates, J. E., Pettit, G. S., Dodge, K. A., & Ridge, B. (1998). The interaction of temperamental resistance to control and parental discipline in the prediction of children's externalizing problems. *Developmental Psychology, 34,* 982–995.

Bearman, P. S., & Moody, J. (2004). Suicide and friendships among American adolescents. *American Journal of Public Health, 94,* 89–95.

Bremner, J. D. (1999). Does stress damage the brain? *Biological Psychiatry, 45,* 797–805.

Breslau, N., Paneth, N. S., & Lucia, V. C. (2004). The lingering effects of low birth weight children. *Pediatrics, 114*(4), 1035–1040.

Bronfenbrenner, U. (1979). *The ecology of human development.* Cambridge, MA: Harvard University Press.

Bronfenbrenner, U. (1989). Ecological systems theory. *Annals of Child Development, 6,* 187–249.

Bronfenbrenner, U. (2001). Growing chaos in the lives of children, youth and families: how can we turn it around?. In J. C. Westman (Ed.), *Parenthood in America* (pp. 197–210). Madison: University of Wisconsin Press.

Bronfenbrenner, U., & Morris, P. A. (1998). The ecology of developmental process. In R. M. Lerner (Ed.), *Handbook of child psychology: Vol. 1. Theoretical models of human development* (5th ed.) (pp. 535–584). Hoboken, NJ: John Wiley & Sons, Ltd.

Chang, K. D., Steiner, H., & Ketter, T. A. (2000). Psychiatric phenomenology of child and adolescent bipolar offspring. *Journal of the American Academy of Child and Adolescent Psychiatry, 39*(4), 453–460.

Cicchetti, D., & Lynch, M. (1993). Toward an ecological/transactional model of community violence and child maltreatment: Consequences for children's development. *Psychiatry, 56,* 96–118.

Crockett, D. (2004). Critical issues children face in the 2000s. *School Psychology Review, 11*(1), 78–82.

Dahl, A., Hoff, K. E., Peacock, G. G., & Ervin, R. A. (2011). The influence of legislation on the practice of school psychology. In M. A. Bray and T. J. Kehle (Eds.), *The Oxford handbook of school psychology* (pp. 745–761). New York: Oxford University Press.

DeHart, G. B., Sroufe, L. A., & Cooper, R. (2004). *Child development: Its nature and course* (5th ed.). New York: McGraw-Hill.

Department for Education and Skills (DfES). (2004). Every child matters: Change for children. Retrieved from https://www.education.gov.uk/publications/standard/publicationDetail/Page1/DfES/1081/2004

Evans, G. W., & Wachs, T. D. (2010). *Chaos and its influence on children's development: An ecological perspective.* Washington, DC: APA.

Fallon, K., Woods, K., & Rooney, S. (2010). A discussion of the developing role of educational psychologists within Children's Services. *Educational Psychology in Practice, 26*(1), 1–23.

Jimerson, S. R., Oakland, T. D., & Farrell, P. T. (Eds.) (2007). *The handbook of international school psychology.* Thousand Oaks, CA: Sage.

Nastasi, B. K., & Varjas, K. (2011). International development of school psychology. In M. A. Bray & T. J. Kehle (Eds.), *The Oxford handbook of school psychology* (pp. 810–828). New York: Oxford University Press.

Norwich, B., Richards, A., & Nash, T. (2010). Educational psychologists and children in care: Practices and issues. *Educational Psychology in Practice: Theory, Research and Practice, 26*(4), 375–390.

O'Connor, T. G., Rutter, M., Beckett, C., Keaveney, L., Kreppner, J. M. & The English and Romanian Adoptees Study Team. (2000). The effects of global severe deprivation on cognitive competence. Extension and longitudinal follow-up. *Child Development, 71,* 376–390.

Reschly, D. J., & Ysseldyke, J. E. (1995). School psychology paradigm shift. In A. Thomas & J. Grimes (Eds.), *Best practices in school psychology – III* (pp. 17–31). Washington, DC: NASP.

Rutter, M. (1989). Isle of Wight revisited: Twenty-five years of child psychiatric epidemiology. *Journal of the American Academy of Child and Adolescent Psychiatry, 28*(5), 633–653.

Sameroff, A., & Chandler, M. (1975). Reproductive risk and the continuum of caretaking casualty. In F. D. Horowitz (Ed.), *Child development research,* vol. 4 (pp. 187–244). Chicago: University of Chicago Press.

Sroufe, L. A., & Rutter, M. (1984). The domain of developmental psychopathology. *Child Development, 55,* 17–29.

US Department of Education. (2001). No Child Left Behind Act. Retrieved from http://www2.ed.gov/policy/elsec/leg/esea02/index.html.

Wachs, T. D., & Evans, G. W. (2010). Chaos in context. In G. W. Evans & T. D. Wachs (Eds.), *Chaos and its influence on children's development: An ecological perspective* (pp. 3–13). Washington, DC: APA.

Williams, S., Anderson, J., McGee, R., & Silva, P. A. (1990). Risk factors for behavioral and emotional disorder in preadolescent children. *Journal of the American Academy of Child and Adolescent Psychiatry, 29,* 413–419.

Wohlwill, J. F. (1970). The emerging discipline of environmental psychology. *American Psychologist, 25*(4), 303–312.

Woods, K. (1994). Towards national criteria for special educational needs. *Educational Psychology in Practice, 10*(2), 85–92.

World Health Organization (WHO). (1992). *The ICD-10 classification of mental and behavioural disorders. Clinical descriptions and diagnostic guidelines.* Geneva: Author.

World Health Organization (WHO). (2005). *Atlas: Child and adolescent mental health. Global concerns: Implications for the future.* Geneva: Author.

2

Theoretical Models

Chapter preview and learning objectives

Developmental changes can be shaped by a variety of contextual influences (heredity and environment) and interpreted from a number of theoretical perspectives. Within this chapter, the nature of developmental change will be viewed from the vantage point of five important theoretical models: the biological model, the cognitive and behavioral models, the psychodynamic model (attachment), and the parenting practices and

Clinical and Educational Child Psychology, First Edition. Linda Wilmshurst.
© 2013 John Wiley & Sons, Ltd. Published 2013 by John Wiley & Sons, Ltd.

family systems model (including theories of parenting style and practices). Ultimately, a transactional ecological bio-psycho-social model will be discussed as the over-arching framework. Information presented in this chapter will provide readers with a better understanding of:

- how different models contribute to our knowledge of developmental change;
- the role of contextual influences in shaping the course of development;
- important neurological and physiological changes that occur in childhood;
- behavior as a learned response;
- the role of cognition in maladaptive thinking;
- the role of parenting practices and attachment styles in outcomes for child development;
- the importance of theoretical models in guiding the development of intervention programs.

Although the child was once seen as a passive recipient of information, we now know that interactions between the child, the caregiver, and other environmental factors are not only bidirectional but represent a complex, dynamic, and on-going process. These influences can alter the trajectory for growth, for better or worse, and shape the course of future development. Contemporary theorists emphasize the **transactional** nature of the developmental process as it unfolds in an environment that may place the child at increased risk or provide him or her with increased opportunities for growth. The transactional process will be discussed in greater detail later in this chapter.

Theoretical models: an introduction

Theoretical models can provide a framework for organizing information, and can assist in understanding the etiology of child and adolescent problems. The case example cited in the text box provides an opportunity to view one disorder, in this case depression, as it might be envisioned by therapists who represent a number of different theoretical (psychodynamic, behavioral, cognitive, and biological) orientations.

In the eye of the beholder

Cecile is concerned about her six-year-old son Jason's increasingly noncompliant behavior; every request turns into a major battlefield. She seeks counsel from four different therapists who all agree that Jason has oppositional and defiant behaviors, but all provide different reasons and suggestions for improvement. The psychodynamic therapist suggests that noncompliance represents an internal and unconscious conflict which is causing anxiety and suggests that struggles represent the conflict between Jason's needs for dependence and autonomy which are at the core of the problem. He recommends conjoint play therapy so that mother and son can work through these conflicts. The behavioral therapist states that noncompliance is being rewarded because the mother gives up after several requests, and then completes the chores herself, and the suggestion is for a program that rewards Jason's compliance with requests. The cognitive therapist states that Jason's noncompliance results from maladaptive thought processes, resulting from Jason's belief that he cannot do anything right to please his mother and has stopped trying as a result (learned helplessness). The biological therapist suggests that the problems between Cecile and Jason relate to their temperaments and that there is not a "goodness of fit" between the two. Basically, Cecile is highly strung and a bit of a perfectionist, while her son Jason is more prone to avoid any emotional tension. Given this mix, Cecile pushes when Jason tries to withdraw and problems escalate into a battle of wills. Training in relaxation exercises will help both to reduce the tension and help them deal with the issues in a calm and reasonable manner.

It is important to recognize, however, that a model can also represent a set of inherent biases and assumptions that can influence the nature of inquiry, the method and target of observations (behaviors that are emphasized and those that are minimized), and the conclusions resulting from the inquiry. As a result, based on the particular model employed, one observer may emphasize how a given behavior is learned through environmental contingencies (according to the *behavioral model*), while another observer may be more likely to evaluate the underlying thought processes and faulty reasoning that are responsible for the same behavior (according to the *cognitive model*). It is evident that each model contributes a given set of assumptions about the behavior based on a unique conceptual framework that will ultimately shape the expectations for future outcomes (social, emotional, cognitive, physical, behavioral), and guide the course of treatment and intervention. From a biological perspective, inherited traits might be the first line of insight into the problem areas, while, if needed, medication might be a therapeutic option if the problem was related to some form of chemical imbalance. From a behavioral or cognitive perspective, programs designed to change existing behaviors or reframe maladaptive thoughts might be the most appropriate course of action.

While it is important to know the contributions that each of these perspectives adds to the overall picture, contemporary theorists have increasingly focused their attention on achieving a better understanding of the relationships between or among the various models and how certain perspectives can provide building blocks and better inform us about how the various aspects of the total child fit the bigger picture. A schematic of the different theoretical models discussed in this book and their predominant focus is presented in Figure 2.1.

The biological model: physical and neurological development

The biological model emphasizes the "nature" side of the heredity and environment equation, and addresses how biological, genetic, and physiological factors contribute to human behavior. From this perspective, causes of behavioral and developmental change can be traced to abnormalities in the **brain** (*anatomy or chemical function/malfunction*) or **genetics** (*heredity and the influence of potential genetic risk factors*). Since brain chemistry can be linked to various mood states (such as

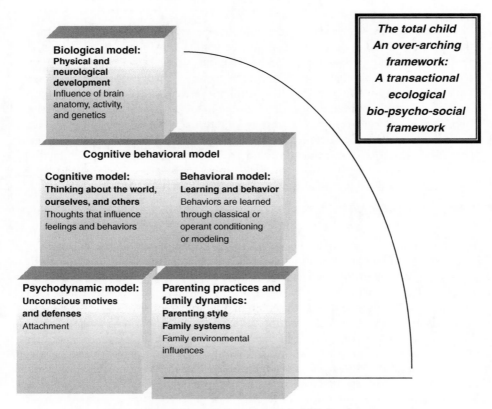

Figure 2.1   Theoretical models and child development.

depression and anxiety), clinicians often rely on a biological answer to explain etiology and provide direction for medical treatment to restore the appropriate chemical balance (neurotransmitter function) and brain function.

Historical advances   Initially, autopsies on humans and research with animals were the only available methods of localizing functions such as memory and sensory receptors in the brain. Increased knowledge from technical advances, such as functional magnetic resonance imagining (fMRI), have provided opportunities to localize activity levels in the brain. As a result, our knowledge of abnormal brain activity in populations with different disorders (dyslexia, attention deficit disorder, schizophrenia, and so on) has increased substantially.

Different brain activity can signal different problems

Children with attention deficit hyperactivity disorder (ADHD) often demonstrate reduced activity in the frontal lobes, while those with dyslexia exhibit over-stimulation of the inferior frontal gyrus (Shaywitz, 1998).

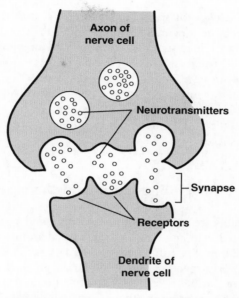

Figure 2.2 Chemical activity in the brain: neurotransmitters send messages across the synapse.

Neurological development

Neurological development refers to brain anatomy, location of function, and chemical responses to activation of neural impulses (neurotransmitters) and responses from the endocrine system (corticosteroids).

Neurons and glial cells The brain and spinal cord make up the **central nervous system** (CNS) which is comprised of: **neurons**, cells that send and receive messages; and **glial cells**, cells that provide support, nutrition, insulation, and maintenance (clean-up of dead neurons). There are three types of neurons that specialize in transmitting different types of messages: **sensory neurons** (which transmit messages to the five senses); **motor neurons** (which transmit messages of fine and gross motor movements), and **interneurons** (which are located in the cerebral cortex, and act as a link between the sensory and motor neurons).

Growth and development of the brain's neurons and the number of **synapses** (gaps between neurons where messages are transmitted) created escalates during the first two years of life. The neurons transmit messages to other neurons by releasing chemicals called **neurotransmitters** into the synapse. The chemical responses and synaptic activity are depicted in Figure 2.2.

Neurotransmitters Neurotransmitters are chemicals that send messages to *excite* or *inhibit* responses. For example, **GABA** (gamma-aminobutyric acid) sends a message to inhibit responses; however, when a malfunction occurs, anxiety can be the result. Too little, or too much, of a neurotransmitter in the system can result in shifts in moods and behaviors (e.g., low serotonin levels can result in depression).

Development and efficiency of message transfer Within the first two years of life, the brain constructs new neural networks and enhances the efficiency of the transmission of the neural messages, by **pruning** and **myelination**. Until middle adolescence, periods of prolific creation of connections are followed by periods of clever housekeeping (pruning). During this period, connections that are frequently used will be strengthened, while the least-used connections will be eliminated. Since formation of neural pathways is dependent on the number and variety of experiences that a toddler is exposed to, early intervention programs are essential in increasing opportunities for later success.

One language or two: bilingualism and the brain

Although some parents are concerned that learning two languages may have an adverse effect on the developing brain, research has demonstrated the opposite. Native bilingual children (Spanish-English bilingual) were found to outperform monolinguals (English) or peers in the second-language immersion kindergarten on tasks of cognitive flexibility, such as executive function tasks requiring the management of conflicting attentional demands (Carlson & Meltzoff, 2008).

During the first two years of life glial cells are instrumental in regulating the production and maintenance of **myelin**, a fatty sheath that coats the nerve fibers. The process of **myelination** increases the conductivity of neural impulses to create more efficient message transmission.

Other chemical messengers

While neurons send excitatory or inhibitory messages by releasing chemicals into the brain (neurotransmitters), hormones released into the bloodstream by the endocrine system also send messages to excite or inhibit responses.

Brain anatomy and brain function Three weeks after gestation, cells begin to differentiate into three regions that will form the hindbrain, the midbrain, and the forebrain.

Hindbrain The **hindbrain** is the lowest portion of the brain, consisting of the **medulla, cerebellum**, and **pons**. The hindbrain links the spinal cord to the brain and regulates respiration (*medulla*), consciousness, arousal (*pons*), and the coordination of smooth muscle movements (*cerebellum*). The medulla is the area where the nerves cross over from the left side of the body to the right side of the brain and the right side of the body to the left side of the brain.

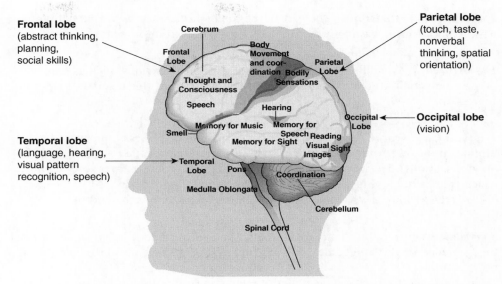

Figure 2.3 Parts of the brain.

Midbrain The midbrain is located between the hindbrain and the forebrain and contains the **reticular activating system (RAS)** which is responsible for habitual patterns of behavior such as walking and sleeping.

Forebrain The forebrain contains structures of the highest and most complex functioning which separates humans from chimpanzees and other animals. The forebrain contains such structures as the **limbic system**, which is responsible for learning, emotion, memory, and motivation. The major parts of the brain can be seen in Figure 2.3.

The brain and survival

The **brain stem**, which is the most primitive part of the brain, includes the hindbrain (excluding the cerebellum) and the midbrain. The brain stem is responsible for basic survival functioning, such as determining the level of alertness/consciousness and regulating breathing, heartbeat, and blood pressure (Rollenhagen & Lubke, 2006).

The cortex and structures under the cortex The cerebral cortex ("cortex" is Latin for "bark") is the convoluted grey mass that covers the brain, consisting of many tightly packed interneurons. The limbic system is located just under the cortex and contains the thalamus, hypothalamus, hippocampus, and amygdale.

Thalamus   The **thalamus** is the part of the forebrain that acts as a relay station for sensory information, passing it on to the cerebral cortex from the sensory organs.

Hypothalamus   In addition to regulating normal body functions, such as temperature and metabolism, the **hypothalamus** also regulates fear, thirst, sexual drive, and aggression.

Hippocampus   Our ability to remember and form new memories is influenced by the **hippocampus** (e.g., our ability to compare our perceptions of sensory information to our expectations). The hippocampus is also rich in the neurotransmitter **acetylcholine** which is associated with memory and muscle control. Individuals with Alzheimer's disease register lower levels of acetylcholine in the hippocampus than normal.

Amygdale   Our recall for emotional events, fear, and memory for fear are all under the influence of the **amygdale**, as is our ability to interpret nonverbal emotional expressions.

Given the specific functions of each of these brain structures, it is not surprising to see how individuals who sustain brain injury or trauma (e.g., due to closed head injury or stroke) can lose specific function in one area but are able to maintain functioning in other areas that are not compromised.

There are two symmetrical cerebral hemispheres (halves) which are separated by a deep fissure that contains a strip rich in neural fibers (**corpus callosum**). There are four major areas (lobes) found in each hemisphere, responsible for specific functions: **occipital lobes** (vision), **parietal lobes** (sense of touch, movement, and location of objects/body in space), **temporal lobes** (auditory discrimination and language), and **frontal lobes** (attention, planning and social skills, abstract reasoning, and memory). The frontal lobes house the **executive functions** which are responsible for managing, directing, and controlling problem-solving activity. The executive functions are discussed at length in *Chapter 8*. (See Figure 2.3 for a graphic illustration of where the lobes are located.)

Genetics and heritability

Closely tied to a discussion of brain development, anatomy, and chemistry is the concept of genetic inheritance. Our understanding of the heritability of certain characteristics has increased significantly due to studies that have focused on twins reared together or twins reared apart (adopted into different households). Genetic transmission can be traced in **monozygotic (MZ) twins**, *identical twins*, compared to **dizygotic (DZ) twins**, *fraternal twins*.

A study of MZ twins and DZ twins provides a comparative analysis of the influence of genetic factors, while controlling for environmental factors. It is also possible to compare MZ twins reared together with those reared apart to evaluate the influence of environmental factors on development. As a result, recent longitudinal studies have revealed that although environmental factors, such as child maltreatment, can increase the risk of antisocial behavior in adulthood, negative outcomes may be moderated by genetic factors, such as an individual's genotype (Caspi et al., 2002; Caspi et al., 2003).

Twins and DNA

The difference between *monozygotic (MZ) twins* or identical twins and *dizygotic (DZ) twins* or fraternal twins is that MZ twins develop from the same ovum which splits after fertilization, while two different ova are fertilized for DZ twins. As a result, MZ twins share identical DNA, while DZ twins share similarities in DNA, comparable to that of other siblings.

Phenotypes and genotypes

Children inherit 23 chromosomes from each parent (22 autosomes and 1 sex chromosome). **Phenotype** refers to those inherited characteristics which are visible, such as eye color and curly or straight hair, while **genotype** refers to inherited characteristics which are not visible (DNA code).

More recently, studies have focused on **endophenotypes** (phenotypical markers or systems that are thought to underlie a given psychological disorder) such as clusters of traits that may come together to explain the existence of certain behavioral tendencies. Lahey, Moffitt, and Caspi (2003) found a certain cluster of **endophenotypes** that place individuals at greater risk of engaging in antisocial behaviors, including: frontal lobe hyperarousal, fearlessness, callousness, and negative emotionality.

Genes can influence how we interact with the environment, but can environment influence genes?

Studies of infants exposed to prolonged trauma (Beers & De Bellis, 2002) have demonstrated changes in the brain's responses to subsequent stressors (hyperarousal), providing support for the theory of a bidirectional influence between heredity and environment (**epigenesis**) where environmental influences can actually be responsible for changes in genetic make-up.

Temperament as a genetic trait   In infancy and early development, **temperament** refers to the general behavioral style that is relatively constant across situations. Although personality traits or characteristics can be learned, there is support for the genetic transmission of a number of traits, such as *general activity level, ease of distress,* and *inhibition or wariness* (Kagan, 1992; Plomin, 1994; Rothbart, Ahadi, & Evans, 2000). Although infants can show a wide range of responses to their environments, by 12 months of age caregivers describe infants as having a unique individual style, with some children being more social and approachable and others being more irritable and emotionally reactive (DeHart, Sroufe, & Cooper, 2004).

One of the earliest research teams to investigate temperament was Thomas and Chess (1977) who rated infants (on a scale from 1 to 10) on the relative strength of the following nine behavioral traits: activity, intensity of response, distractibility, persistence of attention, rhythmicity (biological regulation of function, such as sleeping and eating patterns), adaptability, sensory threshold, mood, and approach-avoidance.

Studies have suggested that *difficult babies* are associated with a greater number of negative outcomes than their easy-going peers. Contemporary researchers have also investigated the need to consider the **"goodness of fit"** between a parent's style and the child's response style, which may be instrumental in promoting stability, or serve to exacerbate problems. For example, Patterson, DeBaryshe, and Ramsey (1989) found that children with "difficult temperament traits" tend to have parents who are themselves highly reactive and punitive. However, the nature of the interaction remains unclear and the question remains: are the parent and child responses similar due to genetic transmission, or environmental influence, or are these similarities an example of what Scarr and McCartney (1983) have described as "evocative" gene–environment interactions?

Easy baby...

Based on the intensity and combination of characteristics, Thomas and Chess (1977) found that 60% of infants could be classified into one of three categories: **easy babies** (high in rhythmicity, approach, positive mood, and adaptability), **difficult babies** (low in rhythmicity and adaptability, and high in avoidance, intensity, and negative moods), and **slow-to-warm-up babies** (mid-range rhythmicity, mild negative reactions to new experiences, adaptive over time).

Bio-physiological responses to stress and threat

In the chapters that follow, discussions of how children respond to perceptions of threat or stress, will focus on physical, emotional, cognitive, and behavioral responses. When a stressful event occurs, the **hypothalamus** places two important systems on alert: the **autonomic nervous system (ANS)** and the **endocrine system**. In response to the alert, there are two pathways that mobilize responses of arousal and fear: the **sympathetic nervous system pathway** and the **hypothalamic–pituitary–adrenal (HPA) pathway**. The two pathways are presented graphically in Figure 2.4.

Sympathetic nervous system pathway   The ANS regulates the involuntary activities of organs, such as pupil dilation, respiration, and heart rate, through two complementary systems: the **parasympathetic nervous system** and the **sympathetic nervous system**. When the ANS receives a message of alert from the hypothalamus, this message is relayed to the sympathetic nervous system, and nerve impulses are sent to the organs to inhibit or stimulate functioning. When the threat has passed, the parasympathetic nervous system returns the system to normal (heart rate and breathing slow down).

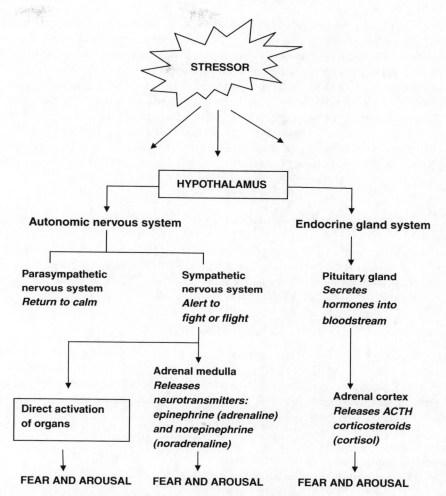

Figure 2.4 Hypothalamus relays stress alert through the sympathetic nervous system pathway and the hypothalamic–pituitary–adrenal (HPA) pathway.

Hypothalamic–pituitary–adrenal (HPA) pathway   The endocrine system controls the **endocrine glands** which secrete **hormones** into the bloodstream. The **HPA** pathway has been implicated in biological explanations for adjustment problems, anxiety, stress disorders, and mood disorders. In response to danger or threat, the hypothalamus activates the pituitary gland which causes the adrenal glands to release **corticosteroids**, a group of stress hormones, such as **cortisol**, into the system in order to mobilize vital organs to respond to the stressful situation, or pending threat.

Summation: the biological model

The biological model contributes to our understanding of child development in a number of significant ways. First, the model provides an understanding of how neurological development should proceed developmentally, and also informs us of the underlying brain structures associated with specific functions. Second, it increases our awareness of the importance of early stimulation in the formation of new neural pathways. Third, understanding the bio-physiological response pathways enhances our awareness of the impact of stress on children at a very early age. Information gathered from twin studies has provided an increased appreciation of the role of genetics in such disorders as dyslexia, learning disabilities, autism, bipolar disorder, anxiety, and schizophrenia. In addition, we are becoming increasingly aware of the complex nature of the interplay between genetics and environmental influences (e.g., that the environment can shape the brain and vice versa). Based on evidence of the role of early experiences in shaping our behaviors and the ability to predict adult characteristics based on childhood traits, the importance of early stimulation and intervention becomes increasingly apparent.

Cognitive and behavioral models

Many therapists combine the use of cognitive and behavioral methods in what is referred to as **cognitive-behavioral therapy (CBT)**. To assist with better understanding how each of these components contributes to CBT, this discussion begins with an in-depth look at each of the models individually.

Behavioral models

While theorists from a biological perspective look to brain function, structure, and genetics to help explain the nature of development, theorists rely on a behavioral model to explain how certain behavior patterns are learned. The principles of learning will assist in predicting how behavior develops and is maintained in three important ways:

- classical conditioning;
- operant conditioning;
- modeling or observational learning.

Classical conditioning   The **classical conditioning** paradigm is very helpful to our understanding and treatment of **irrational fears** or **specific phobias** (sometimes called simple phobias) which are actually quite common in children.

Pavlov and the salivating dogs

Although Ivan Pavlov has become famous for his theory of classical conditioning, his discovery of the phenomenon was really by coincidence. Pavlov was actually studying salivation in dogs, when he made an important discovery. Pavlov noticed that the dogs began to salivate (a reflex response) in response to the sounds of the food being prepared before the dogs received any food. He later introduced a bell to announce the food and the dogs quickly began to salivate in response to the bell.

Table 2.1 The classical conditioning paradigm explains how little Albert was conditioned to fear the rat

Prior to conditioning:		
Stimulus		Response
White rat	⟶	**Mild interest or curiosity**
Neutral stimulus (NS)		Neutral response (NR)
Conditioning phase:		
White rat (NS)	**Loud noise**	**Fear and crying**
	Unconditioned stimulus (US)	Unconditioned response (UR)
After conditioning:		
White rat	⟶	**Fear and crying**
Conditioned stimulus (CS)		Conditioned response (CR)

In the experiment described in the box, Pavlov reasoned that the dogs had learned to associate the sound of the bell with the actual food and thereby had been **conditioned to salivate (conditioned response: CR)** to the bell, which had become the **conditioned stimulus (CS)**. In this scenario, the food is the **unconditioned stimulus (US)** which elicits salivation naturally, and salivation is the **unconditioned response (UR)**.

In a study that would be deemed highly unethical today, Watson and Raynor (1920) successfully conditioned a small child (Little Albert) to fear a white rat by pairing presentations of the white rat with a loud and frightening noise. Although Little Albert was initially curious about the rat, the loud noise ultimately caused Albert to become fearful of the rat. Over time, Albert became fearful of many fur-like objects, including his mother's fur coat and Santa's white beard, through a process of **stimulus generalization** (conditioning generalizes to stimuli that resemble the original). The classical conditioning paradigm is presented in Table 2.1.

Systematic desensitization   Based on the underlying premise that one cannot be anxious/fearful and relaxed at the same time, Wolpe (1958) devised a technique to dissipate a fear or phobia gradually over a number of trials.

Systematic desensitization

The program consists of three steps:

1. Develop a **fear hierarchy**, a list of increasingly fearful images or activities related to the fear, based on the individual's **subjective units of distress (SUDs)**.
2. Train the individual in **deep relaxation**.
3. Beginning with the fear at the lowest level in the hierarchy, pair each of the fears in the hierarchy with a relaxation response until the fear is mastered at each level.

Systematic desensitization is one of a number of different **exposure techniques** that have been developed based on principles of conditioning and learning. Another successful technique is that of **exposure and response prevention (ERP)** which can be used to treat individuals who engage in compulsive ritualistic behaviors. In this treatment, individuals are exposed to their fears (such as fear of germs or contamination) and are prohibited from engaging in the compulsive ritual (such as excessive hand washing, or cleaning rituals). Exposure techniques will be discussed at length in *Chapter 10*, as they relate to the treatment of fears, phobias, and anxieties in children and adolescents.

Operant conditioning   While classical conditioning explains how we develop conditioned responses involving involuntary reflexes (salivation/eyeblink) or intense emotional reactions (fears and phobias), operant conditioning provides the framework for understanding responses that are voluntary in nature. According to behavioral principles of operant behavior, there are two possible explanations for increasing or maintaining behavior: **positive reinforcement** and **negative reinforcement**.

   Reinforcements are consequences that have a positive outcome and, as a result, always <u>increase</u> the likelihood that a behavior will be repeated, since associations (contingencies) are formed linking the behaviors to these positive consequences. Consequences are **positive** if:

1. they **add a positive** outcome (*positive reinforcement*; for example, "when your chores are finished you can watch television"), or:
2. they **remove a negative** outcome, thereby allowing the individual to *avoid/escape* a negative consequence (*negative reinforcement*; for example, "if you come home on time, you will not be grounded"). Negative reinforcement is often confused with punishment; however, recall that reinforcement always increases behavior, while punishment has the opposite effect.

Punishments are consequences that have negative outcomes and always <u>decrease</u> the likelihood that a behavior will be repeated.

   Consequences are **negative**, if:

a. they **add a negative** outcome (*positive punishment*; for example, "you are late and you are grounded"), or
b. they **remove a positive** outcome and a penalty is levied (*negative punishment*; for example, "if you stay out past midnight, I will take away your car keys").

The positive and negative implications of the reward and punishment paradigm are presented in Table 2.2.

   If a behavior stops being rewarded altogether, or if it is severely punished, the behavior will likely terminate, a condition known as **extinction**.

Behavior modification   We can use principles of reinforcement and punishment, as outlined in Table 2.2, to replace undesirable behaviors with behaviors that are more acceptable. There are several methods that can be used to change or shape behaviors and to sustain the improved behaviors over time, such as a **token economy** (e.g.,

Table 2.2 Operant conditioning: reinforcement and punishment paradigm

Goal	Add	Remove
Increase behavior *(for example, increase homework behavior)*	***Positive reinforcement*** Add a positive *If you do your homework, I will buy you a pizza.*	***Negative reinforcement*** Remove a negative *If you do your homework, you will not have to do the dishes.*
Decrease behavior *(for example, decrease off-task behavior)*	***Positive punishment*** Add a negative *If you don't do your homework, you will have to stay after class, until it is done.*	***Negative punishment*** Remove a positive *If you don't do your homework, you cannot go outside to play with your friends.*

tokens are given for good behavior and can be exchanged for prizes at the end of the day).

On the surface, behavior may not always be what it seems to be, as is evident in the case of Erik (see box). In Erik's case, a **functional behavioral assessment (FBA)** could provide insight into what is causing and sustaining the behavior. Behavioral techniques will be further addressed throughout the book as they relate to specific problems discussed and in *Chapter 5*, where specific applications of FBA are discussed at greater length.

The case of Erik: punishment gone awry

When Erik acts out in the classroom, his teacher "*punishes*" him by sending him to the administrator's office. Erik has been there three times this week. So why is the punishment not working? For Erik, being sent to the office means that he can avoid (escape) class work (*negative reinforcement*), and also reap the benefit of added attention from office staff who chat with him (*positive reinforcement*). It can be predicted that both consequences would serve to increase, rather than decrease, his "acting out" behaviors in the future.

Modeling or observational learning In a classic experiment conducted by Bandura, Ross, and Ross (1961), researchers witnessed young children abuse a "Bobo doll" (an inflatable doll with sand feet, like a punching bag) after observing an adult acting aggressively towards the doll. Peers who did not observe the aggressive adult, did not demonstrate aggressive behaviors. Bandura and colleagues found that children's observations of behaviors could involve **delayed imitation**, where the child would not respond immediately, but could carry forward earlier lessons observed. **Observational learning** represents the third type of learning where information is observed and later modeled or imitated.

Factors that increase the likelihood of observational learning

Bandura (1986) has listed a number of elements that can increase the likelihood that observational learning will occur, including:

- *attention* (the action must be noticeable);
- *memory* (the action must be memorable and retained in memory);
- *imitation* (the learner must be able to imitate the action and sequence of actions observed);
- *motivation* (the desire to perform the action must be present).

A summation of the behavioral models   The cardinal feature of the behavioral model is that outcomes are based on the principles of learning. Within this context, a child's behavior has been either conditioned (if the response is an intense emotional one, such as a phobia), or reinforced (positively reinforced or negatively reinforced, since both serve to increase and sustain behaviors), or the child has observed the behavior in others (i.e., the child is modeling the behavior). Behavioral interventions are particularly well suited to children of younger ages, since teachers and adults can monitor the programs and provide rewards for compliance, while children can benefit from clear boundaries and an established set of rules to guide their behaviors. The behavioral perspective provides a systematic approach to the analysis of problem behaviors and the development of appropriate intervention programs. In some cases, such as fears and phobias, behavioral methods are often the treatment of choice, while in other cases behavioral programs can provide an effective adjunct to other treatments.

Cognitive models

The cognitive model provides insight into the nature and development of thinking skills and how thoughts can influence behavior. Based on astute observations of his own children, Jean Piaget (1896–1980) proposed a comprehensive theory of cognitive development that identified competencies, and limitations in reasoning ability, based on faulty logic and inaccurate assumptions that exist at certain stages of development. While Piaget focused on stages of innate understanding, and how children construct their own reality about their physical world, Lev Vygotsky (1896–1934) was most interested in the social and cultural context in which the child's cognitive skills originated and how mentors could enrich the child's understanding, by **scaffolding** or guiding them to the next level of understanding. Theorists who support an **information processing model** to explain how we attend to and recall information have used a computer framework to explain how information goes from the *input stage* (sensory registers), to **short-term memory** and **longer-term memory** (Atkinson & Shiffrin, 1968).

Social cognitive theorists have adapted the information processing model to explain how faulty social information processing can lead to inappropriate behaviors based on incorrect assumptions about others (Dodge, 1991). In the field of clinical psychology, cognitive theorists such as Aaron Beck (1976, 1997) have developed highly successful programs for the treatment of depression and anxiety disorders based on re-framing maladaptive thoughts and assumptions into healthy alternatives. Finally, the field of cognitive neuroscience has made significant advances in the understanding of the role of **executive functions** (the system that manages higher order cognitive processes, such as attention, cognitive flexibility, planning, abstract thinking, and the initiation of appropriate responses while inhibiting inappropriate actions). Russell Barkley (1997) has written extensively concerning the role of central executive function and problems of **disinhibition** in his model, developed to explain the breakdown of these underlying processes in children who experience problems due to impulsivity and/or hyperactivity.

Cognitive neuroscience and executive functions   The role of executive functions has received increasing attention in the explanation of child problems encountered in academic and social settings connected to specific learning disabilities, problems of attention and impulsivity, memory impairment, and a wide combination of other problems. Barkley (1997) has developed a model to increase our understanding of the crucial role that **behavioral inhibition** (the child's ability to inhibit a response, or block a distractor) can exert on the success of executive functioning processes. According to Barkley, if a child does not have the capacity for behavioral inhibition, then behavior is executed (stimulus → response) without the benefit of input from the executive processes (working memory, internalization of speech, self-regulation of affect, and reconstitution) that are required to guide, plan, problem solve, and monitor reactions. As a result, the child is unable to engage in goal-directed persistence or re-engage in tasks when interrupted. The development of techniques to measure executive function, such as the **Behavior Rating Inventory of Executive Function: BRIEF** (Gioia, Isquith, Guy, & Kenworthy, 2000), has advanced our understanding about the potential processes involved and the nature of their impact on behavior. In the development of the BRIEF, Goia et al. (2000) identified eight subdomains of executive function. Five subdomains cluster together to provide a score for the **Metacognition Index** (initiate, working memory, plan/organize, organization of materials, and self-monitoring), and three subdomains provide the composite score for the **Behavioral Regulation Index** (inhibit, shift, and emotional control). Implications of the executive functions for problems in a wide variety of areas will be addressed, as they apply, throughout the book.

Social cognitive models   Bandura's (1977, 1986) contribution to the field of social cognition stems from his early work on social learning processes that were previously discussed under modeling and observational learning. As a result of Bandura's (1977) studies of the nature of social learning, we have developed an increased appreciation of the positive consequences (nurturing and empathic caring behaviors) or negative outcomes (aggressive responses, for example, after witnessing domestic violence) that can result. Furthermore, Bandura's concept of **triadic reciprocity** advanced our understanding of the complex nature of the interrelationships between people, behaviors, and the environment. The social cognitive model links the world of mental representations and problem solving to tasks where the goal is the increased understanding of the self and others.

Social information processing   Dodge and colleagues (Coie & Dodge, 1998; Crick & Dodge, 1996; Dodge, 1991, 2000) have outlined six steps that occur when processing social information in a given social situation, including:

- *encoding social clues* (selectively attending to social cues);
- *mentally representing and interpreting the cues* (linking cues to previous experiences);
- *clarifying social goals*;
- *searching for possible social responses* (either from memory or formulation of new response possibilities);
- *making a response decision* (selecting a response based on an evaluation of probable outcomes);
- *acting out selected responses, monitoring their effects and adjusting accordingly*.

Researchers have found that some children with learning disabilities or aggressive behaviors do not process social cues accurately, either by failing to consider information at one or more of the six steps, or by misreading social cues, such as inaccurately attributing hostile intentions to others in ambiguous situations (**hostile attribution bias**).

As a result, these children demonstrate weaker competence in social interactions compared to their peers. The social information processing model will be revisited in later chapters, as we discussion social skills problems and possible solutions and interventions.

A summation of the cognitive models   Understanding children's cognitive limitations from a developmental perspective is essential to appreciating how children may misconstrue events, and how to provide treatment programs that are suitable for a child's cognitive level. Furthermore, understanding the role of social cognition and social information processing in strengthening or weakening social exchange is fundamental to positive intervention. Researchers have identified a number of behaviors that indicate attempts at **social exchange**, or **affective sharing** and **social referencing** (looking to the caregiver for cues in ambiguous situations) in normally developing toddlers (Emde, 1992; Moses, Baldwin, Rosicky, & Tidball, 2001). These behaviors are conspicuously absent in children with **autism spectrum disorders** who do not engage in affective exchange due to deficits in social reciprocity and social pragmatics. The impact of lack of reciprocity on development will be discussed at length in the chapter on neurodevelopmental disorders (*Chapter 7*).

Cognitive behavioral therapy (CBT)

Cognitive behavioral therapy (CBT) is a form of therapy that is based on a theoretical approach founded on models of cognitive (thoughts) and behavioral (actions) interventions. CBT is one of the most highly researched models of therapeutic intervention, as will become evident in the extensive references to CBT and its application to numerous disorders throughout this book. Since the importance of this therapeutic approach is evident in its application to a variety of disorders, further discussion of this approach will be addressed as it relates to specific applications, as they are presented throughout this book.

Psychodynamic models and attachment

Freud and the Neo-Freudians

Sigmund Freud developed his theories of repressed sexual urges as the basis for psychic trauma based on his conversations with females during the Victorian era who presented with many symptoms of hysteria (later labeled as conversion disorders). As a result, Freud developed his **psychosexual theory of development** wherein he described three parts of the personality that become integrated during five stages of development.

Freud's theories on personality development and psychosexual stages   The following provides a brief overview of Freud's theories on personality formation and psychosexual development.

Personality formation   Freud's structural model of personality formation was based on conflict between desires, dictates of the conscience, and constraints of reality. The model consists of three parts: the **id** (primitive sexual and aggressive urges seeking gratification through the **pleasure principle**); the **ego** (the conscious part of our self system driven by the **reality principle** and whose goal is to keep the id impulses under conscious control); and the **superego** (our conscience that develops between three and six years of age based on moral values internalized from our interactions with our parents). Within this mode, it is the ego's function to maintain a healthy balance of compromises between the demands of the id and superego. Freud believed the ego protected itself from battles between the id and the superego through the use of **defense mechanisms** which are unconscious mental processes developed to alleviate anxiety or bolster self-esteem. These defense mechanisms add depth to our understanding of more primitive child defenses, such as denial, or more socially constructive defenses, such as humor.

Psychosexual stages   Freud constructed his developmental model which linked libidinal drive to different **erogenous zones** (regions of the body that generate sexual pleasure) based on his belief that libidinal drive (sexual pleasure) was the key to personality development. Freud's model contains five stages, each representing a different erogenous zone and the conflict or concerns generated at each stage. The stages, and conflicts/concerns, are presented in Table 2.3.

Freud believed that too little or too much satisfaction or conflict might result in adult forms of **fixations** or **regressions** based on earlier unresolved stages of conflict. Freud's **psychosexual stages** provide potential insight into unconscious drives and conflicts which may influence the underlying dynamics of certain pathologies and will be revisited within the context of the different disorders discussed in this book. Historically, psychodynamic applications have been difficult to support empirically; however, influenced by Bowlby's theories of self-development and attachment, recent research

Table 2.3   Stages of psychosexual (Freud) and psychosocial (Erikson) development

Age range	Freud's psychosexual stage *Issues and conflicts*	Erikson's psychosocial stages *Task to be mastered*
0–18 months	Oral stage *Dependency issues*	Trust vs mistrust *Satisfaction of basic needs*
2–3 years	Anal stage *Orderliness, control, compliance*	Autonomy vs shame and doubt *Increased physical independence*
4–6 years	Phallic stage *Identification with parent of same sex (resolution of Oedipus Complex)* *Superego evolves*	Initiative vs guilt *Increased independence and emotional control, curiosity and exploration*
7–11 years	Latency stage *Sexual and aggressive impulses are sublimated*	Industry vs inferiority *Increased productivity, self-concept and competence*
12 + years	Genital stage *Mature sexuality and relationship*	Identity vs role confusion *Sense of self and own identity*

has demonstrated empirical support for play therapy programs that integrate psycho-dynamic concepts within the practice of **psychodynamic developmental therapy for children (PDTC)** (Fonagy & Target, 1996; Lieberman, Ippen, & Marans, 2009). Working through the medium of play, therapists assist children to develop skills in the self-regulation of impulses and enhanced awareness of others. Lefebre-Mcgevna (2007) applied a play therapy technique for traumatized children based on methods of *Dialectical Behavior Therapy* (DBT), a hybrid of psychodynamic and cognitive-behavioral methods, and reported preliminary success with this procedure. Previously, DBT has been found to be successful in treating adults with borderline personality disorder (Linehan, 1987; Linehan & Dexter-Mazza, 2008).

Erikson's psychosocial stages   Erik Erikson (1902–1994) also supported the notion of stages. However, unlike Freud, Erikson's **psychosocial stages** were based on *socio-emotional tasks* requiring mastery at various stages of development, in order to promote positive growth across the lifespan, and contributing to our overall goal of understanding ourselves and others, and our role in society. Erikson believed that psychosocial development continued over the course of our lifetime and he divided the lifespan into eight different stages of man. Although we will only be discussing those stages that relate to child and adolescent behavior, it is interesting to know that Erikson's theory contained three stages beyond adolescence, including: early adulthood (intimacy vs. isolation), middle adulthood (generativity vs. stagnation), and late adulthood (ego-integrity vs. despair). Erikson's psychosocial stages, along with Freud's psychosexual stages, can be seen in Table 2.3. Psychosocial stages will be discussed further as they relate to different milestones in development.

Mahler and object relations theory   Crucial to the development of an individual identity is the need to recognize that one must separate from the caregiver and assume a separate identity. Mahler, Pine, and Bergman (1975) describe this process of **separation-individuation** occurring in the first three years of life, as a process that evolves from an initial lack of differentiation between caregiver and infant (*normal autism*), to an increasing awareness of an individual identity and sense of self, moving through several stages: the *symbiotic phase*, the *differentiation phase*, and the *practicing phase*, culminating in the *rapprochement phase* at two years of age. In this phase, toddlers must solve the dilemma of how to be independent without feeling vulnerable. Finally, the young child achieves a sense of **object constancy** knowing intuitively that a caregiver is available, if not in the moment, but on a constant basis. Based on our understanding of different types of caregiver practices, it is readily apparent that some children in situations of abuse or neglect may never achieve a sense of object constancy with the caregiver. Next, Bowlby's theory and Ainsworth's studies of attachment provide a greater understanding of the types of caregiver relationships that can ultimately thwart the development of object constancy.

Attachment theory and models of attachment

Bowlby and adaptation theory John Bowlby (1907–1990) incorporated ideas from several theories (ethology, systems theory, cognitive theory, and psychoanalysis) into his theory of attachment which provided a framework for understanding the child's social emotional development based on the degree of comfort and security available in the first seven to eight months of the attachment relationship. Influenced by Freud's concept of internal working models and Darwin's survival theories, Bowlby believed that the infant is "pre-wired" with a set of responses (crying, looking, clinging) to ensure survival, providing *proximity maintenance* (closeness to the caregiver), *a secure base*, and a *safe haven*. A sensitive caregiver responds to an infant's calls of distress by soothing the infant and alleviating the infant's stress, which sets the stage for the development of the infant's ability to self-soothe in times of stress. As a result, a secure attachment provides a secure base for exploration resulting in increased self-confidence, and provides the prototype for the infant's **internal working model** (IWM) for defining future social and emotional relationships as dependable and caring.

Attachment Bowlby believed that attachments formed within the first two years of life carried a profound influence throughout the lifespan, as an internal working model (IWM) for all future relationships. Mary Ainsworth, a student of Bowlby, explored attachment issues using a procedure called the **strange situation** to observe individual differences in the reactions of infants to their caregiver's leaving and return (Ainsworth, Blehar, Waters, & Wall, 1978). Based on the infant's unique behavioral responses, Ainsworth described a number of different attachment patterns for infants who were **securely attached** or who demonstrated **insecure attachment** patterns. In these studies, although securely attached infants would be distressed upon separation from their mothers, they were able to be soothed by the caregiver upon return. However, some infants demonstrated insecure attachment patterns such as **anxious–resistant attachment**, also referred to as *ambivalent attachment* (distressed upon leaving and unable to be soothed upon return) or **anxious–avoidant attachment** patterns (ignoring the caregiver's leaving and return). Researchers have determined that infants with both avoidant and ambivalent attachments demonstrate more irritable (fussy) behaviors than their securely attached peers (Pederson, Gleason, Moran, & Bento, 1998).

Table 2.4 Patterns of attachment

Attachment pattern	Reactions to maternal separation	Reactions to maternal reunion
Secure attachment		
	Child is distressed at mother leaving	Child welcomes mother's return; child is readily calmed by mother
Insecure attachment		
Anxious–resistant or ambivalent	Child is very distressed at mother leaving	Child wants to be close to mother but is angry and irritable; child cannot be calmed by mother
Anxious–avoidant	Child ignores mother leaving	Child ignores mother's return
Disorganized–disoriented	Child appears dazed and confused	No predictable pattern; may engage in rocking behaviors, disoriented

Later, Main and Solomon (1990) discovered a fourth type of attachment evident in their population of children of abusive parents. Children who demonstrated a **disorganized–disoriented attachment** style displayed no consistent pattern of response but rather acted as if they were conflicted between an approach and an avoidance pattern, appearing dazed and confused. The authors suggest that this disorganized attachment pattern results from inconsistent parenting which does not provide the opportunity for infants to develop consistent internal working models of how to relate to significant others. The different attachment patterns and likely response to parent separation and reunion are illustrated in Table 2.4.

Strange situation experiments (Ainsworth et al., 1978)

In this procedure, infant behaviors are observed in a laboratory equipped with one-way glass. There are eight steps to the experiment and behaviors are recorded as the infant is separated from the caregiver on two different occasions:

- Baby and mother are alone in the lab play room.
- Stranger enters.
- Mother and stranger chat, briefly, and mother leaves.
- Stranger leaves after a few minutes, leaving infant alone.
- Mother returns and attempts to comfort the child.
- Mother leaves again.
- Stranger returns and attempts to comfort the child.
- Mother returns and attempts to comfort the child.

Attachment theory emphasizes early infant experiences and the degree to which the child is able to seek comfort from a caregiver in times of distress, thereby constructing an IWM which becomes the underlying foundation for socio-emotional development. In a secure attachment relationship, the infant's IWM predicts that distress is a temporary state and the infant develops increasing skills in self-regulatory behaviors, based on the premise that distress can be soothed and others can be depended on. Securely attached infants are more independent and better problem-solvers than their insecurely attached peers (Sroufe, 2002), while those who do not have consistent access (physically or emotionally) to their primary caregiver are at risk for developing self-representations as "unlovable and unworthy" (Cicchetti & Toth, 1998).

Parenting practices and family dynamics

Parenting style

In addition to early attachment patterns, researchers have also studied the impact of parenting style on subsequent emotional and social development and parent effectiveness based on three areas: the degree of acceptance of the child and engagement in the parenting process; the amount of control exercised; and the amount of autonomy granted to the child (Hart, Newell, & Olsen, 2003). Based on her factor analysis of parenting styles, Baumrind (1991, 2005) found two predominant categories of delineation: *responsiveness* and *demandingness*. According to Baumrind (2005), *responsiveness* refers to the extent to which parents foster individuality and self-assertion by being attuned, supportive, and acquiescent to the children's requests; it includes warmth, autonomy support, and reasoned communication. *Demandingness* refers to the claims parents make on children to become integrated into society by behavior regulation, direct confrontation, and maturity demands (behavioral control) and supervision of children's activities (monitoring). Behavioral control and monitoring are modified in their expression and effect on children's development by parental support, reflection-enhancing communication, and psychological control (Baumrind, 2005, pp. 61–62).

Baumrind (1991) isolated four parenting styles related to the degree of structure (demandingness) and warmth (responsiveness) inherent in the style. The **authoritative parenting** style provides strong feelings of warmth toward the children and provides a good deal of structure and guidance. Those using an **authoritarian parenting** approach are overly controlling and rigid, and lack warmth in their harsh parenting practices. **Permissive parenting** is associated with child indulgence, minimal structure or guidance, and few limits. **Uninvolved parenting** describes parents who provide low structure and low warmth. Researchers have found that the different parenting styles can predict different child outcomes. Parenting practice patterns are summarized in Table 2.5.

Family systems theory

While the majority of theories evaluate child psychopathology from the perspective of individual differences, theorists within **family systems theory** emphasize the family unit as the focus of assessment and intervention, relating to several subsystems, such as parent/child, marriage partners, siblings, or extended family. Within this context, the focus is on the **identified problem** (often the child referred for behavioral problems) as it relates to dynamics inherent in issues related to **boundaries**, **alliances**, and **power**. If the spousal system is dysfunctional, then the response may be "scapegoating

Table 2.5 Parenting styles

Parenting style	Child outcomes	Structure or control	Warmth	Acceptance
Authoritative	Positive self-concept	High structure Adaptive	High	High
Authoritarian	Anxiety and hostility	High structure Overly rigid and coercive	Low	Low
Permissive	Demandingness	Low structure Overindulgent	High	High
Uninvolved	Dependency	Lacking in structure Negligent	Low	Low

of children or co-opting them into alliances with one partner against the other" (Goldberg, Goldberg, & Goldberg Plavin, 2011, p. 420).

Boundaries are the imaginary lines that serve to define the various subsystems. Often a family's degree of dysfunction can be predicted by characteristics of boundary formation, which can manifest as weak limit-setting resulting from inconsistent or **loosely defined boundaries**, or as lack of family engagement due to very **rigid boundaries**. Children growing up in situations of loose boundaries may be privy to information that is well beyond their years, in a family environment where family members are **enmeshed** and overly involved in each other's lives (Minuchin, 1985; Minuchin, Nichols, & Lee, 2006). However, children who grow up in families where boundaries are overly rigid may experience a sense of detachment where family members are **disengaged**. Within the family system, therapists often look for family assigned roles (rescuer, victim, scapegoat, and so on) and how the balance of power is aligned. In cases of conflict, often the dynamic of **triangulation** will be evident, as the balance of power is weighted for two family members who align against a third member (e.g., mother and father vs. child, siblings vs. parents, mother and child vs. father).

Coercion theory Patterson, Capaldi, and Bank (1991) developed the concept of **coercion theory** to account for the impact of coercive parenting practices on exacerbating children's negative behaviors. In a theoretical framework that bridges the behavioral and family systems models, Patterson et al. (1991) suggest that parents who confront and then eventually yield to a child's negative behaviors and demands actually serve to increase the negative behaviors over time. Negative behaviors increase because the behaviors are **positively reinforced** by the parent (the parent complies and the child gets what he or she wants), while at the same time, the parent is **negatively reinforced** for their own compliance (the child's negative behavior, such as whining or tantrum behavior, ceases momentarily).

Coercion theory and reinforcement

Recall that **positive reinforcement** (the behavior is rewarded by a positive consequence) and **negative reinforcement** (the behavior is rewarded because it removes a negative event) both serve to increase behaviors. In this case, the parent's compliance is rewarded because the negative behavior stops (in the short term) and the child's negative behaviors (demands) are rewarded because the goal is achieved. Parent and child become locked into a coercive cycle of positive and negative reinforcement.

Therapeutically, the parent would be made aware of the dynamics inherent in this reinforcement cycle and would be advised not to yield to the child's demands and to be consistent in not complying with unreasonable child demands. Over time, this would serve to extinguish the child's negative behaviors and break the coercive cycle.

The total child: an over-arching framework

Although it is important to recognize the various theoretical models that can be applied to child psychopathology, it is equally important to see how these perspectives can converge to provide an all-encompassing system that incorporates different models into one over-arching framework.

A transactional ecological bio-psycho-social framework

Although debate in the past contrasted nature with nurture, contemporary researchers are well aware that the contexts surrounding development can have a powerful influence on the degree to which human potential is realized. Urie Bronfenbrenner's (1979) **ecological systems theory** has been a crucial force in bringing about awareness of the importance of contextual influences on human development, and provides the necessary organizational format for addressing information from the major theoretical perspectives in one over-arching framework.

Bronfenbrenner and the contexts of development   Bronfenbrenner's bioecological theory provides an ideal framework for discussing the interaction between *child characteristics* (genetics, temperament, neurological development) and *environmental characteristics* (proximal and distal sources) as seen in various levels of influence. In this system, the child is depicted as the central figure in a series of concentric circles of influence that emanate between the individual and the environment.

Within this model, Bronfenbrenner envisioned the layers of influence as *bidirectional* and *interacting influences*, characterized by their dual nature (i.e., influences are in two directions – both away from the child and toward the child). For example, a given parenting approach may affect a child's behaviors (poor limit-setting may increase the child's acting out behaviors). However, a child's behaviors may also influence parenting style (increased limit-setting to reduce acting out behaviors). More recently, Bronfenbrenner has suggested that his model might best be characterized as a **bioecological model**, in order to emphasize how the child's biological characteristics interact with the different environmental factors (Bronfenbrenner, 2001; Bronfenbrenner & Morris, 1998). Bronfenbrenner's model is depicted graphically in Figure 2.5.

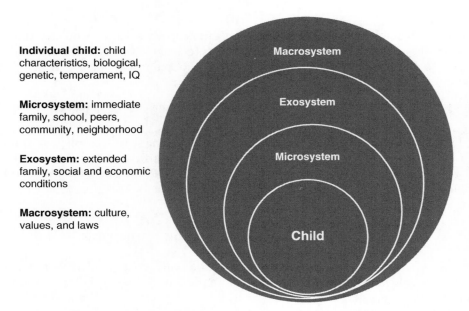

Individual child: child characteristics, biological, genetic, temperament, IQ

Microsystem: immediate family, school, peers, community, neighborhood

Exosystem: extended family, social and economic conditions

Macrosystem: culture, values, and laws

Figure 2.5   Bronfenbrenner's bioecological model.

The ecological-transactional model (Bronfenbrenner, 1979; Cicchetti & Lynch, 1993) provides an over-arching framework for conceptualizing ecological contexts "consisting of a number of nested levels with varying degrees of proximity to the individual" (Lynch & Cicchetti, 1998, p. 235). Within this model, beyond the individual there are three levels of environmental influence: the microsystem, the exosystem, and the macrosystem.

Individual   The *individual* child is at the core of the model, and internal factors emanating from biological and genetic sources contribute to strengths or vulnerabilities that can enhance or inhibit a child's interaction with all other levels/layers in the system. In a transactional model, child characteristics influence, but are in turn shaped or modified in an on-going way by, the external factors. The biological model addresses potential risk and protective factors, such as: maternal prenatal health and nutrition; any medications or drug/alcohol use during the embryonic period; and family history of psychopathology). Risks and protective factors will be discussed throughout the book as they apply to the disorders discussed.

Microsystem   The **microsystem** represents the primary relationships and interactions that a child experiences in his or her immediate surroundings. At this level, bi-directional influences of family, school, neighborhood, and child care are seen to exert the strongest and most direct influence on the developing child. The family context is a primary source of influence during the early years and sets the parameters for a child's concept of family and the roles of mother, father, and siblings. In various cultures what defines the "family" can differ widely from the inclusion of friends in the family circle to the exclusion of all but the immediate family. In many African American families, grandmothers play a major role in child-rearing (Cain &

Combs-Orme, 2005), while in Asian families female family members (grandmothers and aunts) and older siblings may play an increasing role in care-giving over time (Kurrien & Vo, 2001). Furthermore, the influence of **individualism** versus **collectivism** (Hofstede, 1980) can play a major role in whether the family dynamics support the individual (independence, autonomy) versus the group (fostering group cohesion and cooperation).

Individualism versus collectivism

In an individualistic society, independence and autonomy are revered, and individuals relate to those outside the family, usually in loose associations through shared interests and activities. In a collective society, in addition to very strong loyalty and ties to family, individuals have strong ties to "in groups," such as extended family. Group participation outside the family is limited to a select few permanent groups. Within this context, the United States and the United Kingdom would be considered individualistic societies, while Asia and Central America would be considered collectivistic.

Family systems are also subject to change, with the advent of new siblings and the possible dissolution of a marriage. The impact of a chaotic environment at the microsystem level will be discussed in *Chapter 6*, as it relates to child and adolescent adjustment difficulties experienced due to family dynamics, psychosocial turmoil, and problems in the school environment.

The quality of the child's school day care setting (e.g., primary school) can have an important influence on development, as can the peer group that the child relates to within these settings. In North America, formal schooling begins at age six and children will spend six hours a day during the week in their school setting. In Western Europe and Japan the time spent in school is even longer. The transition to primary school and high school can be a difficult time for most children and adolescents, since it marks the entrance into a new set of circumstances and influences. Finally, the neighborhood itself (access to resources and recreation, neighbors, safety, and quality of neighborhood upkeep) can also influence the developing child, for better or worse. The influence of school transitions, as well as other challenges, such as peer group affiliations, and quality of neighborhood will be addressed in *Chapter 6*. Within the microsystem, the degree of communication or compatibility between the structures can strengthen or undermine the influence of either factor. Bronfenbrenner used the term **mesosystem** to refer to the degree of connection/communication between factors in the microsystem.

Mesosystem effects

The quality of communication between individuals in the child's microsystem can have important effects on development. For example, if parents (home) and teachers (school) communicate regularly and share the same goals for the child, the potential for academic success will increase significantly, since the two factors support each other. Conversely, poor communication between home and school has been associated with increased risk for academic difficulties.

Although the microsystem represents the most proximal source of influence, interactions at more distal levels can also impact the inner structures positively or negatively.

Exosystem　The **exosystem** consists of factors related to the social and economic context, such as a parent's employment situation, and the socioeconomic status of the family, and the extended family. Although this level does not impact the child directly, one can readily imagine how a parent's work stress might impact a child, or conversely, how a child's ill health might impact on a parent's work situation (increased absenteeism due to child care needs). Studies have demonstrated that poor access to community resources can also have a negative effect on development and place children at risk for negative peer relationships (Jones & Offord, 1989).

Macrosystem　The outer sphere of influence is the **macrosystem** which involves cultural values, customs, and laws, and can have a ripple effect of a cascading influence throughout the inner spheres. For example, a change in education law can ultimately have a direct impact on educational instruction for a child with special needs. Similarly, a parent's rigid adherence to cultural values that conflict with an adolescent's peer group in a new country may cause significant turmoil for the child and his family.

A transactional ecological bio-psycho-social framework: a summation　Ultimately, the quality of these contexts and interactions will influence the nature of child and adolescent development and the learning and acquisition of skills necessary for successful adaptation and communication. Increased understanding of the on-going and transactional nature of the process of development brings with it an appreciation of how changes within the child can result in transformations in the environment at all levels depicted above, and that conversely, changes at all levels of influence can impact the growing child.

Our knowledge of skill development in cognitive, emotional, and social areas and our understanding of predicted patterns of behavior not only provides a blueprint for change, but also gives the necessary benchmarks required to evaluate the degree to which an individual's developmental trajectory adheres to or deviates from the norm. In the next chapters, we will take a closer look at milestones for cognitive, emotional, and social development as they unfold during early and later childhood (*Chapter 3*) and adolescence (*Chapter 4*).

References

Ainsworth, M. D. S., Blehar, M. C., Waters, E., & Wall, S. (1978). *Patterns of attachment.* Hillsdale, NJ: Erlbaum.

Atkinson, R. C., & Shiffrin, R. M. (1968). Human memory: A proposed system and its control processes. In K. W. Spence & J. T. Spence (Eds.), *Advances in the psychology of learning and motivation*, vol. 2 (pp. 90–195). New York: Academic Press.

Bandura, A. (1977). *Social learning theory.* Englewood Cliffs, NJ: Prentice Hall.

Bandura, A. (1986). *Social foundations of thought and action: A social cognitive theory.* Englewood Cliffs, NJ: Prentice Hall.

Bandura, A., Ross, D., & Ross, S. A. (1961). Transmission of aggression through imitation of aggressive models. *Journal of Abnormal and Social Psychology, 63*, 575–582.

Barkley, R. A. (1997). Behavior inhibition, sustained attention and executive function. *Psychological Bulletin, 121*, 65–94.

Baumrind, D. (1991). The influences of parenting style on adolescent competence and substance use. *Journal of Early Adolescence, 11*, 56–95.

Baumrind, D. (2005). Patterns of parental authority and adolescent autonomy. *New Directions for Child and Adolescent Development: Special Issue: Changing Boundaries of Parental Authority during Adolescence*, 61–69.

Beck, A. T. (1976). *Cognitive therapy and emotional disorders.* New York: International University Press.

Beck, A. T. (1997). Cognitive therapy: Reflections. In J. K. Zeig (Ed.), *The evolution of psychotherapy: The third conference* (pp. 55–64). New York: Brunner/Mazel.

Beers, S. R., & De Bellis, M. (2002). Neuropsychological function in children with maltreatment-related posttraumatic stress disorder. *American Journal of Psychiatry, 159*, 483–486.

Bronfenbrenner, U. (1979). *The ecology of human development.* Cambridge, MA: Harvard University Press.

Bronfenbrenner, U. (2001). Growing chaos in the lives of children, youth and families. How can we turn it around? In J. C. Westman (Ed.), *Parenthood in America* (pp. 197–210). Madison: University of Wisconsin Press.

Bronfenbrenner, U., & Morris, P. A. (1998). The ecology of developmental processes. In R. M. Lerner (Ed.), *Handbook of child psychology;* Vol. *1. Theoretical models of human development* (5th ed.) (pp. 535–584). New York: John Wiley & Sons, Ltd.

Cain, D. S., & Combs-Orme, T. (2005). Family structure effects on parenting stress and practices in the African American family. *Journal of Sociology and Social Welfare, 32*(2), 19–40.

Carlson, S. M., & Meltzoff, A. N. (2008). Bilingual experience and executive functioning in young children. *Developmental Science, 11*(2), 282–298. doi:10.1111/j.1467-7687.2008.00675.x

Caspi, A., McClay, J., Moffitt, E. E., Mill, J., Martin, J., Craig, I. W., Taylor, A., & Poulton, R. (2002). Role of genotype in the cycle of violence in maltreated children. *Science, 297*, 851–854.

Caspi, A., Sugden, K., Moffit, T. E., Taylor, A., Craig, I. W., Harrington, H., . . . Poulton, R. (2003). Influence of life stress on depression moderation by a polymorphism in the 5-HTT gene. *Science, 18*, 386–389.

Cicchetti, D., & Lynch, M. (1993). Toward an ecological/transactional model of community violence and child maltreatment: Consequences for children's development. *Psychiatry, 56*, 96–118.

Cicchetti, D., & Toth, S. L. (1998). The development of depression in children and adolescents. *American Psychologist, 53*(2), 221–241.

Coie, J. D., & Dodge, K. A. (1998). Aggression and antisocial behaviour. In W. Damon & N. Eisenberg (Eds.), *Handbook of child psychology; Vol. 3. Social, emotional, and personality development* (5th ed.) (pp. 779–862). Hoboken, NJ: John Wiley & Sons, Ltd.

Crick, N. R., & Dodge, K. A. (1996). Social information-processing mechanisms in reactive and proactive aggression. *Child Development, 67*, 993–1002.

DeHart, G. B., Sroufe, L. A., & Cooper, R. (2004). *Child development: Its nature and course* (4th ed.). New York: McGraw-Hill.

Dodge, K. A. (1991). The structure and function of reactive and proactive aggression. In D. J. Pepler and K. H. Rubin (Eds.), *The development and treatment of childhood aggression* (pp. 201–218). Hillsdale, NJ: Erlbaum.

Dodge, K. A. (2000). Conduct disorders. In A. Sameroff, M. Lewis, & S. Miller (Eds.), *Handbook of developmental psychopathology* (2nd ed.) (pp. 447–466). New York: Plenum.

Emde, R. N. (1992). Social referencing research: Uncertainty, self, and the search for meaning. In S. Feinman (Ed.), *Social referencing and the social construction of reality in infancy* (pp. 79–92). New York: Plenum Press.

Fonagy, P., & Target, M. (1996). A contemporary psychoanalytical perspective: Psychodynamic developmental therapy. In E. D. Hibbs and P. S. Jensen (Eds.), *Psychosocial treatments for child and adolescent disorders: Empirically based strategies for clinical practice* (pp. 619–638). Washington, DC: APA.

Gioia, G. A., Isquith, P. K., Guy, S. C., & Kenworthy, L. (2000). *Behavior Rating Inventory of Executive Function (BRIEF). Professional manual.* Odessa, FL: Psychological Assessment Resources.

Goldberg, I., Goldberg, H., & Goldberg Plavin, E. (2011). Family therapy. In R. J. Corsini & D. Wedding (Eds.), *Current psychotherapies* (9th ed.) (pp. 417–453). Belmont, CA: Brooks Cole.

Hart, C. H., Newell, L. D., & Olsen, S. F. (2003). Parenting skills and social-communicative competence in childhood. In J. O. Greene & B. R. Bulreson (Eds.), *Handbook of communication and social interaction skills* (pp. 753–797). Mahwah, NJ: Erlbaum.

Hofstede, G. H. (1980). *Culture's consequences, international differences in work-related values.* Beverly Hills, CA: Sage Publications.

Jones, M. B., & Offord, D. R. (1989). Reduction of antisocial behaviour in poor children by nonschool skill-development. *Journal of Child Psychology and Psychiatry, 30*(5), 737–750.

Kagan, A. E. (1992). Yesterday's promises, tomorrow's promises. *Developmental Psychology, 28*, 990–997.

Kurrien, R., & Vo, E. D. (2001). Who's in charge? Coparenting in South and Southeast Asian families. *Journal of Adult Development, 11*, 207–219.

Lahey, B., Moffitt, E. E., & Caspi, A. (Eds.). (2003). *Causes of conduct disorder and juvenile delinquency.* New York: Guilford Press.

Lefebre-Mcgevna, J. A. (2007). A developmental attachment-based play therapy: A new treatment for children diagnosed with reactive attachment and developmental trauma disorders. *Dissertation Abstracts International. B: The Sciences and Engineering, 67*, 4715.

Lieberman, A. F., Ippen, C., & Marans, S. (2009). Psychodynamic therapy for child trauma. In E. B. Foa, T. M. Keane, M. J. Friedman et al. (Eds.), *Effective treatments for PTSD: Practice guidelines from the International Society for Traumatic Stress Studies* (2nd ed.) (pp. 370–387). New York: Guilford.

Linehan, M. M. (1987). Dialectical behavior therapy for borderline personality disorder: Theory and method. *Bulletin of the Menniger Clinic, 51*, 261–276.

Linehan, M. M., & Dexter-Mazza, E. T. (2008). Dialectical behavior therapy for borderline personality disorder. In D. H. Barlow (Ed.), *Clinical handbook of psychological disorders: A step-by-step treatment manual* (4th ed.) (pp. 365–420). New York: Guilford Press.

Lynch, M., & Cicchetti, D. (1998). An ecological-transactional analysis of children and contexts: The longitudinal interplay among child maltreatment, community violence, and children's symptomatology. *Development and Psychopathology, 10,* 235–257.

Mahler, M. S., Pine, F., & Bergman, A. (1975). *The psychological birth of the human infant.* New York: Basic Books.

Main, M., & Solomon, J. (1990). Procedures for identifying infants as disorganized/disoriented during the Ainsworth Strange Situation. In M. T. Greenberg, D. Cicchetti, & E. M. Cummings (Eds.), *Attachment in the preschool years* (pp. 121–160). Chicago: University of Chicago Press.

Minuchin, P. (1985). Families and individual development: Provocations from the field of family therapy. *Child Development, 56,* 289–302.

Minuchin, S., Nichols, M. P., & Lee, W. (2006). *Assessing families and couples: From symptom to system.* Boston: Allyn & Bacon.

Moses, L., Baldwin, D., Rosicky, J., & Tidball, G. (2001). Evidence for referential understanding in the emotions domain at twelve and eighteen months. *Child Development, 72,* 718–735.

Patterson, G. R., Capaldi, D., & Bank, L. (1991). An early starter model for predicting delinquency. In D. Pepler & K. H. Rubin (Eds.), *The development and treatment of childhood aggression* (pp. 139–168). Hillsdale, NJ: Erlbaum.

Patterson, G. R., DeBaryshe, B. D., & Ramsey, E. (1989). A developmental perspective on antisocial behavior. *American Psychologist, 44,* 329–335.

Pederson, D. R., Gleason, K. E., Moran, G., & Bento, S. (1998). Maternal attachment representations, maternal sensitivity, and the infant–mother attachment relationship. *Developmental Psychology, 34*(5), 925–933.

Plomin, R. (1994). *Genetics and experience: The interplay between nature and nurture.* Thousand Oaks, CA: Sage.

Rollenhagen, A., & Lubke, J. H. (2006). The morphology of excitatory central synapses: From structure to function. *Cell Tissue Research, 326,* 221–237.

Rothbart, M. K., Ahadi, S. A., & Evans, D. E. (2000). Temperament and personality: Origins and outcomes. *Journal of Personality and Social Psychology, 78*(1), 122–135.

Scarr, S., & McCartney, K. (1983). How people make their own environments. *Child Development, 54,* 424–435.

Shaywitz, S. E. (1998). Current concepts: Dyslexia. *New England Journal of Medicine, 338*(5), 307–312.

Sroufe, L. A. (2002). From infant attachment to promotion of adolescent autonomy: Prospective, longitudinal data on the role of parents in development. In J. Borkowski, S. Ramey, & M. Bristol-Power (Eds.), *Parenting and the child's world* (pp. 187–202). Mahwah, NJ: Lawrence Erlbaum.

Thomas, A., & Chess, S. (1977). *Temperament and development.* New York: Brunner/Mazel.

Watson, J. B., & Raynor, R. R. (1920). Conditioned emotional reactions. *Journal of Experimental Psychology, 3,* 1–14.

Wolpe, J. (1958). *Psychotherapy by reciprocal inhibition.* Stanford, CA: Stanford University Press.

3

Developmental Milestones: Early and Middle Childhood

Clinical and Educational Child Psychology, First Edition. Linda Wilmshurst.
© 2013 John Wiley & Sons, Ltd. Published 2013 by John Wiley & Sons, Ltd.

Chapter preview and learning objectives

Although it is recognized that development continues across the lifespan with on-going change in mental health and lifelong learning, it has also been acknowledged that growth in the latter stages of development (early, middle, and late adulthood) progresses at a significantly slower pace than in childhood or adolescence. Further-more, changes in later life often focus on the consolidation of previously acquired foundation skills, rather than the acquisition of new skills and competencies.

This chapter focuses on the initial years of the **acquisitive stage** (Schaie & Willis, 1993), which spans childhood and adolescence; a time when the major task is to amass information that will be effectively applied in later stages of development. Rapid rates of growth in these formative years can produce significant changes that can have profound influences on a child's responsiveness to the environment and, ultimately, the social and emotional lessons learned along the way. It is important that practitioners working with children have a good understanding of expected time-lines for the acquisition of different competencies and skills, or they risk missing valuable opportunities for early intervention initiatives, and for designing programs that are developmentally appropriate.

This chapter focuses on the milestones in development that provide benchmarks of increasingly complex skills, in cognitive, affective, and social development, in early and middle childhood. Adolescent milestones will be discussed in *Chapter 4*. After reading this chapter, readers will have a greater appreciation of:

- biological influences on the neurological and physical/motor development of the child;
- brain anatomy, structure, and function relative to child development;
- milestones and gender differences in physical maturation;
- the role of genetics and heritability in individual differences in development;
- milestones in cognitive development from the dual perspectives of stage theory and information processing;
- expectations for increased self-awareness and self-control across the developmental spectrum;
- milestones in understanding emotions in the self and others in the developing child;
- the role of attachment in social, emotional, and affective development;
- the impact of parenting practices on outcomes for child development.

Biological beginnings

Neurological and physical/motor development

Neurological development

Brain development   The infant's brain weighs approximately 350 grams, which is equal to about 25% of its adult weight (Morgan & Gibson, 1991). By two years of age, the child's brain will have tripled in weight (70% of its adult weight) and by six years of age, the brain will reach 90% of its adult weight (Thatcher, Lyon, Rumsey, &

Krasnegor, 1996). As was discussed in *Chapter 2*, initially, the brain is actively involved in creating new neural networks and **pruning** pathways that are no longer useful or stimulated. In the first two years, **glial cells** produce **myelin**, a fatty sheath that coats the neural fibers and increases the efficiency of the message transfer between neurons. As a result, preschoolers rapidly improve their skills in a wide variety of areas, including coordination, perception, attention, memory, and language.

Between three and six years of age there is rapid growth in the **frontal-lobe** areas of the brain associated with planning and organization. During the preschool and school years, increased impulse control, planning ability, and problem solving are related to development in the prefrontal cortex. Initially, the brain is highly **plastic**, which means that the cerebral cortex has not yet designated different hemispheres for specialized functions, a process which is called **lateralization**. For example, studies of early brain damage have demonstrated that regardless of where the injury is located (the left or right side of the brain), language delays can result, and remit by early school entrance, suggesting that language is not lateralized in very young brains. However, damage to the right hemisphere (spatial processing) can result in long-term disabilities in processing visual spatial information (Stiles, 2008), such as the type of processing deficits that are experienced by children with nonverbal learning disabilities (Rourke et al., 2002) which will be discussed in *Chapter 8*.

Lefty or righty?

There is heightened activity in the left hemisphere of the brain between three and six years of age, when language acquisition is at its peak. Activity in the right hemisphere (which deals with spatial abilities) continues to increase throughout middle childhood (Thompson et al., 2000). Hand preference is clearly established in 90% of children by five years of age (Ozturk et al., 1999). Studies have revealed that right-handed dominance is primarily associated with a dominant left hemisphere. However, for those who are left-handed (10% of the population), language functions are often shared between the two hemispheres (Knecht et al., 2000). As a result, left- or mixed-handed children are more likely than their right-handed peers to develop superior verbal and mathematical skills, likely due to the use of both hemispheres to process cognitive information (Flannery & Liederman, 1995).

Other brain functions   The **cerebellum**, responsible for smooth muscle movements, continues to myelinate until the child is approximately four years of age, which is evident in increased balance and control (Tanner, 1990). Myelination of the **reticular formation** continues throughout this period and into adolescence, providing increased attention and concentration. Throughout childhood and into adolescence, myelination increases the efficiency of the **corpus callosum**, which integrates information from many sources, including memories, attention, perception, language, and problem solving (Thompson et al., 2000).

Physical and motor development   Physical growth is dramatic during the early years, with **gross motor skills** (large muscle movement, such as throwing a ball) developing prior to **fine motor skills** (smaller movements, such as holding a pencil). By their third birthday, children have amassed a number of motor skills, including jumping, hopping, and skipping. By five years of age, most children can master the ability to ride a bicycle, climb a ladder, and engage in athletic activities such as skiing, skating, soccer, and baseball. School-aged children have increased control over their muscles and demonstrate enhanced gross motor coordination in their agility, flexibility, balance, and force (Cratty, 1986).

Fine motor skills also continue to improve with practice and mastery of fine motor movements. What started as a scribble at 18 months, can be perfected into a drawing of a circle and square by three years of age, and a recognizable person by four years of age. By six years of age, most children have mastered the ability to print the letters of the alphabet, the numbers from one to 10 and their initial and last names. Drawings take on increasing sophistication, and by nine to 10 years of age, drawings are more complex in detail and begin to integrate concepts of depth perception and perspective.

Assessments of developmental functioning in young children often include instruments to evaluate perceptual and motor skills, such as the *Beery-Buktenica Developmental Test of Visual-Motor Integration* (VMI-6; Beery, Beery, & Buktenica, 2010) which is now in its sixth edition. The test requires the child to reproduce a number of increasingly complex designs which can be scored to determine how the child meets developmental expectations.

Gender and physical maturation   Until approximately 10 years of age, boys and girls demonstrate similar rates of physical and motor growth evident in increased motor control and coordination, as well as enhanced physical strength and agility. Sexual differentiation begins soon after conception, as the presence or absence of the male hormones (*androgens*) determines whether male or female sex organs develop. Androgen levels remain relatively constant throughout early childhood but begin to rise again in middle childhood in preparation for the physical development that accompanies puberty.

Genetics and heritability   A significant question that has its roots in the nature/ nurture controversy is the degree to which traits and characteristics such as brain structure, chemistry, and function are inherited. Twin and adoption studies have provided information about the risks of inheriting a genetic vulnerability to developing depression, anxiety, attention/concentration problems, or learning difficulties such as dyslexia.

Is intelligence a product of nature or nurture?

Gardner (1999) addresses this question, suggesting that it is primarily a question generated by Western societies, since collectivistic Eastern societies downplay the role of individual differences. However, based on twin studies, IQ is predicted by intellectual scores obtained by birth parents, not adoptive parents.

There is growing research support of the interaction between genetics and the environment, such as the finding that prolonged exposure to trauma and abuse in infants can impact how the brain is genetically wired for future hyper-responsiveness to stress (Beers & DeBellis, 2002). In *Chapter 6*, common stressors and developmental responses to stress will be addressed.

The role of temperament   Allport (1961) noted that **temperament** was "dependent on constitutional make-up and (was) therefore largely hereditary in nature" (p. 34). Since that time, there has been considerable controversy over whether temperament is determined more by heredity or environment. Temperament, like personality, defines consistent patterns of behavior (strength, speed, and nature of response, and so on) that predict how an individual is likely to respond in a given situation. Furthermore, most behavioral traits are considered to be relatively stable by the end of the infant stage. Although some traits can be learned, researchers have found support for a genetic basis for some characteristics, like wariness/shyness (Kagan, 1992), or being inhibited and experiencing negative emotions (Plomin, 1994). In studies of "high reactive" and "low reactive" infants, these characteristics are considered to be biologically based (Kagan & Fox, 2006; Kagan & Snidman, 2004) and related to level of excitation in the amygdale and associated structures.

Is biology our destiny?

Kagan poses this question in a film clip featuring his work on temperament and infant responsiveness to stimulation (http://www.youtube.com/watch?v = CGjO1KwltOw). He states that although we may be born with tendencies to react in certain ways, parents can guide the wary child with a gentle push to be more social, and can improve their potential for social engagement.

Milestones in cognitive development

Piaget and cognitive stage theories

Piaget identified five periods of development based on competencies and limitations in thinking and problem solving.

Sensorimotor period   The **sensorimotor period** spans the first two years of life, and ushers in a number of significant cognitive milestones, such as **object permanence**, an understanding that objects continue to exist even when they are out of sight. This awareness paves the way for symbolic learning and early representational thought evident in the child's increased ability to demonstrate deferred imitation and engage in make-believe play. In *Chapter 7*, readers will find that children diagnosed with pervasive developmental disorders (PDD), such as the autism spectrum disorders (ASD), demonstrate a qualitative impairment in communication which is often lacking in spontaneous, make-believe, or imitative play. The major milestones and limitations during the sensorimotor and preoperational periods are summarized in Table 3.1.

Table 3.1   Cognitive milestones: early childhood (birth to seven years of age)

Developmental period	Milestones/ limitations
Birth–2 years *Piaget: sensorimotor* *period*	**Object permanence** *(objects continue to exist when hidden)* **Intentional goal-directed behavior** **Deferred imitation** **Make-believe play**
Information processing	**Recognition memory** *(known as familiar)* **Perceptual organization** *(categorization by perceptual features)* **Recall memory** *(mental image)* **Conceptual organization** *(organize by category, usage)*
2 –7 years *Piaget: preoperational* *period, early stage*	**Milestones:** **Sociodramatic play** (include others in make-believe play) **Can sort objects into familiar categories** **Limitations in thinking:** **Egocentrism** (inability to take viewpoint of another) **Animism** (inanimate objects given real-life qualities) **Illogical thinking** (cannot solve class inclusion problems) **Centration** (inability to consider more than one factor at a time) **Conservation** (inability to conserve; lack of irreversibility) **Appearance/reality** (inability to distinguish)
Preoperational period, *later stage*	**Milestones:** **Increased understanding in all above areas** **Can perform conservation of number tasks**
Information processing	**Increased attention span** **Numbers: simple addition, subtraction, and counting** **Can repeat 4 digits** **Formation of autobiographical memories**

Preoperational period   Despite significant cognitive advances, children in the early stages of the **preoperational period** (approximately 2–6/7 years) have several limitations in their thinking, including **egocentrism** which is the inability to take the perspective of another. Early studies focused on the child's inability to predict what another would see from a given perceptual vantage point (matching the correct view of three mountains from where a doll was sitting); however, later studies expanded this notion to include the child's inability to take another's social or emotional viewpoint (i.e., empathy).

A second major limitation at this stage is the child's inability to solve problems involving principles of **conservation**. These problem-solving tasks require the child to reason that actual properties of number, mass, length, and volume remain constant despite changes in physical appearance. Examples of conservation experiments are available in Table 3.2.

In the first example in Table 3.2, children in the preoperational stage will respond that the row with the blocks stretched out has more blocks, even if they responded that the rows were the same, earlier. Piaget reasoned that children in the preoperational period make this error in judgment due to their inability to **decenter** *(focus on more than one aspect of the array at a time)*. As a result, the child is unable to reason that

Table 3.2   Examples of Piaget's conservation tasks

Type of conservation	Method Initial presentation	Method Transformation	Age of mastery
Conservation of number	Is there the same number of blocks in each row?	Is there the same number of blocks in each row? If not, which one has more?	6–7 years
Conservation of liquid	Is there the same amount of water in each glass?	Is there the same amount of liquid in each glass, or does one have more?	6–7 years
Conservation of length	Is each of these sticks just as long as the other one?	Are the two sticks each as long, or is one longer than the other?	7–8 years
Conservation of mass	Is there the same amount of clay in each ball?	Do they still have the same amount of clay, or does one have more?	7–8 years

objects or situations remain stable (are conserved) despite alterations in their superficial or visual appearance.

The curious case of Maynard: the cat who became a dog

In a landmark study by DeVries (1969), children (three to six years of age) were asked to identify if Maynard was a cat or dog prior to playing with the animal. As would be anticipated, all the children correctly identified Maynard as a "cat." However, following the play period, the researcher placed a dog mask on Maynard and asked the children, once again, if Maynard was a cat or a dog. Almost all of the three-year-olds now claimed that Maynard was a "dog."

Table 3.3 Cognitive milestones: school age to pre-adolescence

Developmental period	Milestones/limitations
7–11 years	**Mastery of conservation tasks:**
Piaget: concrete operational period	*Substance/mass (7–8 years), length (7–8 years), area (8–9 years), weight (9–10 years)*
	Classification and class inclusion
	Seriation (*order objects by length or weight*)
	Theory of mind
	Increased understanding of metacognition
Information processing 7–8 years	**Improved selective attention**
	Rehearsal as a spontaneous memory strategy
	Can repeat 5 digits
	Increased use of classification skills
	Increased flexibility of attention
9–11 years	**Increased planning**
	Metamemory: memory strategies increase (*organization, elaboration*)
	Can repeat 6 digits
	Increases in cognitive self-regulation
	(*monitoring progress towards a goal, readjusting plan accordingly*)
	Increased speed and efficiency of processing

The inability to consider more than one dimension simultaneously also accounts for problems experienced with issues of **appearance and reality**.

Faulty logic is also demonstrated in problems involving **class inclusion** because children at this stage do not understand that a subcategory cannot contain more items than the superordinate category. For example, if a child is shown a picture of cows and horses in a field, and the cows (10) clearly outnumber the horses (2), when asked if there are more cows or animals in the field, the child at this stage will answer "more cows."

Concrete operational period   Following a transition period (between five and seven years), when children are prone to make inconsistent responses, school-age children can respond to the majority of conservation tasks correctly, with a good degree of confidence in their responses, and can provide a rationale based on observable facts (e.g., glasses contain the same amount of liquid, since only the shape of the container has changed). However, even at this stage, children are still limited by what is observable and concrete and they cannot engage in problem solving of a hypothetical nature. Milestones for the concrete operational stage are available in Table 3.3.

Formal operations   Finally, entrance into the stage of **formal operations** places the adolescent within the realm of adult reasoning and logic. For Piaget, the ability to think in the abstract is the cornerstone of this period which allows the adolescent to perform tasks requiring **hypothetical** and **deductive reasoning**, which will be discussed in *Chapter 4*.

Stages of moral reasoning   For Piaget, moral reasoning evolves over the course of two broad developmental stages. The first stage, **heteronomous morality** or **moral**

realism (ages five to 10), is dominated by a sense that rules are created by authority; laws are not changeable and obedience is essential. At this stage, children do not consider "*intention*" and focus exclusively on the outcome. Based on developmental responses to a series of moral dilemmas, Kohlberg (1976) proposed a stage theory of moral development that is closely aligned with Piaget's ideas that moral reasoning is closely tied to limitations in cognition. Kohlberg's first stage of moral reasoning, **preconventional morality**, reflects early childhood concepts of doing the right thing, based on the consequences; for example, we want to avoid punishment or obtain a reward. Later on, in middle childhood, the concept of morality is represented by what Kohlberg labeled **conventional morality**, where the correct moral response is dictated by what is the expected response given the standards prescribed by the group; that is, doing the right thing and maintaining the status quo. For Kohlberg, the final level, postconventional morality, which will be discussed in the next chapter, was achieved by a select few. Kohlberg's stages of moral development are available in *Chapter 4*, Table 4.1.

Accident or purposeful act?

John is helping his mother set the table and he accidently breaks five plates.
George is upset and throws his plate on the floor, breaking it.
Which child is naughtier, John or George?
A young child would not consider the intent and would say that John is naughtier
    because he broke *more* plates.

Strengths and limitations of cognitive stage theories   Although there is agreement that stages occur in the sequence Piaget suggested, rates may vary; for example, the pace may be accelerated (in the case of giftedness) or slower (in the case of cognitive delay). In addition, while Piaget believed that cognitive development was universal, there is growing evidence that children in different cultures develop skills in different ways (Chavajay & Rogoff, 1999; Rogoff & Chavajay, 1995). For example, Piaget's stages apply more to children who attend traditional schools, compared to tribal children without formal schooling (Fahrmeier, 1978). Piaget's theory is also criticized by researchers who believe that several of the milestones occur much earlier than originally thought. For example, using a technique that focuses on **impossible events**, Baillargeon and colleagues (Aguilar & Baillargeon, 2002; Baillargeon, 1993, 2008) have demonstrated the existence of object permanence in infants as young as five months of age.

Kohlberg's theories of moral development have also been criticized for not recognizing gender differences in moral thinking. Gilligan (1982) has suggested that females are more prone to make moral decisions based on the perspective of "care" (affection and mutual trust), while males are more likely to make their moral judgments based on "justice," although these suggestions have not been supported by research (Turiel, 2006).

Vygotsky and facilitated learning

Although Piaget focused primarily on learning through self-discovery, Vygotsky believed that learning could be enhanced by social facilitation and such strategies as **scaffolding**, where the adult or mentor provides **guided participation** (Rogoff, 2003) to raise performance to the next level. Children demonstrate improved skills in planning and problem solving when more skilled mentors (adult or peer) are involved (Kobayashi, 1994). For optimum learning to take place, those providing the assistance to the learner should have an understanding of the child's **zone of proximal development (ZPD),** or the optimum level of intervention that is just within the child's grasp (not too difficult or too easy). Within this context, it is also important to know when to withdraw assistance to allow the child time to consolidate the newly acquired skills (Tudge & Rogoff, 1999). When parents use scaffolding techniques, children demonstrate an increased capacity to concentrate and focus at an early age, and greater social and academic maturity later on (Bono & Stifter, 2003; Ruff & Capozzoli, 2003).

Milestones in information processing

Studies of information processing focus on the child's growing capacity in attention, memory, and problem-solving skills. Selective attention, concentration, and flexibility in engaging and disengaging attention from the task at hand improve over the course of childhood. In *Chapter 8*, the discussion focuses on children and youth who experience problems with attention and concentration due to executive functioning deficits that impair their ability to inhibit responses and sustain goal-directed behaviors. Individuals with attention deficit hyperactivity disorder (ADHD) have less activity in the prefrontal area of their brain, which is associated with planning ability and the ability to shift attention between different tasks (Barkley, 1998).

As early as three to five years of age, children who are able to inhibit responses perform better on tasks of math and reading achievement later on (Blair & Razza, 2007). Studies using functional magnetic resonance imaging (fMRI) techniques have found increased activation of the prefrontal cortex (associated with planning ability) at this stage of development when young children are engaged in tasks that require the need to inhibit inappropriate responses (Bartgis, Lilly, & Thomas, 2003).

Increasing awareness of the **theory of mind** (awareness that others have their own thoughts and perceptions), **metacognition** (thinking about thinking), and **metamemory** (awareness of the different strategies available to assist recall) all contribute to a refined ability to process information over the course of development.

Children with autism spectrum disorders (ADS), which will be discussed in *Chapter 7*, experience significant difficulty with theory of mind problems (also known as the false belief test), although those with higher functioning autism (HFA) may acquire the ability at a later stage of development.

Children develop an increased capacity for **cognitive self-regulation** (the ability to monitor and alter strategies when needed in order to meet one's goals). Young children who use private speech (or self-directed speech) on challenging tasks perform better than peers who do not (Winsler, Naglieri, & Manfra, 2006). The use of private speech eventually lessens with age; however, children who experience learning and behavior problems tend to engage in self-directed speech beyond their age-mates, most likely in an effort to sustain their focus in light of their attention and processing problems. Children who do not increase their cognitive self-regulation skills are at risk for negative outcomes in all areas of functioning, including: learning, academic performance, and social/emotional development. Milestones in information processing are available in Tables 3.1 and 3.3.

Theory of mind

Brenda and Meredith are sharing crayons from the wooden crayon box at the play table. The teacher asks the girls to put the crayons back in the box and close the lid. Brenda is sent out of the classroom to do an errand. While Brenda is gone, the teacher replaces the crayons with chalk and asks Meredith the following question: *When Brenda returns to the room, what will she say is in the wooden box?* If Meredith has acquired a theory of mind, she will state "crayons," because Brenda was not privy to information about the exchange. However, if Meredith does not yet have a theory of mind, her response will be that Brenda will say there is chalk in the box.

Milestones in self-awareness and self-control

Development of self-awareness

An examiner places red rouge on a child's nose; at what age will the child first touch his nose when viewing his image in the mirror? Lewis and Brooks (1978) found that approximately 75% of children between the ages of 21 and 24 months will respond to their own nose, rather than the reflection in the mirror, indicating a sense of visual self-concept (**perceptual self**) or self-recognition. Self-recognition is related to cognitive development and is delayed in children with Down syndrome (Cicchetti & Beeghly, 1990).

Toddlerhood   Erikson recognized the major task for mastery at this stage of psychosocial development was **autonomy versus shame and doubt**. In this stage, children can be non-compliant and negative, traits that have come to define the "terrible twos." However, opposition is less evident in families that practice warm parenting and guidance (Kochanska, Tjebkes, & Forman, 1998). Self-descriptions, at this stage, usually contain references to age, gender, and physical size.

Preschool and early childhood   During this stage (three to six years), Erikson believed the major task was **initiative versus guilt** as preschoolers develop a sense of purposefulness and **self-efficacy** (Bandura, 1995) resulting from increased experiences of mastery. However, overconfidence can be an issue, as children tend to overestimate their abilities and underestimate the difficulty of the task (Harter, 1998). Preschoolers develop a sense of **self–representation** based on their own sense of personal attributes (Eder & Mangelsdorf, 1997) and often describe themselves in terms of their physical activities (*"I like to run"*) and possessions (*"I have a new red truck"*). The development of **self-concept** (attributes, competencies, values) evolves over the course of childhood and eventually is accompanied by a sense of **self-esteem** (evaluations of one's own worth and the associated feelings). The impact of parenting practices and attachment style on the child's developing sense of self-esteem will be discussed at greater length later in this and the following chapter.

In early childhood, children begin to associate themselves with concrete categories and in addition to providing information about their possessions (*"I have a new red bike"*) and their abilities (*"I can make a car out of Lego"*), they now add being part of a group to their description (*"I go to preschool and I live with my mommy and sister"*).

Middle childhood   Erikson saw this as a time to master **industry versus inferiority**, which becomes evident as there is an increased tendency to include the **social self** (Damon & Hart, 1988) in self-reports (e.g., *"I am a girl scout and I am a member of the soccer team"*) and to use **social comparison** to gauge performance. At this stage (seven to 10 years of age), children describe themselves by reference to their internal attributes (thoughts, feelings) as well as their external characteristics and abilities (Harter, 1998). For example, when asked to describe herself, Monica might say: *"I have blonde hair and blue eyes. I am a great speller. I don't do math very well. I am a kind person and I can sing a lot better than my brother."* Middle childhood is a time when gender differences contribute to individual variations in self-perceptions; for example, boys tend to rate themselves equally along dimensions of social, scholastic conduct, appearance, and athletics, while girls tend to rate themselves lower for categories of appearance and athletics than males (Bukatko & Daehler, 2004).

Development of self-control or behavioral self-regulation

Children who demonstrate **self-regulation** have an ability independently to monitor and control their behaviors appropriate to the given situation (Grolnick & Farkas, 2002). Children's *"effortful control"* or ability to regulate their behaviors (**behavioral self-regulation**) and their emotions (**emotion regulation**) increases dramatically between two-and-a-half and three years of age due to rapid development of the prefrontal cortex (Rothbart & Bates, 2006; Thompson & Goodvin, 2007). This development also results in more consistent responses to environmental stressors through increases in the inhibition of impulses and increases in attentional control (Li-Grining, 2007).

Early childhood to preschool   Temper tantrums peak at three years of age, then dissipate as children develop increased coping skills which allow for increased maturation in **frustration tolerance**. At the same time, willfulness and non-compliance are increasingly replaced by cooperative behaviors generated to please adults, as children begin to internalize parental values and are motivated to gain their parents' approval (Kochanska, Aksan, & Keonig, 1995). **Delay of gratification** is also improving, aided by children's ability to use a number of self-initiated strategies, such as **self-distraction** (*looking away, self talk, singing*) to alleviate the frustration of waiting to obtain a coveted reward, such as opening a present or eating a treat (Wolf, 1990). Researchers have found that girls, who have more advanced development of attention and language skills, perform at a higher level than boys, evidencing greater self-control in these tasks (Else-Quest, Hyde, Goldsmith, & Van Hulle, 2006).

Caregivers can increase their child's ability to regulate behaviors by encouraging patience and rewarding compliance, especially in the case of young children who tend to be more reactive. Kochanska, Aksan, and Carlson (2005) found that when caregivers used encouragement and assurance with reactive toddlers, their skills improved when assessed again, several months later; however, if parents were impatient, these toddlers' reactive behaviors intensified on later evaluation. Researchers have consistently found that the **goodness of fit** between a child's temperament and environmental conditions (such as parenting style) can have positive outcomes (increased compliance and self-regulation) or negative outcomes (increased anxious and reactive responses and reduced self-regulation) for the developing child (Feldman, 2007).

The importance of self-regulation of emotions and behaviors cannot be overstated, as will become evident in future discussions of adaptive and maladaptive responses to frustration, aggression, and learning, and in the context of social situations. When these milestones are not achieved, this can result in many negative outcomes, academically, socially, and emotionally. Children who achieve these milestones continue along a path of increased maturity and social acceptance, while those who do not become at increased risk for social isolation, peer rejection, and depression.

Summation   The rapid development of the prefrontal cortex during the latter half of the toddler period and in the preschool years provides the foundations for increased ability to regulate behaviors and emotions (Rothbart & Bates, 2006). This increased capacity within the context of a supportive environment helps prepare the child for primary school with a sense of confidence, competence, and readiness to be successful in school both academically and socially.

However, some children enter primary school ill-equipped to face the challenges in their school environment due to poor ability to regulate their emotions or behaviors, and an inability to focus and attend to the tasks at hand. These children can become readily overwhelmed by their lack of success on a daily basis, and are at greatest risk for developing the disorders of childhood and adolescence which are the focus of Part Two of this book.

Ego resiliency

Ego resiliency (*the ability to monitor and alter behavior to suit the situation*) also emerges with greater consistency during the latter half of the toddler period and the preschool years, as self-control leads to increased management of behavioral outcomes that are situation-specific (e.g., the knowledge that behaviors on the playground are not appropriate in the home).

Milestones in emotional development

Understanding emotions

During the toddler period, the **self-conscious emotions** begin to emerge and become increasingly refined throughout the preschool period (Saarni, Campos, Camras, &

Witherington, 2006). Unlike the basic emotions (such as happiness, sadness, anger, and fear), these emotions require an element of cognitive appraisal regarding one's intention and an understanding of social roles, and include an understanding of more subtle emotions such as **positive self-evaluation** (an early form of **pride**) and **shame**. Toddlers also develop an increased sensitivity to others in distress, which is an early precursor to feelings of **empathy** which may be evident in such gestures as offering a toy, blanket, or hug to soothe another child (Moreno, Klute, & Robinson, 2008). Children whose parents encourage them to express and label their emotions develop an increased emotional vocabulary and are better able to recognize emotional cues in others (Cole, Armstrong, & Pemberton, 2010; Taumoepeau & Ruffman, 2006).

Compared to toddlers, preschoolers will use words increasingly to communicate feelings and to comfort peers in distress (Eisenberg, Fabes, & Spinrad, 2006). However, for some children who are reactive and have poor emotion regulation, witnessing a peer in distress can result in a contagion effect, where they become increasingly overwhelmed due to increased activation of the right central hemisphere, the part of the brain that regulates negative emotions (Jones, Field, & Davalos, 2000). As with other aspects of emotion regulation, caregivers can be instrumental in assisting their child to cope with their responses to the feelings of others in ways that are sensitive and caring, rather than fearful, angry, or punitive (Eisenberg, 2003).

Due to their enhanced cognitive capacity, school-age children increasingly associate success with pride and failure with guilt relative to their own self-doing and self-concept (Saarni et al., 2006). Although toddlers tend to overestimate their abilities and underestimate task demands, school-aged children tend to take their failures personally, and if lack of success is met with harsh criticism, they are more likely to respond with an increased sense of shame, self-criticism, anger, and withdrawal (Mills, 2005). During this age span (six to 12 years) children are also able to increase their understanding of ambivalent emotions; for example, understanding that a child may be happy that the team won the game, but upset that she struck out at bat.

Emotional problem solving   *Chapter 6* focuses on adjustment problems in children and adolescents which are temporary responses (such as anxiety or depression) to environmental stressors. Towards the end of the school-aged period (around 10 years of age) advances in cognitive development provide children with the ability to problem solve in emotional situations. When faced with a stressor, individuals can meet the challenge in two important ways: **problem-focused coping** or **emotion-focused coping**. While problem-focused coping involves looking for information to help solve a problem (e.g., "*What materials do I need? Who can I get them from?*"), emotion-focused coping involves the need to change how the person actually feels about the situation or to change the reaction to the stressor (Eschenbeck, Kohlmann, & Lohaus, 2007). A child may be very upset and write her thoughts in a journal to help calm herself down. Another way of emotional coping is to use a defense mechanism, such as humor or rationalization.

Emotions and interpersonal aggression

Normally, aggressive outbursts, like temper tantrums, reach their peak at three years of age; the same time that aggressive behaviors typically begin to decline. Initially, aggression takes the form of **instrumental aggression**, where a toddler will push a child to gain access to a desired object or activity (Sammy pushes Joey off the tricycle because it is his turn to ride). More serious forms of aggression involve **hostile aggression** or **interpersonal aggression** where the intent is to injure another. The research predicts that children who remain aggressive after the toddler stage, or who increase their aggressive behaviors, have increasingly poor outcomes across a number of areas (Loeber, Green, Lahey, Frick, & McBurnett, 2000; Patterson & Yoerger, 2002). Growing emphasis has been placed on the types of aggressive behaviors that can be exhibited. Some children primarily demonstrate patterns of **reactive aggression**, also known as "hot-blooded aggression"; these children lack emotional and behavioral self-control (emotion dysregulation) and respond to frustration internally by high levels of activation of their autonomic nervous system (the "flight or flight response"). On the other hand, some children are more prone to patterns of **proactive aggression**, also known as "cold-blooded aggression"; these children participate in planned acts of aggression, such as bullying, domination, or teasing, without demonstrating any emotional response. About half of aggressive children vacillate between the two forms of aggression. However, about one-third will be primarily reactive, while only 15% will engage exclusively in proactive forms of aggression (Dodge, Lochman, Harnish, Bates, & Pettit, 1997).

Several factors have been implicated in placing children at risk for developing aggressive behaviors (biological factors, cognitive factors, social learning, and parenting practices). Increased levels of the **hormone testosterone** (Dabbs & Morris, 1990) and having a parent with **anti-social personality disorder** have been suggested as potential biological markers for increased aggressive responses (APA, 2000). Females who are aggressive have tendencies to engage in **relational aggression** often including emotions of jealousy, betrayal, and conflict (Werner & Crick, 2004) with the goal of damaging another girl's "social status" or increasing "feelings of exclusion" for the target of the aggression (Keenan, Coyne, & Lahey, 2008). Children who come from an abusive home, or who experience harsh parenting practices, are more likely to demonstrate reactive forms of aggression, although this can also trigger patterns of proactive aggression (Vitaro, Barker, Boivin, Brendgen, & Tremblay, 2006). It is possible that for some children growing up in a harsh and punitive environment causes excess activation of the autonomic nervous system (resulting in reactive aggression), while for others, modeling these punitive and aggressive behaviors may result in patterns of proactive aggression. The different forms of aggression will be discussed at greater length in *Chapter 9*.

Milestones in psychosocial development

Understanding others and social exchange

Social referencing   In situations of ambiguity, toddlers as young as 12 months will look to the caregiver for clues to guide their behavior, a condition referred to as **social referencing** (Moses, Baldwin, Rosicky, & Tidball, 2001). Studies have demonstrated that shortly after their first birthday, children will approach or avoid an ambiguous toy based on their mother's facial expressions. Furthermore, the tendency to look to others to endorse or avoid ambiguous situations or toys increases significantly between one and two years of age (Emde, 1992).

Early social exchange   Although Piaget believed that the preoperational child was unable to take the perspective of another, Repacholi (1998) found that after observing an experimenter's dislike for crackers (disgusted expression) versus broccoli (pleased expression), toddlers as young as 18–19 months offered the preferred food. Also by two years of age, toddlers have a basic understanding of the rules of social exchange in such games as hide and seek. **Social exchange** or **affective sharing** (Emde, 1992) in toddlers is evident as they share their experiences with adults (pointing, bringing the object to the adult). Children with autism spectrum disorders do not engage in affective exchange due to deficits in social reciprocity and social pragmatics. The impact of this lack of reciprocity on development will be discussed at length in *Chapter 7*.

Social competence   During early childhood, relations with peers take on increasing importance, since the majority of children are enrolled in school programs. Peer group experiences can have a positive or negative effect on the development of self-concept and **social competence** (the ability to engage and respond in peer interactions that are positive). Children who are socially competent are better liked and more popular than children who act aggressively or display negative emotions (Arsenio, Cooperman, & Lover, 2000).

Bandura (1985) demonstrated the power of observational learning and modeling on subsequent aggressive behaviors in children, while Coie and Dodge (1998) applied social information processing to children's aggressive responses and suggested that some children are prone to misinterpret ambivalent cues (such as facial and physical expressions) in others as "hostile" and respond aggressively as a result, a concept referred to as the hostile attribution bias.

Children who act out or those who are withdrawn can benefit from interventions to increase positive interactions with others. Discussions of specific intervention programs will be addressed throughout this book as they relate to specific types of problems children may encounter when relating to their peers. Children who have successful peer relationships do better academically than those who struggle socially due to poor self-regulation and lack of social skills (Ladd, Buhs, & Seid, 2000). Children who are successful in conflict resolution demonstrate good ability to process social information and **social problem-solving skills**, evident in their ability to: read social cues appropriately; formulate a plan; respond; and monitor the reactions of others (Coie & Dodge, 1998). Children with poor social problem-solving skills may misread a social situation and commit a number of social blunders, such as attempting to gain entry to a peer group activity at a totally inappropriate time and being rejected as a result. Other equally ineffective strategies (avoidance of social situations, aggressive reactions) serve to alienate the child even further (Dodge, Coie, & Lynam, 2006).

Researchers can use a technique called a **sociogram** to determine a child's status among his or her peers (Asher & Wheeler, 1985). Children's responses to a number of questions about their classmates (*Who would you invite to your party? Who would you not invite? Who is the most popular?*) can provide insight into the social dynamics of the classroom. Researchers have isolated five potential categories: popular, rejected, neglected, average, and controversial. Studies have shown that acceptance or rejection by peers can have a number of positive or negative consequences. Dodge et al. (2006) have identified two types of rejected children: **rejected–aggressive** (who are often involved in conflict, aggressive, impulsive, have poor ability to interpret social cues, and frequently use the hostile attribution bias); and **rejected–withdrawn** (who avoid interactions with peers, and display anxious fears of being victimized). Eventually, the rejected–aggressive child often takes on the role of bully, while the rejected–withdrawn type is more likely to become the victim (Putallaz et al., 2007). Children who are rejected and withdrawn often also demonstrate poor academic progress, which can have long-term consequences (Buhs & Ladd, 2001; Veronneau, Vitaro, Brendgen, Dishion, & Tremblay, 2010). Buhs, Ladd, and Herald (2006) tracked children from kindergarten through fifth grade and found that early peer rejection led to poor classroom participation, and school avoidance. Later on, rejection took the form of peer exclusion or chronic peer abuse, resulting in direct verbal or physical, or indirect (relational), victimization.

Children who are **controversial** display both positive and negative behaviors and can be confusing for peers who are drawn to them but fear them at the same time. Although it was once thought that **neglected** children would suffer dire consequences of being ignored by their peers, research has shown that these children tend to retreat from the social arena, are shy, and tend to do well academically. Neglected children have **low social impact scores** (low on social visibility).

Social skills training programs can enhance social problem solving through direct instruction and practice in working through different social scenarios. A number of these programs will be discussed in future chapters, as they relate to children with specific learning disabilities (*Chapter 8*), and children with behavior problems (*Chapter 9*).

Attachment, parenting style, and child outcomes

The attachment process

Theories of attachment and attachment styles were introduced in *Chapter 2*. Recall that Ainsworth, Blehar, Waters, and Wall (1978) conducted the **strange situation experiments** and found patterns of **secure attachment** (60%), and two variants of **insecure attachment**, namely: **anxious–avoidant attachment** (20%) (the child ignores the mother's departure and ignores her return); and **anxious–resistant or ambivalent attachment** (10–15%) (the child is upset at the mother leaving, but is unable to be consoled upon her return). Main and Solomon (1990) found a **disorganized–disoriented attachment** pattern in their study of abused infants who displayed a number of confused and contradictory behaviors (rocking, appearing dazed). These disorganized responses continue during the first two years of life (Barnett, Ganiban, & Cicchetti, 1999) and have been associated with increased risk for hostility and aggression in the preschool and primary school years (Lyons-Ruth, 1996).

Child outcomes associated with attachment patterns   Research has linked attachment patterns to socio-economic status (SES), finding securely attached and stable patterns in middle-SES families, with greater risk for insecure and shifting patterns of insecurity in low-SES families (Vondra, Hommerding, & Shaw, 1999). Although longitudinal studies have produced mixed results (Thompson et al., 2000), some studies have found that preschool teachers rated children who were "securely attached" as higher in self-esteem, social skills, and popularity than their insecurely attached peers (Elicker, Englund, & Sroufe, 1992). At 10 years of age, camp counselors rated children as more socially competent if they were securely attached as infants (Shulman, Elicker, & Sroufe, 1994).

Can early attachment patterns influence later outcomes?

There is research support for Bowlby's thesis of individual differences in the security of the attachment process and the development of internal working models. Not only are attachment patterns stable over time (Weinfield, Whaley, & Egeland, 1999), but patterns can predict future outcomes, such as enthusiasm in solving problems, peer relations, and self-esteem (Sroufe, 2002).

Studies of cross-cultural attachment patterns have found that when asked to rate characteristics of the securely attached child and the ideal child, experts and mothers produced very similar ratings for these two classifications, regardless of whether the raters were from collectivistic or individualistic countries (Posada et al., 1995).

Amidst the controversy of whether a secure attachment represents the universal ideal, Crittenden (2000) suggests that the terms "secure" and "insecure" may not be the best ways to categorize attachment patterns when taking different contexts into consideration. Instead Crittenden contends that terms such as "adaptive" and "mal-adaptive" might be more appropriate when describing different attachment patterns, especially within the context of different cultures.

Attachment and culture

Although secure attachment is considered the gold standard in most countries, some cultures prefer to promote different attachment styles in their children. German mothers promote avoidant attachment as the ideal, since it instills early independence (Grossmann, Grossmann, Spangler, Suess, & Unzer, 1985), while Japanese children demonstrate high rates of anxious ambivalent attachment, fostering a strong sense of dependence in this collectivist society (Miyake, Chen, & Campos, 1985).

Attachment and intervention

Until recently, the majority of intervention programs for child issues of attachment and maltreatment have targeted changes in the caregiver's attitude and parenting behaviors (Cicchetti & Valentino, 2006; MacMillan et al., 2009). Many of these programs have delivered services as home visitations from nurses (Olds, Sadler, & Kitzman, 2007), and other health care professionals (Dozier et al., 2006), offered on a short-term (one to four months) or long-term basis (five months to a year).

Bakermans-Kranenburg, vanIJzendoorn, and Juffer (2003) successfully helped mothers to modify their behavior using video feedback from taped sessions, which increased their consistency and warmth in later sessions. Longer-term programs reveal that long-lasting improvements can be made in maternal sensitivity, warmth, infant mental development, and reduced risk for future child behavior problems (Olds et al., 1997, 2007).

Moss et al. (2011) evaluated the efficacy of a short-term (eight-week) home-visiting program in enhancing maternal sensitivity, child attachment, and reducing child behavioral concerns in maltreated children. The study involved 67 caregivers reported for maltreatment and their children, randomly assigned to the intervention or control group. Intervention involved eight, weekly 90-minute visits conducted by clinical workers who engaged the parent in a sequence of activities, involving: discussion of the problem for that week (20 minutes); videotaping of parent–child interaction (10 to 15 minutes); video feedback session (20 minutes); and wrap-up session (10 to 15 minutes). Attachment was measured using the strange situation procedure (Ainsworth et al., 1978) for infants up to two years of age, and the *Preschool Separation–Reunion Procedure* (Cassidy, Marvin, & the MacArthur Working Group on Attachment, as cited in Moss et al., 2011) for children two to six years of age. Results revealed that significantly more children in the intervention group moved to the secure and organized categories on post-test than the control group. This study demonstrates the effectiveness of intervention in changing attachment security and organization in older, preschool children and infants, and the success of video feedback in assisting parents to be more sensitive to their child's behaviors, and in enhancing their ability to read social and emotional cues related to anxiety and insecurity.

Since maltreated children tend to exhibit more problems in the preschool period, Moss et al. (2011) suggest that intervention during this period may assist maltreated children to increase their ability to regulate their emotions in periods of distress, and reduce emotional dysregulation which has been associated with increased risk for internalizing and externalizing behaviors (Toth, Cicchetti, & Kim, 2002). Issues of maltreatment are discussed at length in *Chapter 12*.

Parenting style and child outcomes

Baumrind's four parenting styles and child outcomes   Baumrind (1991, 2005) investigated parenting styles relative to the degree and nature of parent warmth/acceptance (responsiveness), or control/monitoring (demandingness), and found four different parenting styles: **authoritative** (high in responsiveness and demandingness); **authoritarian** (low in responsiveness, high in demandingness); **permissive** (high in responsiveness, low in demandingness); and **uninvolved** (how in responsiveness and demandingness). Initially, it was thought that the authoritative style was the universal "gold standard" for parenting style because it was associated with the most positive outcomes for children (see *Chapter 2* for more background information on parenting styles).

Is the authoritative parenting style a universal gold standard?

Studies have found that the harsh discipline associated with the authoritarian parenting style may be of benefit in some situations, such as environments where there are increased opportunities for youth to engage in high-risk behaviors in dangerous neighborhoods (Bradley, 1998; Kelley, Power, & Wimbush, 1992).

However, other researchers suggest that punitive practices may signal acceptance of violence and encourage youth to model these behaviors (Raymond, Jones, & Cook, 1998).

Authoritative style The *authoritative style* fosters many child qualities, including: increased self-control, positive mood and self-esteem, task persistence, social competence, and academic performance (Herman, Dornbusch, Herron, & Herting, 1997; Luster & McAdoo, 1996). In middle childhood, school-age children raised by authoritative parents tend to score higher in **agency** (the tendency to take initiative) and **self-assertion** (Baumrind, 1989).

Authoritarian style Parents who employ an *authoritarian style* tend to use harsh coercive practices and demonstrate minimal warmth. Children raised in this manner are more likely to be anxious and unhappy, and to have low frustration tolerance, and can be passive aggressive (Baumrind, 1991). Boys tend to be aggressive with peers, while girls may be overly dependent and easily overwhelmed (Hart et al., 2000).

Permissive style Lacking in guidance, children raised in *permissive* and indulgent households tend to be impulsive, lacking in self-reliance, and demanding, with boys at risk for dependence and low achievement (Barber & Olsen, 1997).

Uninvolved style In its extreme form, *uninvolved* parents can be guilty of child neglect, with far-reaching negative consequences for development in cognitive, social, and emotional areas. Children raised by indifferent parents tend to be dependent and moody with minimal self-control or social skills. The majority of uninvolved parents are emotionally unavailable to their children due to life stressors (Maccoby & Martin, 1983).

Child outcomes for parenting styles are summarized in Table 3.4.

Culture, SES, and parenting styles

Parenting styles and culture Parenting styles may also reflect different cultural expectations. Joshi and MacLean (1997) compared maternal expectations for child development for 45 tasks, in mothers from India, Japan, and England. Japanese mothers demonstrated higher expectations than British mothers in areas of education, self-care, and environmental independence, while Indian mothers had lower expectations than Japanese and British mothers in all areas except environmental independence.

Su and Hynie (2011) evaluated the effects of life stress, social support, cultural beliefs, and social norms on parenting style for mothers of preschool children two to six years of age, for mainland Chinese (MC), European Chinese (EC), and Chinese Canadian (CC) mothers. Results revealed that the mothers' level of stress moderated parenting style, with mothers being more authoritative when less stressed and when their parenting beliefs were less traditional (i.e., more individualistic). In this study, the use of an authoritarian parenting style increased, especially for CC and MC mothers,

Table 3.4   Parenting style and child outcomes

Parenting style	Child outcomes	Child autonomy	Child independence
Authoritative	Good self-concept and self-esteem Task persistence Higher academic performance Higher agency	Child is able to negotiate and make decisions within appropriate limits	Independent
Authoritarian	Fearful, anxious, and unhappy Low frustration tolerance Boys: aggressive Girls: dependent	Minimal opportunity for autonomy Parent makes the decisions with minimal or no input from child	Lack of independence
Permissive– indulgent	Demanding Few boundaries Low self-reliance Boys: dependent, low achievement	Permissive and indulgent Child makes decisions without guidance or direction	Excessive independence Indulged
Permissive– uninvolved	Dependent Moody Unpredictable based on nature of "acquired" role models Low self-control Poor social skills	Parents are indifferent to child's concerns or issues	Indifferent

when they were under the most stress. Sumer, Orta, and Ankara (2010) conducted a meta-analysis of 34 studies conducted in Turkey regarding parenting style and child outcomes. Based on their results, studies consistently endorsed the authoritative parenting style, versus the authoritarian parenting style, for producing the most positive outcomes in areas of increased self-esteem, less aggressiveness, academic success, lower anxiety, and higher self-acceptance.

Parenting styles and SES   Although children develop behavioral problems through the interaction of multiple influences, low family SES has long been acknowledged as a risk factor for many child and adolescent problems, including: behavior, academic, and social problems (Dodge, Pettit, & Bates, 1994). Parenting styles that are more negative (Grant et al., 2003) have been associated with lower levels of SES and higher levels of child problems. However, as Callahan and Eyberg (2010) report, the importance of maternal education is often not included in studies of low SES and as a result valuable information has been lost, since in their study higher levels of maternal education were associated with increased maternal warmth and responsiveness. In their studies, the inclusion of factors such as maternal income, education, and occupation provided much more predictable indicators of higher maternal prosocial verbalizations and potential resources for child resiliency in these low SES populations.

Parenting practices, parenting styles, and child outcomes In addition to parenting styles, researchers have also studied the impact of various **parenting practices** on a number of child outcomes, including school achievement, child behavior, and behavior problems, as well as the mediational links between parenting styles and SES, as was discussed. While parenting practices refer to the goals parents set for "socializing" their children based on their expectations and beliefs, parenting style is related more to the prevailing "attitude and climate" embedded in the manner in which parents achieve these goals (Darling & Steinberg, 1993).

School achievement Positive relationships have been found between parenting practices, such as parental engagement, expectations, and beliefs, and children's academic outcomes (Bronstein, Ginsburg, & Herrera, 2005; Davis-Kean, 2005; Spera, Wentzel, & Matto, 2009). In a meta-analysis of the influence of parenting practices on children's academic success, Jeynes (2010) reported that parental expectation was the single leading contributor to academic achievement for both elementary school and secondary school students. With respect to parenting style, the authoritative style (high in responsiveness, high in demandingness/monitoring) was significantly related to elementary and secondary school achievement; however, while responsiveness consistently was related in a positive way, monitoring (e.g., checking homework) was not significantly related to achievement for either elementary or secondary school students (Jeynes, 2010). As a result of this analysis, Jeynes (2010) has recommended that educational programs aimed at enhancing parental involvement focus more on the subtle factors such as encouragement and communication, rather than tasks such as monitoring of homework and attending school functions.

Based on a large sample from Statistics Canada, Areepattamannil (2010) surveyed over 6,000 households regarding school achievement (parents' reports of school grades), parenting style (encouragement and monitoring), parenting practices (expectations and beliefs), and family SES. Results of this study were consistent with results from previous research and indicated that children from families higher in SES had higher educational achievement scores, and that both components of the authoritative parenting style (responsiveness and demandingness/monitoring) were significantly related to academic achievement, but not in the expected direction for monitoring. While responsiveness and encouragement were related to academic success in a significant and positive direction, as parental monitoring increased academic achievement decreased. The latter result supports findings of other researchers (Niggli et al., and Rogers et al., as cited in Areepattamannil, 2010) who reason that excessive monitoring of academic activities in the form of checking homework, monitoring time, and setting rules may actually increase academic pressure, lower academic self-concept, and result in weaker achievement. As a result, "parental monitoring in the form of parental pressure and control can decrease children's intrinsic motivation and may undermine the learning process and children's sense of personal value and responsibility" (Areepattamannil, 2010, p. 287).

Given that parental beliefs and encouragement can have a strong impact on a child's academic success, there is a need for educators to enhance parental engagement in their child's academic orientation. One of the most successful parental involvement programs in the United Kingdom (Sure Start) has been successful in enhancing parent involvement through home visitations which are an integral part of the program (Garbers, Tunstill, Allnock, & Akhurst, 2006).

Social and emotional development   In the previous discussions regarding attachment, it was apparent that the parent-child relationship serves as a prototype for future relationships and sets the stage for the nature of increasing socialization. It is not surprising to see that researchers such as Baumrind (1991, 2005) have found that parenting styles have a direct impact on child development in many areas, including social and emotional development. However, while most studies have focused on maternal responses, or combined maternal and paternal responses, Rinaldi and Howe (2012) examined the separate roles of mothers' and fathers' parenting styles on child behavior patterns in toddlers. Results revealed that fathers' authoritarian parenting style (use of physical coercion, verbal hostility, and lack of reasoning with children) predicted externalizing and internalizing problems in the toddlers, while mothers' permissive parenting style predicted externalizing behaviors. The authoritative parenting style for all parents predicted the most adaptive behaviors.

References

Aguiar, A., & Baillargeon, R. (2002). Developments in young infants' reasoning about occluded objects. *Cognitive Psychology, 45*(2), 267–336.

Ainsworth, M. D. S., Blehar, M., Waters, E., & Wall, S. (1978). *Patterns of attachment.* Hillsdale, NJ: Erlbaum.

Allport, G. W. (1961). *Pattern and growth in personality.* New York: Holt.

American Psychiatric Association (APA). (2000). *Diagnostic and statistical manual of mental disorders* (4th ed., text revision). Washington, DC: Author.

Areepattamannil, S. (2010). Parenting practices, parenting style and children's school achievement. *Psychology Studies, 55*(4), 283–289. doi:10.1007/s12646-010-0043-0

Arsenio, W., Cooperman, S., & Lover, A. (2000). Affective predictors of preschoolers' aggression and peer acceptance: Direct and indirect effects. *Developmental Psychology, 36*(4), 438–448.

Asher, S. R., & Wheeler, V. A. (1985). Children's loneliness: A comparison of rejected and neglected peer status. *Journal of Consulting and Clinical Psychology, 53*, 500–505.

Baillargeon, R. (1993). The object concept revisited. New directions in the investigation of infants' physical knowledge. In C. E. Granrud (Ed.), *Visual cognition and perception in infancy* (pp. 265–315). Hillsdale, NJ: Erlbaum.

Baillargeon, R. (2008). *Perspectives on Psychological Science. Special Issue: From philosophical thinking to psychological empiricism, 3*(1), 2–13.

Bakermans-Kranenburg, M. J., van IJzendoorn, M. H., & Juffer, F. (2003). Less is more: Meta-analyses of sensitivity and attachment interventions in early childhood. *Psychological Bulletin, 129*, 195–215.

Bandura, A. (1985). A model of causality in social learning theory. In M. Mahony and A. Freeman (Eds.), *Cognition and therapy* (pp. 81–99). New York: Plenum Press.

Bandura, A. (1995). *Self-efficacy in changing societies.* New York: Cambridge University Press.

Barber, B. K., & Olsen, J. A. (1997). Socialization in context: Connection, regulation, and autonomy in the family, school, and neighborhood, and with peers. *Journal of Adolescent Research, 12*, 287–315.

Barkley, R. A. (1998). *Attention deficit hyperactivity disorder: A handbook for diagnosis and treatment* (2nd ed.). New York: Guilford.

Barnett, D., Ganiban, J., & Cicchetti, D. (1999). Maltreatment, negative expressivity, and the development of Type D attachments from 12 to 24 months of age. In J. I. Vonda & D. Barnett (Eds.), *Atypical attachment in infancy and early childhood among children at developmental risk, Monographs of the Society for Research in Child Development, 64*(3), 97–118.

Bartgis, J., Lilly, A. R., & Thomas, D. G. (2003). Event-related potential and behavioral measures of attention in 5-, 7-, and 9-year-olds. *Journal of General Psychology, 130,* 311–335.

Baumrind, D. (1989). Rearing competent children. In W. Damoin (Ed.), *Child development today and tomorrow* (pp. 349–378). San Francisco: Jossey-Bass.

Baumrind, D. (1991). The influences of parenting style on adolescent competence and substance use. *Journal of Early Adolescence, 11,* 56–95.

Baumrind, D. (2005). Patterns of parental authority and adolescent autonomy. *New Directions for Child and Adolescent Development, 108,* 61–69.

Beers, S. R., & DeBellis, M. (2002). Neuropsychological function in children with maltreatment-related posttraumatic stress disorder. *American Journal of Psychiatry, 159,* 483–486.

Beery, K. E., Beery, N. A., & Buktenica, N. A. (2010). *The Beery-Buktenica developmental test of visual motor integration (Beery-VMI6, Manual).* Bloomington, MN: Pearson.

Blair, C., & Razza, R. P. (2007). Relating effortful control, executive function and false belief understanding to emerging math and literacy ability in kindergarten. *Child Development, 78*(2), 647–663.

Bono, M. A., & Stifter, C. A. (2003). Maternal attention-directing strategies and infant focused attention during problem solving. *Infancy, 4,* 235–250.

Bradley, R. C. (1998). Child rearing in African American families: A study of the disciplinary practices of African American parents. *Journal of Multicultural Counseling and Development, 26,* 273–281.

Bronstein, P., Ginsburg, G. S., & Herrera, I. S. (2005). Parental predictors of motivational orientation in early adolescence: A longitudinal study. *Journal of Youth and Adolescence, 34,* 559–575.

Buhs, E. W., & Ladd, G. W. (2001). Peer rejection as an antecedent of young children's school adjustment: An examination of mediating processes. *Developmental Psychology, 37,* 550–560. doi:10.1037//OO12-1649.37.4.55

Buhs, E. W., Ladd, G. W., & Herald, S. L. (2006). Peer exclusion and victimization: Processes that mediate the relation between peer group rejection and children's classroom engagement and achievement. *Journal of Educational Psychology, 98,* 1–13. doi:10.1037/00220663.98.1

Bukatko, D., & Daehler, M. W. (2004). *Child development* (5th ed.). New York: Houghton Mifflin.

Callahan, C. L., & Eyberg, S. M. (2010). Relations between parent behavior and SES in a clinical sample: Validity of SES measures. *Child and Family Behavior Therapy, 32,* 125–138. doi:10.1080/07317101003776456

Chavajay, P., & Rogoff, B. (1999). Cultural variation in management of attention by children and their caregivers. *Developmental Psychology, 35*(4), 1079–1091.

Cicchetti, D., & Beeghly, M. (1990). *Down syndrome: A developmental perspective.* Cambridge: Cambridge University Press.

Cicchetti, D., & Valentino, K. (2006). An ecological–transactional perspective on child maltreatment: Failure of the average expectable environment and its influence on child development. In D. Cicchetti & D. J. Cohen (Eds.), *Developmental psychopathology: Vol. 3. Risk, disorder, and adaptation* (2nd ed.) (pp. 129–201). Hoboken, NJ: John Wiley & Sons, Ltd.

Coie, J. D., & Dodge, K. A. (1998). Aggression and antisocial behavior. In W. Damon and N. Eisenberg (Eds.), *Handbook of child psychology: Vol. 3. Social, emotional, and personality development* (5th ed.) (pp. 779–862). Hoboken, NJ: John Wiley & Sons, Ltd.

Cole, P. M., Armstrong, L. M., & Pemberton, C. K. (2010). The role of language in the development of emotion regulation. In S. D. Calkins & M. A. Bell (Eds.), *Child development at the intersection of emotion and cognition* (pp. 59–77). Washington, DC: APA.

Cratty, B. J. (1986). *Perceptual and motor development in infants and children* (3rd ed.). Englewood Cliffs, NJ: Prentice-Hall.

Crittenden, P. M. (2000). A dynamic-maturational exploration of the meaning of security and adaptation: Empirical, cultural and theoretical considerations. In P. M. Crittenden & A. H. Claussen (Eds.), *The organization of attachment relationships: Maturation, culture and context* (pp. 358–383). New York: Cambridge University Press.

Dabbs, J., & Morris, R. (1990). Testosterone, social class and antisocial behavior in a sample of 4,462 men. *Psychological Science, 1,* 209–211.

Darling, N., & Steinberg, L. (1993). Parenting style as context: An integrative model. *Psychological Bulletin, 113*(3), 487–496.

Damon, W., & Hart, D. (1988). *Self-understanding in childhood and adolescence.* Cambridge: Cambridge University Press.

Davis-Kean, P. E. (2005). The influence of parent education and family income on child achievement: The indirect role of parental expectations and the home environment. *Journal of Family Psychology, 19*(2), 294–304.

DeVries, R. (1969). Constancy of generic identity in the years three to six. *Monographs of the Society for Research in Child Development, 34* (serial no. 127).

Dodge, K. A., Coie, J. D., & Lynam, D. (2006). Aggression and antisocial behavior in youth. In N. Eisenberg (Ed.), *Handbook of child psychology: Vol. 3. Social, emotional, and personality development* (6th ed.) (pp. 719–788). Hoboken, NJ: John Wiley & Sons, Ltd.

Dodge, K. A., Lochman, J. E., Harnish, J. D., Bates, J. E., & Pettit, G. S. (1997). Reactive and proactive aggression in school children and psychiatrically impaired chronically assaultive youth. *Journal of Abnormal Psychology, 106,* 37–51.

Dodge, K. A., Pettit, G. S., & Bates, J. E. (1994). Socialization mediators of the relation between socioeconomic status and child conduct problems. *Child Development, 65,* 649–665.

Dozier, M., Peloso, E., Lindhiem, O., Gordon, M. K., Manni, M., Sepulveda, S., & Ackerman, J. (2006). Developing evidence-based interventions for foster children: An example of a randomized clinical trial with infants and toddlers. *Journal of Social Issues, 62,* 767–785.

Eder, R., & Mangelsdorf, S. (1997). The emotional basis of early personality development: Implications for the emergent self-concept. In R. Hogan, J. A. Johnson, & S. R. Briggs (Eds.), *Handbook of personality psychology* (pp. 209–241). Orlando, FL: Academic Press.

Eisenberg, N. (2003). Prosocial behavior, empathy, and sympathy. In M. H. Bornstein & L. Davidson (Eds.), *Well-being: Positive development across the life course* (pp. 253–265). Mahwah, NJ: Erlbaum.

Eisenberg, N., Fabes, R. A., & Spinrad, T. L. (2006). Prosocial development. In N. Eisenberg (Ed.), *Handbook of child psychology: Vol. 3. Social, emotional, and personality development* (6th ed.) (pp. 646–718). Hoboken, NJ: John Wiley & Sons, Ltd.

Elicker, J., Englund, M., & Sroufe, L. A. (1992). Predicting peer competence and peer-relationships in childhood from early parent–child relationships. In R. D. Parke & G. W. Ladd (Eds.), *Family-peer relationships; Modes of linkage* (pp. 77–106). Hillsdale, NJ: Erlbaum.

Else-Quest, N. M., Hyde, J. S., Goldsmith, H. H., & Van Hulle, C. A. (2006). Gender differences in temperament: A meta-analysis. *Psychological Bulletin, 132,* 33–72.

Emde, R. N. (1992). Social referencing research: Uncertainty, self and the search for meaning. In S. Feinman (Ed.), *Social referencing and the social construction of reality in infancy* (pp. 79–92). New York: Plenum Press.

Eschenbeck, H., Kohlmann, C. W., & Lohaus, A. (2007). Gender differences in coping strategies in children and adolescents. *Journal of Individual Differences, 28*(1), 18–26.

Fahrmeier, E. D. (1978). The development of concrete operations among the Hausa. *Journal of Cross-Cultural Psychology, 9*(1), 23–44.

Feldman, R. (2007). Maternal versus child risk and the development of parent–child and family relationships in five high-risk populations. *Development and Psychopathology, 19*, 293–312.

Flannery, K. A., & Liederman, J. (1995). Is there really a syndrome involving the co-occurrence of neurodevelopmental disorder, talent, non-right handedness and immune disorder among children? *Cortex, 31*, 503–515.

Garbers, C., Tunstill, J., Allnock, D., & Akhurst, S. (2006). Facilitating access to services for children and families: Lessons for Sure Start local programmes. *Child and Family Social Work, 11*, 287–296.

Gardner, H. (1999). Who owns intelligence? *Atlantic Monthly, 283*(2), 67–76.

Gilligan, C. (1982). *In a different voice*. Cambridge: Harvard University Press.

Grant, K. E., Compas, B. E., Stuhlmacher, A., Thurm, A. E., McMahon, S. D., & Halpert, J. A. (2003). Stressors and child and adolescent psychopathology: Moving from markers to mechanisms of risk. *Psychological Bulletin, 129*, 447–466.

Grolnick, W. S., & Farkas, M. (2002). Parenting and the development of children's self-regulation. In M. H. Bornstein (Ed.), *Handbook of parenting: Vol. 5. Practical issues in parenting* (pp. 89–110). Mahwah, NJ: Erlbaum.

Grossmann, K., Grossmann, K. E., Spangler, S., Suess, G., & Unzer, L. (1985). Maternal sensitivity and newborn attachment orientation responses as related to quality of attachment in northern Germany. In I. Bretherton & E. Waters (Eds.), *Growing Points of Attachment Theory, Monographs of the Society of Research in Child Development, 50* (1-2 serial no. 209).

Hart, C. H., Yang, C., Nelson, L. J., Robinson, C. C., Olsen, J. A., Nelson, D. A., . . . Olsen, S. F. (2000). Peer acceptance in early childhood and subtypes of socially withdrawn behavior in China, Russia and the United States. *International Journal of Behavioral Development, 24*, 73–81.

Harter, S. (1998). The development of self-representation. In W. Damon & N. Eisenberg (Eds.), *Handbook of child psychology: Vol. 3. Social, emotional, and personality development* (5th ed.) (pp. 553–617). New York: John Wiley & Sons, Ltd.

Herman, M. R., Dornbusch, S. M., Herron, M. C., & Herting, J. R. (1997). The influence of family regulation, connection, and psychological autonomy on six measures of adolescent functioning. *Journal of Adolescent Research, 12*, 34–67.

Jeynes, W. H. (2010). The salience of the subtle aspects of parental involvement and encouraging that involvement: implications for school-based programs. *Teachers College Record, 112*, 747–774.

Jones, N. A., Field, T., & Davalos, M. (2000). Right frontal EEG asymmetry and lack of empathy in preschool children of depressed mothers. *Child Psychiatry and Human Development, 30*, 189–201.

Joshi, S. M., & MacLean, M. (1997). Maternal expectations of child development in India, Japan, and England. *Journal of Cross-Cultural Psychology, 28*(2), 212–234.

Kagan, A. E. (1992). Yesterday's promises, tomorrow's promises. *Developmental Psychology, 28*, 990–997.

Kagan, J., & Fox, N. A. (2006). Biology, culture and temperamental biases. In N. Eisenberg (Ed.), *Handbook of child psychology: Vol. 3. Social, emotional, and personality development* (6th ed.) (pp. 167–225). Hoboken, NJ: John Wiley & Sons, Ltd.

Kagan, J., & Snidman, N. (2004). *The long shadow of temperament*. Cambridge, MA: Belknap Press.

Keenan, K., Coyne, C., & Lahey, B. B. (2008). Should relational aggression be included in DSM-V? *Journal of the American Academy of Child and Adolescent Psychiatry, 47*(1), 86–93.

Kelley, M., Power, T. G., & Wimbush, D. D. (1992). Determinants of disciplinary practices in low-income black mothers. *Child Development, 63*, 573–582.

Knecht, S., Draeger, B., Deppe, M., Bobe, L., Lohmann, H., Floel, A., . . . Henningsen, H. (2000). Handedness and hemispheric language dominance in healthy humans. *Brain, 123,* 2512–2518.

Kobayashi, Y. (1994). Conceptual acquisition and change through social interaction. *Human Development, 37,* 233–241.

Kochanska, G., Aksan, N., & Carlson, J. J. (2005). Temperament, relationships, and young children's receptive cooperation with their parents. *Developmental Psychology, 41,* 648–660.

Kochanska, G., Aksan, N., & Koenig, A. L. (1995). A longitudinal study of the roots of preschoolers' conscience: Committed compliance and emerging internalization. *Child Development, 66*(6), 1752–1769.

Kochanska, G., Tjebkes, T. L., & Forman, D. R. (1998). Children's emerging regulation of conduct: Restraint, compliance, and internalization from infancy to the second year. *Child Development, 69,* 1378–1389.

Kohlberg, L. (1976). Moral stages and moralization: Cognitive-developmental approach. In R. Lickona (Ed.), *Moral development and behaviour: Theory, research and social issues* (pp. 31–53). Chicago: Rand McNally.

Ladd, G. W., Buhs, E. S., & Seid, M. (2000). Children's initial sentiments about kindergarten: Is school liking an antecedent of early classroom participation and achievement? *Merrill-Palmer Quarterly, 46,* 255–279.

Lewis, M., & Brooks, J. (1978). Self-knowledge and emotional development. In M. Lewis & L. Rosenblum (Eds.), *The development of affect* (pp. 205–226). New York: Plenum Press.

Li-Grining, C. P. (2007). Effortful control among low-income preschoolers in three cities: Stability, change and individual differences. *Developmental Psychology, 43,* 208–221.

Loeber, R., Green, S. M., Lahey, B. B., Frick, P. J., & McBurnett, K. (2000). Findings on disruptive behavior disorders from the first decade of the Developmental Trends Study. *Clinical Child and Family Psychology Review, 3,* 37–60.

Luster, T., & McAdoo, H. (1996). Family and child influences on educational attainment: A secondary analysis of the High/Scope Perry Preschool data. *Developmental Psychology, 32,* 26–39.

Lyons-Ruth, K. (1996). Attachment relationships among children with aggressive behavior problems: The role of disorganized early attachment patterns. *Journal of Consulting and Clinical Psychology, 64,* 64–73.

Maccoby, E. E., & Martin, J. A. (1983). Socialization in the context of the family: Parent–child interaction. In E. M. Hetherington (Ed.), *Handbook of child psychology: Vol. 4. Socialization, personality, and social development* (4th ed.) (pp. 1–101). New York: John Wiley & Sons, Ltd.

MacMillan, H. L., Wathen, C. N., Barlow, J., Fergusson, D. M., Leventhal, J. M., & Taussig, H. N. (2009). Interventions to prevent child maltreatment and associated impairment. *Lancet, 373,* 250–266.

Main, M., & Solomon, J. (1990). Procedures for identifying infants as disorganized/disoriented during the Ainsworth Strange Situation. In M. T. Greenberg, D. Cicchetti, & E. M. Cummings (Eds.), *Attachment in the preschool years* (pp. 121–160). Chicago: University of Chicago Press.

Mills, R. S. (2005). Taking stock of the developmental literature on shame. *Developmental Review, 25,* 26–63.

Miyake, K., Chen, S., & Campos, J. J. (1985). Infant temperament, mother's mode of interaction and attachment in Japan. An interim report. In I. Bretherton & E. Waters (Eds.), *Growing points of attachment theory, Monographs of the Society of Research in Child Development, 50* (1-2, serial no. 209).

Moreno, A. J., Klute, M. M., & Robinson, J. L. (2008). Relational and individual resources as predictors of empathy in early childhood. *Social Development, 17,* 613–637.

Morgan, B., & Gibson, K. R. (1991). Nutrition and environmental interactions in brain development. In K. R. Gibson & A. C. Petersen (Eds.), *Brain maturation and cognitive development: Comparative and cross-cultural perspective* (pp. 91–106). New York: Aldine De Gruyter.

Moses, L., Baldwin, D., Rosicky, J., & Tidball, G. (2001). Evidence for referential understanding in the emotions domain at twelve and eighteen months. *Child Development, 61,* 929–945.

Moss, E., Dubois-Comtois, K., Cyr, C., Tarabulsy, M., St. Lauarent, D., & Bernier, A. (2011). Efficacy of a home-visiting intervention aimed at improving maternal sensitivity, child attachment, and behavioural outcomes for maltreated children: A randomized control trial. *Development and Psychopathology, 23,* 195–210.

Olds, D., Eckenrode, J., Henderson, C., Kitzman, H., Powers, J., Cole, R., ... Lucky, D. (1997). Long-term effects of home visitation on maternal life course and child abuse and neglect. *Journal of the American Medical Association, 278,* 637–643.

Olds, D., Sadler, L., & Kitzman, H. (2007). Programs for parents of infants and toddlers: Recent evidence from randomized trials. *Journal of Child Psychiatry and Psychology, 48,* 355–391.

Ozturk, C., Durmazlar, N., Yrakm, B., Karaagaoglu, E., Yalaz, K., & Anlar, B. (1999). Hand and eye preference in normal preschool children. *Clinical Pediatrics, 38,* 677–680.

Patterson, G. R., & Yoerger, K. (2002). A developmental model for early- and late-onset delinquency. In J. B. Reid, G. R. Patterson, & J. J. Snyder (Eds.), *Antisocial behavior in children and adolescents: A developmental analysis and model for intervention* (pp. 147–172). Washington, DC: APA.

Plomin, R. (1994). *Genetics and experience: The interplay between nature and nurture.* Thousand Oaks, CA: Sage.

Posada, G., Gao, Y., Wu, F., Posada, R., Tascon, A., Schoelmerich, A., ... Synnevaag, B. (1995). The secure-base phenomenon across cultures: Children's behavior, mother's preferences and experts' concepts. *Monographs of the Society for Research in Child Development, 60,* 27–48.

Putallaz, M., Grimes, C. L., Foster, K. J., Kupersmidt, J. B., Coie, J. D., & Dearing, K. (2007). Overt and relational aggression and victimization: Multiple perspectives within the school setting. *Journal of School Psychology, 45,* 523–547.

Raymond, J. H., Jones, F., & Cooke, V. (1998). African American scholars and parents cannot blame current harsh physical punishment of black males on slavery: A response to "cultural interpretations of child ellipsis." *Family Journal, 6,* 279–286.

Repacholi, B. M. (1998). Infants' use of attention cues to identify the referent of another person's emotional expression. *Developmental Psychology, 34*(5), 1017–1025.

Rinaldi, C. M., & Howe, N. (2012). Mothers' and fathers' parenting styles and associations with toddlers' externalizing, internalizing and adaptive behaviors. *Early Childhood Research Quarterly, 27*(2), 266–273.

Rogoff, B. (2003). *The cultural nature of human development.* New York: Oxford University Press.

Rogoff, B., & Chavajay, P. (1995). What's become of research on the cultural basis of cognitive development? *American Psychologist, 50,* 859–877.

Rothbart, M. K., & Bates, J. E. (2006). *Temperament.* In N. Eisenberg (Ed.), *Handbook of child psychology: Vol. 3. Social, emotional, and personality development* (6th ed.) (pp. 99–166). Hoboken, NJ: John Wiley & Sons, Ltd.

Rourke, B. P., Ahmad, S., Collings, D., Jayman-Abello, B., Hayman-Abello, S., & Warriner, E. M. (2002). Child clinical/pediatric neuropsychology; Some recent advances. *Annual Review of Psychology, 53,* 309–339.

Ruff, H. A., & Capozzoli, M. C. (2003). Development of attention and distractibility in the first 4 years of life. *Developmental Psychology, 39,* 877–890.

Saarni, C., Campos, J. J., Camras, L. A., & Witherington, D. (2006). Emotional development – action communication and understanding. In N. Eisenberg (Ed.), *Handbook of child psychology: Vol. 3. Social, Emotional, and personality development* (6th ed.) (pp. 226–299). Hoboken, NJ: John Wiley & Sons, Ltd.

Schaie, K., & Willis, S. (1993). Age difference patterns of psychometric intelligence in adulthood: Generalizability within and across ability domains. *Psychology and Aging, 8,* 44–55.

Shulman, S., Elicker, J., & Sroufe, A. (1994). Stages of friendship growth in preadolescence as related to attachment history. *Journal of Social and Personal Relationships, 11,* 341–361.

Spera, C., Wentzel, K., & Matto, H. (2009). Parental aspirations for their children's educational attainment: Relations to ethnicity, parental education, children's academic performance, and parental perceptions of school climate. *Journal of Youth and Adolescence, 38,* 1140–1152.

Sroufe, L. A. (2002). From infant attachment to promotion of adolescent autonomy: Prospective, longitudinal data on the role of parents in development. In J. Borkowski, S. Ramey, & M. Bristol-Power (Eds.), *Parenting and the child's world* (pp. 187–202). Mahwah, NJ: Erlbaum.

Stiles, J. (2008). *Fundamentals of brain development.* Cambridge, MA: Harvard University Press.

Su, C., & Hynie, M. (2011). Effects of life stress, social support and cultural norms on parenting styles among mainland Chinese, European Canadian, and Chinese Canadian immigrant mothers. *Journal of Cross-Cultural Psychology, 42*(6), 944–962.

Sümer, N., Aktürk, E., & Helvaci, E. (2010). Psychological effects of parenting styles and behaviours: A review of studies in Turkey. *Turk Psikoloji Yazilari, 13,* 60–61.

Tanner, J. M. (1990). *Foetus into man: Physical growth from conception to maturity* (revised and enlarged ed.). Cambridge, MA: Harvard University Press.

Taumoepeau, M., & Ruffman, T. (2006). Mother and infant talk about mental states relates to desire language and emotion understanding. *Child Development, 77,* 465–481.

Thatcher, R., Lyon, G., Rumsey, J., & Krasnegor, J. (1996). *Developmental neuroimaging.* San Diego, CA: Academic Press.

Thompson, P. M., Giedd, J. N., Woods, R. P., MacDonald, D., Evans, A. C., & Toga, A. W. (2000). Growth patterns in the developing brain detected by using continuum mechanical tensor maps. *Nature, 404,* 190–192.

Thompson, R. A., & Goodvin, R. (2007). Taming the tempest in the teapot. In C. A. Brownell & C. B. Kopp (Eds.), *Socioemotional development in the toddler years. Transitions and transformations* (pp. 320–341). New York: Guilford.

Toth, S. L., Cicchetti, D., & Kim, J. (2002). Relations among children's perceptions of maternal behavior, attributional styles, and behavioral symptomatology in maltreated children. *Journal of Abnormal Child Psychology, 30,* 487–501.

Tudge, J., & Rogoff, B. (1999). Peer influences on cognitive development: Piagetian and Vygotskian perspectives. In L. Peter & C. Fernyhough (Eds.), *Lev Vygotsky: Critical assessments: The zone of proximal development,* vol. *III* (pp. 32–56). Florence, KY: Taylor and Francis/Routledge.

Turiel, E. (2006). The development of morality. In W. Damon & R. M. Lerner (Eds.), *Handbook of child psychology, Vol. 3. Social emotional and personality development* (6th ed.) (pp. 789–857). Hoboken, NJ: John Wiley & Sons, Ltd.

Veronneau, M., Vitaro, F., Brendgen, M., Dishion, T. J., & Tremblay, R. E. (2010). Transactional analysis of the reciprocal links between peer experiences and academic achievement from middle childhood to early adolescence. *Developmental Psychology, 46,* 773–790.

Vitaro, F., Barker, E., Boivin, M., Brendgen, M., & Tremblay, R. E. (2006). Do early difficult temperament and harsh parenting differentially predict reactive and proactive aggression? *Journal of Abnormal Child Psychology, 34*(5), 685–695.

Vondra, J. I., Hommerding, K. D., & Shaw, D. S. (1999). Stability and change in infant attachment in a low-income sample. In J. I. Vonda & D. Barnett (Eds.), *A typical attachment in infancy and early childhood among children at developmental risk, Monographs of the Society for Research in Child Development, 64*(3), 119–144.

Weinfield, N. S., Whaley, G., & Egeland, B. (2004). Continuity, discontinuity, and coherence in attachment from infancy to late adolescence: Sequelae of organization and disorganization. *Attachment and Human Development, 6*(1), 73–97.

Werner, N. E., & Crick, N. R. (2004). Maladaptive peer relationships and the development of relational and physical aggression during middle childhood. *Social Development, 13*, 495–514.

Winsler, A., Naglieri, J., & Manfra, L. (2006). Children's search strategies and accompanying verbal and motor strategic behavior: Developmental trends and relations with task performance among children age 5 to 17. *Cognitive Development, 21*, 232–248.

Wolf, D. (1990). Being of several minds: Voices and versions of the self in early childhood. In D. Cicchetti & M. Beeghly (Eds.), *The self in transition: Infancy to childhood* (pp. 183–212). Chicago: University of Chicago Press.

4

Developmental Milestones: Adolescence

Chapter preview and learning objectives

Prior to the publication of *Adolescence* (Hall, 1904), few researchers had focused on the period of development marking the transition from childhood to adulthood. Hall (1904) depicted adolescence as a period of *Sturm und Drang* (storm and stress) due to significant changes occurring in physical growth (spurts), sexual maturity (hormonal changes), and emotional development. Today we know that only a minority of adolescents will experience significant difficulties during these years (Arnett, 1999). Yet adolescence does represent a period of increased risk in a number of areas, including: substance use and abuse, eating disorders, delinquent behaviors, depression, and suicide (Cicchetti & Rogosh, 2002).

In this chapter, typical milestones will be discussed that occur in adolescence in neurological, physical, cognitive, and social development. Cross-cultural research will address how these milestones occur in different geographical areas, while gender studies will provide greater insight into how males and females respond to changes in such areas as body image and supportive friendships. Discussions will provide the reader with a better understanding of:

- whether adolescence is universal across all cultures;
- the significant neurological changes (brain chemistry and brain function) that take place during this period of development;
- significant physical changes that accompany this period of development and the impact of gender and culture on attitudes towards these physical changes;
- cognitive advances and limitations during adolescence;
- the development of a more integrated sense of social cognition and thinking about the social world that takes places during this period;
- the changes in self-concept, identity, and social relationships that evolve from the beginning to the end of adolescence;
- the impact of attachment style and parenting style on outcomes in adolescence.

This chapter provides excellent background information in preparation for better understanding why adolescents are at increased risk for substance use/abuse and eating disorders (*Chapter 11*) during this period of development.

Adolescent milestones: an introduction

Is adolescence universal? Whether or not adolescence is universal has been a matter of debate. Prior to the industrial revolution, children often worked and married at very young ages and often bypassed adolescence. Today, most theorists believe that the majority of societies recognize an "*adolescent period*" during life span development (Schlegel & Barry, 1991). However, "adolescence" can vary by culture, gender, and social class, with children of lower classes in some societies working and marrying much earlier, pre-empting the adolescent period (Saraswathi, 1999). Delaney (1995, p. 891) suggests that adolescent **rites of passage** are universal and represent a cross-cultural phenomenon that has four elements:

1. separation from society;
2. preparation or instruction from an elder;
3. a transition (in this case from child to adult);
4. a welcoming back into society with the acknowledgement of changed status.

Although Hall's depiction of "adolescent angst" has been moderated by contemporary research, the idea that adolescence can be a difficult period of development relates to changes evident in three broad areas: parent–youth conflict; the presence of mood swings (particularly depression); and tendencies to engage in high-risk behaviors (Buchanan et al., 1990). Research has confirmed that the frequency of parent–youth conflict peaks during early adolescence but is most intense during mid–adolescence (Laursen, Coy, & Collins, 1998). In addition, adolescents experience significantly more feelings of self-conscious emotions and mood disruptions compared to middle childhood (Larson & Richards, 1994). Tendencies to engage in risky decisions and behaviors can escalate during adolescence (Gardner & Steinberg, 2005). However, even within these patterns, there is wide variability and individual differences in the expression of these behaviors, as well as etiology, based on the inter-relationships among a number of factors, including physical, neurological, and cognitive pubertal changes, and environmental factors (parenting style and practices, as well as peer influences).

Neurological and physical development

Brain development

Prior to the 1960s, it was believed that the brain completed its development early in adolescence. However, we now know that the prefrontal cortex continues to evolve into young adulthood. Studies have provided increasing evidence that **executive functions** (such as *selective attention, decision-making, and response inhibition*) which are primarily located in the prefrontal cortex, show significant development from early to late adolescence (Brocki & Bohlin, 2004, 2006; Casey, Vauss, Chused, & Swedo, 1994). Furthermore, there is some support for the suggestion that frontal lobe circuitry may actually decline with the onset of puberty (11 to 12 years) due to a proliferation of synapses that occur during this time, in the absence of a period of pruning (which occurs later in adolescence), rendering performance less efficient (McGivern, Andersen, Byrd, Mutter, & Reilly, 2002).

In early childhood, the brain is highly flexible; however, it loses **plasticity** in adolescence, as parts of the brain become more specialized in their functions.

Learning a second language in secondary school or university?

Research suggests that children should start to learn a second language in preschool or primary school. The loss of brain plasticity is most evident in studies of second-language learning which demonstrate a gradual decline in abilities from 10 years of age, followed by a sharp drop in the acquisition rate of new language skills from age 12–13 onward (Johnson & Newport, 1989).

Although specialization of brain function gradually evolves over the course of development, **hemispheric specialization** is completed around the onset of puberty. By this time most individuals process certain activities in localized areas of the brain (e.g., using the right side of the brain for visual spatial information, and the left side for language tasks). However, while males tend to use the left side of their brain to process language-based tasks, and the right side of the brain to process emotions, females use both sides of their brains to process language and emotions (Jaeger et al., 1998; Skrandies, Reik, & Kunze, 1999). There is speculation that males and females are socialized to respond in different ways. Girls may be encouraged to bring emotional sensitivity to the problem-solving situation, while males may be programmed to bring logic to the table and leave emotions behind (Fischer, 1993).

Self-regulation, risky choices, and sensation seeking Although there is significant improvement in self-regulation compared to earlier stages of development, studies using functional magnetic resonance imaging (fMRI) techniques have determined that the integration of the prefrontal cortex with other brain areas is not as effective as in the adult brain, and adolescents lag behind adults in their ability to inhibit responses, in planning ability, and in future orientation (Steinberg et al., 2009). The immaturity of the prefrontal network in conjunction with heightened neural activity and excitation during adolescence results in adolescents responding to situations with inflated reactions, whether responding to a distressing (stressful) or pleasurable experience. The intensity of responses coupled with lack of future planning and impulsivity may place youth at increased risk for experimenting with substances, and engaging in high-risk behaviors such as unprotected sex or reckless driving. Adolescence is associated with heightened tendencies to take risks, resulting in statistically more accidents, criminal activity, and suicides occurring during this period (Steinberg et al., 2008). In addition, the sex hormones are also responsible for heightened responsiveness in the prefrontal cortex and amygdale, which are instrumental in our recall of emotional events and interpretation of nonverbal emotional expressions.

In their study of peer influence on risk taking and risky preferences, Gardner and Steinberg (2005) evaluated the responses of individuals in three age groups: adolescents (13–16 years), youth (18–22 years) and adults (24 years and older) on two questionnaires and a risk-taking task. Subjects were randomly assigned to an individual or group (of three same-aged peers) condition. The results revealed that risk taking and risky decision-making declined with age, and that being assigned to the group condition increased risk taking for adolescents and youth. Therefore, not only is adolescence a time of increased vulnerability for engaging in high-risk behaviors, this tendency can be magnified in the company of peers.

Casey, Jones, and Somerville (2011) suggest that neurobiological and cognitive theories have not been able to account for the nonlinear changes that occur during adolescence that make this population so vulnerable to engaging in impulsive behaviors and making risky choices. They argue that adolescent behavior is qualitatively different from that of childhood or adulthood. Based on the theory that cognitive control improves with age, adolescents should be making fewer poor choices relative to their younger peers, but research shows that risky choices and impulsive responses actually increase during the adolescent period (Windle et al., 2008). Although adolescents 15 years of age or younger act more impulsively than older adolescents, even those aged 16–17 years fall short of executing control equivalent to that of adults (Feld, 2008). Casey et al. (2011, p. 22) propose a neurobiological model of adolescence that goes beyond the "exclusive association of risky behavior to the immaturity of the prefrontal cortex," based on their investigation of adolescent transitions in and out of this developmental period. What they suggest is a "perfect storm" based on the "imbalance between a heightened sensitivity to motivational cues (*mature subcortical regions*) and immature cognitive control" (*prefrontal cortical control*) that places the adolescent at risk (Casey et al., 2011, p. 21, emphasis added).

While adolescents are capable of rational decision-making, and are able to articulate inherent risks in the behaviors that they produce (Reyna & Farley, 2008), this does not transfer to situations where they are "caught in the moment." "In emotionally salient situations, subcortical systems will win out (accelerator) over control systems (brakes) given their maturity relative to the prefrontal control system," while in less emotional situations, the cortical control systems are not impaired (Casey et al., 2011, p. 22). As a result, while the ability to inhibit responses improves from childhood to adulthood in a linear progression, risk-taking or reward-seeking behaviors are at their most pronounced in adolescence (Windle et al., 2008) with sensation seeking peaking between 10 and 15 years of age (Steinberg et al., 2009).

Adolescent brain development has also been the focus of inquiry regarding increased risk for alcohol and other drug problems (Bava & Tapert, 2010). It has been suggested that the dual system noted by Casey et al. (2011) may also account for reward seeking and risky choices based on increased activation in subcortical regions of the brain, relative to immaturity in the prefrontal cortex. In their review, Bava and Tapert (2010) discuss the inter-relationships between brain structure and function within the context of socio-emotional processing during adolescence, with adolescents showing heightened activation in the bottom-up emotional processing centers such as the amygdale in the limbic system, and increased efficiency of white matter fibers, in the presence of a slower and more protracted development of the prefrontal cortex (cognitive control). Later on in this chapter, adolescents' tendencies to self-monitor and their sensitivity to evaluation will be discussed; these can also be related to increased activation of the emotional centers in the brain. Increased sensitivity, however, also can lead to increases in behaviors to seek rewards and increased stimulation (sensation seeking).

Neurotransmitter changes, such as increased density of dopaminergic connections during this period, can also impact risk taking and sensation seeking (Tunbridge et al., 2007). In addition, neurotransmitter function is also influenced by hormonal changes (gonadotropic release of hormones in the pituitary gland) heightening sexual and aggressive behaviors (Paus, Keshavan, & Giedd, 2008).

Because adolescents experience heightened activity in the emotional centers of their brains, they are more likely to be influenced by emotions in their decision-making. In addition, youth also demonstrate greater activity (ventral striatal activation) than adults or children when they anticipate a reward (Geier, Terwilliger, Teslovich, Velanova, & Luna, 2010) and greater dopamine release when they experience rewarding circumstances (Koepp et al., 1998). This combination may be responsible for perpetuating engagement in a cycle of reward-driven behavior and increased vulnerability to substance use in adolescence (Bava & Tapert, 2010).

Emotions and mood　Increases in sensitivity and heightened activation of the emotional centers and increases in hormone levels can all result in instabilities in adolescent moods. Studies have demonstrated that adolescents report more dissatisfaction with their mood states, which has been attributed to an increase in stressful life experiences during this period, such as relationship problems, family conflicts, and problems at school (Larson & Ham, 1993).

Physical maturation

Physical development and gender   Until 10 years of age, growth is similar in boys and girls. Females experience a **growth spurt** starting around 10 years of age, with the onset of menstruation (menarche) occurring towards the end of the growth spurt (12 years). For males, the growth spurt occurs around 12 years of age, with sexual maturity occurring about mid-way through the fourteenth year (Tanner, 1990). While early-maturing males seem to reap the benefits of greater athletic prowess and popularity, early onset for females is associated with more negative outcomes, such as increased parental conflict (Ge, Conger, & Elder, 1996, 2001), increased risk for distress and delinquency (Dick, Rose, Viken, & Kaprio, 2000), as well as moodiness and depressive symptoms (Mendle, Turkheimer, & Emery, 2007). Later-maturing boys are at greater risk for insecurity and social awkwardness (Simmons, Burgeson, Carlton-Ford, & Blyth, 1987).

Gender, culture, and the onset of puberty   Adolescence marks the onset of **puberty**, physical changes that occur as the **primary sex characteristics** (maturation of the sex organs) and **secondary sex characteristics** (physical changes) reach their peak. The pituitary gland is responsible for initiating puberty through a feedback system, composed of the hypothalamus, pituitary gland, and gonads, that regulates levels of sex hormones in the system. **Androgens** are produced by the adrenal glands. Under certain conditions (threat, stress, or depression), the hormone **cortisol** is released into the system by the adrenal glands as the **hypothalamus–pituitary–adrenal (HPA) system** sends a "fight or flight" signal. As a result, psychosocial factors such as stress, exercise, and nutrition can all influence the timing of puberty (Ellis, McFayden-Ketchum, Dodge, Pettit, & Bates, 1999).

Eveleth and Tanner (1990) found that female menarche varied widely across cultures, from as early as 12 years of age (middle-class Caracas, Venezuela) to 18 years of age (Bundi highlands of New Guinea). Historically, menarche has been declining, with a drop of approximately 0.3 years per decade in the last 140 years. Several reasons have been suggested for this trend, including: better nutrition (leading to earlier onset), physical exertion (higher activity levels correlate to later onset), and elevation (high altitude regions have later onset).

Gender, culture, and body dissatisfaction   In middle childhood, girls begin to accumulate fat (*adiposity*) in their arms, legs, and trunk in preparation for puberty (Brandao, Lombardi, Nishida, Hauache, & Vieira, 2003). This increase in physical mass coincides with increased **body dissatisfaction** among girls (Stice & Whitenton, 2002), and distress due to a lack of success in dieting (Nowak, 1998).

Research in the 1990s focused on Caucasian upper middle-class women from Western countries and found that 90% of white American teens were dissatisfied with their weight compared to 70% of their African American peers (Parker, Nichter, Vuckovic, Sims, & Ritenbaugh, 1995). Recently, studies have found African American and white American females at comparable risk for eating disorders (Walcott, Pratt, & Patel, 2003; Mulholland & Minz, 2001). Body dissatisfaction and eating disorders appear to be on the increase among Asian American women and among females in many Asian countries (Walcott et al., 2003).

The media message of the Anglo-European beauty ideal has reached worldwide audiences and there is a growing trend for females from ethnic minorities and non-Western cultures to adopt Western images of "beauty" in lieu of their own ethnocultural values (Harris & Kuba, 1997).

Tiggemann and Pickering (1996) suggest a strong link between the media, gender role identity, body stereotype, and body dissatisfaction. The authors found that adolescents who watched more television (especially movies and soap operas) expressed more dissatisfaction with their bodies.

Fiji: before and after the advent of television

Since television was introduced in 1995, eating disorders have increased fivefold among adolescent girls in Fiji. Prior to this time, only 3% of the Fijian teens reported that they had induced vomiting to lose weight, but by 1998, the rate rose to 15%. After viewing American, Australian, and British actresses on television, 62% reported dieting and 74% said they felt fat and wanted to look more like the actresses (Becker, Burwell, Herzog, Hamburg, & Gilman, 2002).

Males entering puberty experience a decrease in fat and an increase in muscle strength. Although male rates for body dissatisfaction lag behind females, there has been increasing body dissatisfaction among males in the past 15 years (Youth Risk Behavior Survey; CDC, 2005). Disorders of body image, such as **body dysmorphic disorder**, once considered rare, are currently evident in 1–2% of Western males (Phillips, 1996). A specific form of the disorder, **muscle dysmorphia** (a preoccupation with muscularity), sometimes referred to as the "Adonis complex," is increasingly found in Western males (Pope, Gruber, Choi, Olivardia, & Phillips, 1997; Pope, Phillips, & Olivardia, 2000b).

Body dysmorphic disorder (BDD)

BDD, also known as **dysmorphophobia**, causes significant distress due to the perception that some aspect of the appearance is flawed or defective. Onset is often in adolescence. One study found that 30% of those diagnosed with BDD became housebound, while 17% had attempted suicide (Phillips, McElroy, Keck, Pope, & Hudson, 1993).

Abuse of **anabolic-androgenic steroids** and other "body image drugs" can be a serious consequence of body image dissatisfaction in males (Blouin & Goldfield, 1995; Kanayama, Pope, & Hudson, 2001); a condition that has been described as the "*flip side*" of anorexia (Smith, 1997). Anabolic steroid abuse has become a major public health concern in the United States, Europe, and Australia (Kindlundh, Isacson, Berglund, & Nyberg, 1999; Kanayama, Pope, Cohane, & Hudson, 2003), although it appears to be rare in non-Western societies (Yang, Gray, & Pope, 2005).

Pope et al. (2000a) conducted male body image studies in the United States, France, and Austria, and found that all males selected an ideal body image that was about 28 pounds (13 kilograms) more muscular than their own physique. Males also overestimated female attraction to an image in excess of their ideal (30 pounds/14 kilograms), although in reality, females selected images closer to the average male. Media influence on body dissatisfaction in males has rarely been studied (Hesse-Biber, Leavy, Quinn, & Zoino, 2006). Pope, Olivardia, Borowiecki, and Cohane (2001) found increasing inclusion of male pictures (from 3% in the 1950s to 35% in the 1990s) in magazines in various states of undress (less clothing than would normally be worn on the street), compared to an increase of only 20% in female pictures, suggesting an increased focus on male body image in the media.

Cognitive and social development

Cognitive milestones

Piaget: the period of formal operations   Piaget called this stage of reasoning the **period of formal operations** to emphasize advances in problem solving, logical thinking, and the ability to combine statements into propositions. A major advance occurs in the adolescent's ability to use abstract reasoning to solve hypothetical problems, or **hypothetico-deductive reasoning**.

Although skills at this level build on earlier skill sets, they are qualitatively different from previous abilities. Inhelder and Piaget (1958) developed a series of experiments to test the acquisition of formal operational skills in adolescents. Their most famous experiment was the **pendulum problem**. In this task, adolescents are given a number of weights that can be tied to a pendulum with string. To derive a solution to the problem, they must rule out *weight*, *height of release*, and *force of push*, to determine that *length of string* is the factor that makes the difference. Adolescents use a systematic approach to solve the problem, while younger children approached the task randomly.

Information processing   **Selective attention** (*ability to ignore distracters*), **divided attention** (*ability to multitask*), **short-term memory**, **long-term memory**, and **metamemory** (*knowledge of memory strategies*) all improve in adolescence (Flavell, Miller, & Miller, 2002). Advances in metamemory result from the understanding that various strategies or **mnemonics** (such as taking notes, highlighting important parts of documents) can assist in managing information (Flavell et al., 2002). Efficiency in accessing information (**automatization**) is also less effortful at this stage (Case, 1998).

Social cognition

Social cognition involves how we think about our social world and how these perceptions influence our behaviors. The immediate environment (friends, family, teachers, neighborhood) can have a powerful impact on our thoughts and behaviors, while the consequences of more distal influences (economic conditions, culture) may be more subtle. The influence of the media on shaping impressionable attitudes towards body shape and substance use during adolescence has been well documented in research.

Adolescent egocentrism   The preschool child views the world from an egocentric perspective because of an inability to take the perspective of another. In adolescence, the ability to think about thinking (**metacognition**) and consider abstract and hypothetical situations can produce a self-conscious framework for analysis. In addition, as was previously discussed, adolescents are highly sensitive to emotional information due to heightened brain activity in the subcortical regions relative to immaturity in the prefrontal cortex. Within this context, **adolescent egocentrism** can result from excessive self-reflection and a preoccupation that they are the focus of everyone's attention.

Two important concepts are fundamental to adolescent egocentrism: imaginary audience and personal fable (Elkind, 1967; Elkind & Bowen, 1979). The **imaginary audience** reflects adolescents' concern that everyone is looking at them, which may cause them to retreat into their own private world, or *perform* for the audience (talking loudly, wearing dramatic clothing, and so on). The **personal fable** is adolescents' belief in their own invulnerability, omnipotence, and personal uniqueness, which supports tendencies to engage in high-risk and reckless behaviors during this period of development.

Eventually, sharing experiences with peers often enhances the understanding that others share similar feelings and concerns. However, adolescents who are isolated from peers may continue to harbor fears of being scrutinized and criticized by others, as well as increased feelings of being misunderstood.

Moral reasoning

Piaget For Piaget, moral reasoning evolves over the course of two broad developmental stages, **heteronomous morality** or **moral realism**, which was discussed in the previous chapter, and **autonomous morality**, a transition that occurs in late childhood and adolescence as youth begin to understand that rules can change if there is agreement among those involved.

Kohlberg's stages of moral understanding Kohlberg's (1976) theories of moral development were also introduced in the previous chapter, and represent six stages of moral understanding across the lifespan, although there are three predominant categories. The stages reflect responses to a series of **moral dilemmas**, vignettes in which an individual is faced with a moral choice. In one scenario, the "Heinz dilemma," Heinz tries desperately to acquire enough money to buy medicine for his dying wife. When unsuccessful, Heinz steals the drug. Kohlberg's level of moral reasoning would be based on a response to the question: *Should Heinz have done that? Why?* Kohlberg's six stages of moral development are available in Table 4.1

Table 4.1 Kohlberg's stages of moral understanding

Morality	Stages/orientation	Motivation
Preconventional morality	Stage 1: Obedience and punishment	Good behavior is based on avoiding punishment
	Stage 2: Instrumental and hedonistic (reward and benefit)	Good behavior results in obtaining a reward
Conventional morality	Stage 3: Good boy; nice girl	Approval of the group
	Stage 4: Authority or law and order	Sense of duty; do the right thing
Postconventional morality, or principled morality	Stage 5: Social contract	Self-respect and respect for rights of others
	Stage 6: Hierarchy of principles; universal ethical principles	Act in accordance with one's own set of principles (conscience)

Kohlberg believed that **preconventional morality** was evident until nine or 10 years of age, and that the majority of adolescents and adults function at the **conventional level**.

Longitudinal studies have supported the order of Kohlberg's stages, with stage 3 reasoning peaking during mid-adolescence, and stage 4 morality continuing to develop into young adulthood (Dawson, 2002). The final stage of morality, **postconventional morality**, was reserved for individuals who endorsed those principles that went above and beyond those prescribed by convention, such as a journalist serving a jail sentence for not divulging a source of information, or women involved in the suffragette movement who chained themselves to railings in order to secure voting rights. Apparently, only about 5% of the population would meet this level of morality (Colby, Kohlberg, & Liberman, 1984).

Gender, culture, and morality   Gilligan (1982) has argued that Kohlberg's model is biased towards the male ideal, since female actions based on affiliation (caring) are rated lower on the hierarchy (stage 3) than actions motivated by duty and justice (stage 4). There is mixed support for Gilligan's claims: themes of justice and caring are evident in responses from both genders (Jadack, Hyde, Moore, & Keller, 1995); however, themes of caring are more prevalent among females (Wark & Krebs, 2000).

Although the sequence of Kohlberg's stages seems to be universal (Snarey, 1995), children and youth in industrialized nations pass through the stages in an accelerated fashion relative to peers in non-industrialized nations (Miller, 1997). In cultures where society is predominant at an early age (e.g., Israeli *kibbutzim*, which are small, closely knit societies), children reach more advanced levels and adolescents often reach stages 4 and 5 (Snarey, Reimer, & Kohlberg, 1985).

A major criticism of Kohlberg's model is that at the highest levels, morality is based on "individual principles and conscience, regardless of the societal laws or cultural customs," which reflects a bias towards individualistic versus collectivistic societies (Matsumoto & Juang, 2008, p. 103).

Collectivistic societies

In **collectivistic societies** (more traditional cultures), the well-being of the group takes precedence over the individual. Loyalty and respect for the group (family, elders, society) are among the highest ideals in such a culture, which would only be seen as level 3 morality in Kohlberg's model.

Identity, self-concept, and awareness of others

Erikson believed the major life task facing adolescents was to emerge from this stage of development with a sense of **identity**; youth who do not master this task face young adulthood unprepared, in a state of **identity confusion**.

Identity and self-concept   Early in adolescence, youth consolidate similar personality traits into more global concepts (e.g., being a good singer and artist may be clustered into the concept of being "*talented*"). However, self–reflection may also point out inconsistencies that may be difficult to reconcile (e.g., *I am fun to be with, but I am also moody sometimes and want to be alone.*) At this stage, self-descriptions take on more abstract and complex attributes (*In some areas I can be very conservative, but in others I can be very liberal*). Ultimately, the ability to see various sides of the self promotes better understanding of individual strengths and weaknesses (e.g., *I excel at math, but do poorly in composition*).

As autonomy increases and dependence on adults declines, adolescents rely increasingly on peers and close friends for information and support. Sharing of information with peers affords the opportunity to compare themselves to others, an integral part of identity formation. Throughout adolescence, social relationships evolve to take on more mature characteristics such as intimacy, mutual understanding, and loyalty (Collins & Madsen, 2006). In addition, increased self-disclosure provides a greater understanding of the complexity involved in relationships and the need to be sensitive to others' needs, preparing the adolescent for romantic partnerships in the future (De Goede, Branje, & Meeus, 2009).

Is there such a thing as too much self-esteem?

In their extensive review of research on aggression, Baumeister, Smart, and Boden (1996) found *high* self-esteem was often related to violence and aggression. Perpetrators of violence can have an inflated sense of self, despite failures at school and in personal relationships. When challenged, these individuals retaliate with anger and aggression, rather than suffer the consequences of loss of self-regard.

Identity status   Marcia (1980) suggests that identity formation in adolescence can take one of four possible directions based on the degree to which the adolescent engages in exploring the available options and their commitment to their role or identity. The four identity statuses are outlined in Table 4.2.

Table 4.2   Identity formation and identity status

Identity status	Exploration	Commitment
Identity achievement	Alternatives have been explored and a decision has been made	Commitment to a definite course of action
Moratorium	In the information gathering stage	Not ready for commitment (on hold)
Identity foreclosure	No exploration of alternatives	Committed to a pre-selected path selected by others (parents, teachers)
Identity diffusion	No exploration of alternatives	Not committed to any course of action

Adolescents with **identity achievement** (exploration and commitment) have the highest levels of self-esteem, are more goal-oriented, and tend to enroll in the most demanding college majors. Individuals with **identity diffusion** (no exploration or commitment) have the lowest self-esteem, and experience the most academic and social difficulties. Adolescents in **foreclosure** (no exploration, but committed) experience the lowest levels of anxiety, while those in **moratorium** (on-going exploration, no commitment) have the highest levels of anxiety (Berzonsky & Kuk, 2000; Kroger, 2000).

The generation gap?

Does the gap between adolescents and parents widen as a result of increasing autonomy and time spent with peers? Although arguments between parents and teens are common on issues of personal choice (such as dress code), parent and teen attitudes are very similar regarding fundamental values, such as social, religious, and political views (Chira, 1994).

Research has also investigated the role of identity formation on mental health and well-being. Youth develop a better sense of selfhood, identity, and cohesion when they shift from a status of diffusion or foreclosure towards taking on more responsibility, evident in moratorium or identity achievement (Snarey & Bell, 2003). Although, as noted earlier, those in moratorium may be more anxious, they are also driven to reduce their anxieties by gathering more information prior to decision-making, which can be an adaptive response in times of uncertainty and result in better problem solving through critical evaluation of alternatives (Berzonsky, 2003). As a result, those in moratorium often transition to a state of identity achievement.

Youth who are in states of foreclosure or diffusion do not fare as well as their peers in moratorium or identity achievement. In contrast to peers who seek out information to help with problem solving for dilemmas, these youth are more passive and either opt to conform to rigid expectations and beliefs espoused by parents (foreclosure), or opt out of the process entirely, avoiding decision-making (diffusion) and taking a "wait and see" attitude (Berzonsky & Kuk, 2000). Youth who adopt a diffuse-avoidant style are at the highest risk for drug abuse and antisocial behaviors, which may also place them at increased risk for a sense of hopelessness and depression (Schwartz, Cote, & Arnett, 2005).

Awareness of others and social relationships Self-understanding paves the way for greater understanding of others. Selman's (1980) seminal work on relationships reveals that our cognitive level dictates how we conceptualize relationships. The adolescent is often painfully aware of how others think and feel and may shrink from being overwhelmed by over-sensitivity to others. In late adolescence, a sense of *mutual understanding* provides the foundation for forming close relationships (Hartup & Stevens, 1999), as the *quantity* of friends is replaced by the *quality* of relationships and "best friends" are valued for their *intimacy* and *loyalty* (Buhrmester, 1996).

Cliques and crowds   Part of adolescent identity formation involves aligning oneself with a smaller group of similar peers (cliques) or larger groups of similar aged peers (crowds). These groups often form a **reference group** for the adolescent, providing a set of shared standards that may be based on activities (such as sports or music) or characteristics (e.g. popular) of the members. According to Newman and Newman (2001), cliques and crowds are important facets of an adolescent's developing understanding of his or her social world; while cliques provide the opportunity for social networking and experimenting with different roles and values, crowds provide a sense of security in a larger context, separate from family.

Social status

Popular or *controversial* adolescents have more close friends, engage in more extracurricular school programs, and are less lonely than less popular peers. By contrast, *rejected* and *neglected* adolescents are more likely to feel lonely, engage in fewer activities, and have fewer friends (Franzoi, Davis, & Vasquez-Suson, 1994).

Gender and friendships   Girls desire more emotional closeness in friendships than boys (Markovits, Benenson, & Dolensky, 2001), while boys seek activity-oriented companions to engage in sports or games (Buhrmester, 1996). However, close emotional ties can have positive and negative outcomes, since girls are twice as likely to report disagreements with friends over interpersonal issues (Hartup & Laursen, 1993).

Attachment and adolescent outcomes

Secure attachment   Attachment has been previously discussed at a theoretical level (*Chapter 2*) and in its relationship to outcomes in early and middle childhood (*Chapter 3*). Attachment theory (Bowlby, 1982) can provide a framework for understanding the development of social-emotional relationships across the lifespan. As previously discussed, adolescence is a time of increased focus and attention on establishing relationships with others, "transferring" attachment styles from parents to peers, partners, and social groups (Allen, 2008). It is a time when adolescents shift their attachment system with parents from *proximity* to *availability*, as parents take on the role of a safe haven or secure base from which to venture out into the social arena (Markiewicz, Lawford, Doyle, & Haggart, 2006). Securely attached adolescents experience more satisfying personal relationships that are based on a system of trust and concern for others' welfare (Larose & Bernier, 2001; Mikulincer et al., 2003) and demonstrate a more coherent sense of identity and positive well-being (Mikulincer, 1995). Longitudinal studies tracking individuals from early childhood until their late twenties have found that secure attachment is related to increased self-reliance, better emotional coping, and enhanced social competence (Sroufe, 2005). Other positive outcomes for adolescents with secure attachments include: fewer internalizing problems (DeKlyen & Greenberg, 2008); less drug use (Schindler, Thomasius, Gemeinhardt, Kustner, & Eckert, 2005); less likelihood of engaging in risky sexual behavior; fewer suicide attempts; and less antisocial behaviors (Allen, Moore, Kuperminc, & Bell, 1998;

Williams & Kelly, 2005). Securely attached adolescents are more successful in school, both socially and academically (Rubin et al., 2004; Simons, Paternite, & Shore, 2001).

Insecure attachment　In their study of attachment styles in adolescents in the United States, Lee and Hankin (2009) suggest that insecure attachment may be a risk factor for the development of later depressive and anxiety disorders. Other studies have supported this suggestion, demonstrating that adolescents with **anxious–avoidant attachment patterns** may become isolated, as they distance themselves from peers at a time when the majority of youth are increasing and strengthening their social relationships (Dozier, Lomax, Tyrrell, & Lee, 2000). Compared to their secure or anxious–avoidant peers, adolescents with an **anxious–resistant attachment pattern** demonstrate poor ability to regulate emotions and cope with distress, resulting in a higher frequency of anxiety disorders, depressive symptoms, and potential for later diagnosis of borderline personality disorder (Cassidy, 1994). Adolescents with this pattern may also experience rejection from peers because they appear too "needy" or due to excessive or inappropriate self-disclosure (Mikulincer, 1995).

In their study of a community sample of youth in early adolescence, Allen, Porter, McFarland, McElhaney, and Marsh (2007) found that insecure attachment was linked to multiple dysfunctional patterns that remained stable over the three-year investigation. Compared to their securely attached peers, insecurely attached youth exhibited more depressive symptoms and increasing levels of externalizing behaviors over the three-year period.

The worst outcomes for psychopathology are evident across the lifespan for youth with a **disoriented–disorganized attachment pattern**, which is often associated with a family history of abuse and inconsistent parenting which does not allow for the development of a consistent internal working model for future relationships. Adolescents with this pattern may demonstrate externalizing disorders (disruptive behaviors such as oppositional defiant disorder or conduct disorder), internalizing disorders (anxiety and depression), or a combination of both (Moss, Cyr, & Dubois-Comtois, 2004).

Attachment and the parent–adolescent relationship　In their study of early adolescent Italian youth, Sarracino, Presaghi, Degni, and Innamorati (2011) found that adolescents were more securely attached to the parent of the same sex, although attachment security to the parent of the opposite sex was predictive of a more moderate social value system, evident in more traditional and conservative beliefs, and fewer problem behaviors.

The role of parents in adolescents' secure attachment has also been investigated in terms of adolescents' relationships with their mothers (Allen et al., 2003) and their fathers (Allen et al., 2007) and conflict resolution. These studies have demonstrated that adolescents who have a secure relationship with their parents are better able to handle negotiations about autonomy compared to their insecure peers. Furthermore, youth with insecure attachment patterns report more harsh methods of conflict management used by fathers, compared to peers who are securely attached (Alber & Allen, 1987). Allen et al. (2007) suggest that their results point to the distinct possibility that "the secure adolescent tends to create relationships characterized by a balance of autonomy and relatedness to create their own secure bases" socially, and that these relationships can serve to buffer the adolescent from "peer pressure to engage in negative behaviours" (p. 1235).

Parenting styles and adolescent outcomes

Bronfenbrenner's (1979, 2001) bioecological model places the family in a pivotal position of influence on child and adolescent development. As a result, the impact of parenting styles on adolescent emotional and social development has attracted the attention of significant research. As was just discussed, adolescents who have an insecure attachment pattern report more harsh parenting tactics than their securely attached peers.

Baumrind (1991, 2005) has investigated the influence of parenting styles on development, especially with respect to autonomy in adolescence. In her studies with adolescents, Baumrind (2005, p. 63) found that "intrusiveness and low parental support" associated with the authoritarian directive approach was related to maladjustment in adolescence. In addition, "demandingness" had a "more beneficial effect when embedded in an authoritative configuration than when embedded in an authoritarian configuration" which conjointly provided "firm behavioral control and monitoring with warmth and autonomy support." Furthermore, Baumrind (2005, p. 63) found that high responsiveness affects children positively when conjoined with high demandingness in an authoritative configuration, but not when conjoined with low demandingness in a permissive pattern. Ultimately, Baumrind (2005, p. 67) suggests that the success of the authoritative parenting style is associated with enhanced adolescent autonomy and is based on the "unique configuration of high warmth, autonomy support and behavioral control and minimal use of psychological control." In this case, psychological control refers to what Barber and Harmon (2002) describe as parent responses of guilt, withdrawal of love, and ignoring, which are perceived by adolescents as intrusive and manipulative. Although authoritative parents assert their power in order to support their directives, they balance this with support for the adolescent's autonomy in their encouragement of the adolescent's ability to engage in critical reflection and reasoning (Baumrind, 1991).

According to domain theory, adolescents will likely take the most issues with parental attempts to control facets of the personal domain versus the prudential domain, resulting in parent–child conflict (Baumrind, 2005). Smetana (1995) studied parenting and its relation to family conflict and found that a less authoritative parent style was related to more frequent adolescent–parent conflict. In this study, parents with an authoritative style were more definitive in selecting issues that they should have control over, and were more likely to be permissive if an issue fell within the adolescent's personal domain.

Give a little, gain a lot

Results from research by Smetana (1995) suggest that it is important to choose your battle ground with adolescents.

Parenting style and other adolescent behaviors   Patock-Peckham, King, Morgan-Lopez, Ulloa, and Filson Moses (2011) investigated the role of parenting style in male and female impulsiveness, and drinking control in emerging adults (university students, 18–21 years of age), and found that lower monitoring by the opposite gender parent was related to impulsivity and alcohol problems. For females, having a permissive father was linked to lower monitoring and increased alcohol problems and impulsive behavior, while for males, having a permissive mother was related to lower monitoring and increased impulsiveness and alcohol problems. Having an authoritative father or mother was linked to fewer alcohol problems and less impulsivity. In another study, involving 16- and 17-year-olds, Ginsburg, Durbin, Garcia-Espana, Kalicka, and Winston (2009) found that compared to teens with uninvolved parents, teens with authoritative parents experienced almost 50% less risk of being in a car accident, while 71% reported that they were less likely to drive while intoxicated, and were less likely to use a cellular phone while driving. Youth with authoritative or authoritarian parents were also twice as likely to wear seat belts and less likely to speed compared to teens with uninvolved parents.

Family parenting styles and adolescent outcomes When Baumrind (1973) conducted her initial research on parenting styles, she only included families (mothers and fathers) who demonstrated the same parenting style (authoritarian, authoritative, indulgent). Fletcher, Steinberg, and Sellers (1999) investigated the impact of different combinations of parenting styles utilized within the same household. Results revealed that having one parent with an authoritative parenting style was related to higher academic competence in adolescents. However, the combination of one authoritative and one authoritarian parent resulted in increased internalizing distress in adolescents. Recently, Simons and Conger (2011) evaluated the relationship of parenting styles (by gender and type for 16 different combinations) to depression, conduct problems, and academic commitment. Results revealed that certain combinations were fairly common, such as authoritative mother and indulgent father, or indulgent mother and uninvolved father, while other combinations were extremely rare (authoritarian mother/authoritative father; indulgent mother/authoritarian father; uninvolved mother/authoritarian father). Family parenting styles associated with the best outcomes were two authoritative parents, or an authoritative parent combined with an indulgent parent. The worst outcomes were associated with an uninvolved mother, combined with an uninvolved or indulgent father, or having two authoritarian parents. Having at least one parent who is authoritative resulted in significant differences for depression, delinquency, and school commitment, although adolescents who had two authoritative parents demonstrated the lowest levels of depression and the highest levels of academic commitment. Although Baumrind (1991) suggested that a typical family might consist of a nurturing mother and controlling father, Simons and Conger (2011) found no evidence to support Baumrind's theory, since virtually no families in their study represented this combination of styles.

Attachment and parenting style: a summation Adolescence is a time of increased individual challenges and a time for negotiation to meet a growing need for autonomy. Youth who are securely attached and have authoritative parents have a more cohesive sense of self, have a better sense of relationships that include both autonomy and relatedness, and are better equipped to handle the challenges of this developmental period and to be successful academically and socially. On the other hand, youth who are insecurely attached often experience a parenting style that is harsh and critical, and are at increased risk for developing depressive symptoms and externalizing behaviors.

References

Alber, J. L., & Allen, J. P. (1987). Effects of maltreatment on young children's socioemotional development: An attachment theory perspective. *Developmental Psychology, 23,* 406–414.

Allen, J. P. (2008). The attachment system in adolescence. In J. Cassidy & P. R. Shaver (Eds.), *Handbook of attachment: Theory, research and clinical applications* (2nd ed.) (pp. 419–435). New York: Guilford.

Allen, J. P., McElhaney, K. B., Land, D. J., Kuperminc, G. P., Moore, C. M., & O'Beirne-Kelley, H. (2003). A secure base in adolescence: Markers of attachment security in the mother–adolescent relationship. *Child Development, 74,* 292–307.

Allen, J. P., Moore, C., Kuperminc, G., & Bell, K. (1998). Attachment and adolescent psychological functioning. *Child Development, 69,* 1406–1419.

Allen, J. P., Porter, M., McFarland, C., McElhaney, K. & Marsh, P. (2007). The relation of attachment security to adolescents' paternal and peer relationships, depression and externalizing behavior. *Child Development, 78,* 1222–1239.

Arnett, J. J. (1999). Adolescent storm and stress, reconsidered. *American Psychologist, 54,* 317–326.

Barber, B. K., & Harmon, E. L. (2002). Violating the self: Parental psychological control of children and adolescents. In B. K. Barber (Ed.), *Intrusive parenting: How psychological control affects children and adolescents* (pp. 15–52). Washington, DC: APA.

Baumeister, R. F., Smart, L., & Boden, J. M. (1996). Relation of threatened egotism to violence and aggression: The dark side of high esteem. *Psychological Review, 103,* 5–33.

Baumrind, D. (1973). The development of instrumental competence through socialization. In A. Pick (Ed.), *Minnesota Symposium on Child Psychology,* vol. 7 (pp. 3–46). Minneapolis: University of Minnesota Press.

Baumrind, D. (1991). The influences of parenting style on adolescent competence and substance use. *Journal of Early Adolescence, 11,* 56–95.

Baumrind, D. (2005). Patterns of parental authority and adolescent autonomy. *New Directions for Child and Adolescent Development, 108,* 61–69.

Bava, S., & Tapert, S. F. (2010). Adolescent brain development and the risk for alcohol and other drug problems. *Neuropsychology Review,* 20, 398–413.

Becker, A. E., Burwell, R. A., Herzog, D. B., Hamburg, P., & Gilman, S. E. (2002). Eating behaviours and attitudes following prolonged exposure to television among ethnic Fijian adolescent girls. *British Journal of Psychiatry, 180,* 509–514.

Berzonsky, M. D. (2003). Identity style and well being: Does commitment matter? *Identity: An International Journal of Theory and Research, 3,* 131–142.

Berzonsky, M. D., & Kuk, L. S. (2000). Identity status, identity processing style, and the transition to university. *Journal of Adolescent Research, 15,* 81–98.

Blouin, A. G., & Goldfield, G. S. (1995). Body image and steroid use in male bodybuilders. *International Journal of Eating Disorders, 18,* 159–165.

Bowlby, J. (1982). *Attachment and loss. Vol. 1. Attachment* (2nd ed.). New York: Basic Books.

Brandao, C. M., Lombardi, M. T., Nishida, S. K., Hauache, O. M., & Vieira, J. G. (2003). Serum leptin concentration during puberty in healthy nonobese adolescents. *Brazilian Journal of Medical and Biological Research, 36,* 1293–1296.

Brocki, K. C., & Bohlin, G. (2004). Executive functions in children aged 6 to 13: A dimensional and developmental study. *Developmental Neuropsychology, 26*(2), 571–593.

Brocki, K. C., & Bohlin, G. (2006). Developmental change in the relation between executive functions and symptoms of ADHD and co-occurring behaviour problems. *Infant and Child Development, 15*(1), 19–40.

Bronfenbrenner, U. (1979). *The ecology of human development.* Cambridge, MA: Harvard University Press.

Bronfenbrenner, U. (2001). Growing chaos in the lives of children, youth and families. How can we turn it around? In J. C. Westman (Ed.), *Parenthood in America* (pp. 197–210). Madison: University of Wisconsin Press.

Buchanan, C. M., Eccles, J. S., Flanagan, C., Midgley, C., Feldlaufer, H., & Harold, R. D. (1990). Parents' and teachers' beliefs about adolescents: Effects of sex and experience. *Journal of Youth and Adolescence, 19*, 363–394.

Buhrmester, D. (1996). Need fulfillment, interpersonal competence, and the developmental contexts of early adolescent friendship. In W. M. Bukowski, A. F. Newcomb, & W. W. Hartup (Eds.), *The company they keep: Friendship during childhood and adolescence* (pp. 158–185). New York: Cambridge University Press.

Case, R. (1998). The development of conceptual structures. In D. Kuhn & R. S. Siegler (Eds.), *Handbook of child psychology: Vol. 2. Cognition, perception and language* (5th ed., series ed. W. Damon) (pp. 745–800). New York: John Wiley & Sons, Ltd.

Casey, B. J., Jones, R. M., & Somerville, L. H. (2011). Breaking and accelerating of the adolescent brain. *Journal of Research on Adolescence, 21*(1), 21–33.

Casey, B. J., Vauss, Y. C., Chused, A., & Swedo, S. E. (1994). Cognitive functioning in Sydenham's chorea: II. *Executive functioning. Developmental Neuropsychology, 10*(2), 89–96.

Cassidy, J. (1994). Emotional regulation: Influence of attachment relationships. In N. A. Fox (Ed.), *The development of emotional regulation: Biological and behavioral considerations, Monographs of the Society for Research in Child Development, 59*, 228–249.

Centers for Disease Control and Prevention (CDC). (2005). YRBS (Youth Risk Behavior Surveillance). *Morbidity and Mortality Weekly Report, 55* (SS55).

Chira, S. (1994, July 10). Teen-agers in a poll report worry and distrust of adults. *New York Times*, pp. *1*, 16.

Cicchetti, D., & Rogosh, F. (2002). A developmental psychopathology perspective on adolescence. *Journal of Consulting and Clinical Psychology, 70*, 6–20.

Colby, A. L., Kohlberg, G., & Liberman, J. (1994). A longitudinal study of moral judgment. In B. Puka (Ed.), *New research in moral development* (pp. 1–124). New York: Garland Publishing.

Collins, W. A., & Madsen, S. D. (2006). Personal relationships in adolescence and early adulthood. In A. L. Vangelisti & D. Perlman (Eds.), *Cambridge handbook of personal relationships* (pp. 191–209). New York: Cambridge University Press.

Dawson, T. L. (2002). New tools, new insights: Kohlberg's moral judgment stages revisited. *International Journal of Behavioural Development, 26*, 154–166.

De Goede, I. H. A., Branje, S. J., & Meeus, W. H. (2009). Developmental changes and gender differences in adolescents' perceptions of friendships. *Journal of Adolescence, 32*, 1105–1123.

DeKlyen, M., & Greenberg, M. T. (2008). Attachment and psychopathology in childhood. In J. Cassidy & R. R. Shaver (Eds.), *Handbook of attachment theory research and clinical applications* (2nd ed.) (pp. 637–665). New York: Guilford.

Delaney, C. H. (1995). Rites of passage in adolescence. *Adolescence, 30*, 891–897.

Dick, D., Rose, R. J., Viken, R. J., & Kaprio, J. (2000). Pubertal timing and substance use: Association between and within families across late adolescence. *Developmental Psychology, 36*, 180–189.

Dozier, M., Lomax, L., Tyrrell, C. L., & Lee, S. W. (2001). The challenges of treatment with clients with dismissing states of mind. *Attachment and Human Development, 3*, 62–76.

Elkind, D. (1967). Egocentrism in adolescence. *Child Development, 38*, 1025–1034.

Elkind, D., & Bowen, R. (1979). Imaginary audience behavior in children and adolescents. *Developmental Psychology, 15*, 38–44.

Ellis, B. J., McFayden-Ketchum, S. A., Dodge, K. A., Pettit, G. S., & Bates, J. E. (1999). Quality of early family relationships and individual differences in the timing of pubertal maturation in girls: A longitudinal test on an evolutionary model. *Journal of Personality and Social Psychology, 77*, 387–401.

Eveleth, P. B., & Tanner, J. M. (1990). *Worldwide variation in human growth* (2nd ed.). Cambridge: Cambridge University Press.

Feld, B. C. (2008). A slower form of death: Implications of Roper v. Simmons for juveniles sentenced to life without parole. *Notre Dame Journal of Law, Ethics, and Public Policy, 22,* 9–65.

Fischer, A. (1993). Sex differences in emotionality: fact or stereotype? *Feminism and Psychology, 3,* 303–318.

Flavell, J. H., Miller, P. H., & Miller, S. A. (2002). *Cognitive development* (4th ed.). Upper Saddle River, NJ: Prentice Hall.

Fletcher, A. C., Steinberg, L., & Sellers, E. B. (1999). Adolescents' well-being as a function of perceived interparental inconsistency. *Journal of Marriage and Family, 61,* 599–610.

Franzoi, S. L., Davis, M. H., & Vasquez-Suson, K. A. (1994). Two social worlds: Social correlates and stability of adolescent status groups. *Journal of Personality and Social Psychology, 67,* 462–473.

Gardner, M., & Steinberg, L. (2005). Peer influence on risk taking, risk preference and risk decision-making in adolescence and adulthood: An experimental study. *Developmental Psychology, 41*(4), 625–635.

Ge, X., Conger, R. D., & Elder, G. H. (1996). Coming of age too early: Pubertal influences on girls' vulnerability to psychological distress. *Child Development, 67,* 3386–3400.

Ge, X., Conger, R. D., & Elder, G. H. (2001). The relation between puberty and psychological distress in adolescent boys. *Journal of Research on Adolescence, 11,* 49–70.

Geier, C. F., Terwilliger, R., Teslovich, T., Velanova, K., & Luna, B. (2010). Immaturities in reward processing and its influence on inhibitory control in adolescence. *Cerebral Cortex, 20*(7), 1613–1629.

Gilligan, C. F. (1982). *In a different voice.* Cambridge, MA: Harvard University Press.

Ginsburg, K. R., Durbin, D. R., Garcia-Espana, J. F., Kalicka, E. A., & Winston, F. K. (2009). Associations between parenting styles and teen driving, safety-related behaviors and attitudes. *Pediatrics, 124*(4), 1040–1051.

Hall, G. S. (1904). *Adolescence.* New York: Appleton.

Harris, D. J., & Kuba, S. A. (1997). Ethnocultural identity and eating disorders in women of color. *Professional Psychology: Research and Practice, 28,* 341–347.

Hartup, W., & Laursen, B. (1993). Conflict and context in peer relations. In C. Hart (Ed.), *Children on playgrounds; Research perspectives and applications* (pp. 44–84). Albany, State University of New York Press.

Hartup, W., & Stevens, N. (1999). Friendships and adaptation across the life span. *Current Directions in Psychological Science, 8,* 76–79.

Hesse-Biber, S., Leavy, P., Quinn, C. E., & Zoino, J. (2006). The mass marketing of disordered eating and eating disorders: The social psychology of women, thinness and culture. *Women's Studies International Forum, 29,* 208–224.

Inhelder, B., & Piaget, J. (1958). *The growth of logical thinking from childhood to adolescence: An essay on the construction of formal operational structures.* New York: Basic Books.

Jadack, R. A., Hyde, J. S., Moore, C., & Keller, M. (1995). Moral reasoning about sexually transmitted diseases. *Child Development, 66,* 167–177.

Jaeger, J. J., Lockwood, A. H., Van Valin, R. D., Kemmerer, D., Murphy, B. W., & Wack, D. S. (1998). Sex differences in brain regions activated by grammatical and reading tasks. *Neuroreport, 9,* 2803–2807.

Johnson, J. S., & Newport, E. L. (1989). Critical period effects in second language learning: The influence of maturational state on the acquisition of English as a second language. *Cognitive Psychology, 21,* 60–99.

Kanayama, G., Pope, H. G., & Hudson, J. I. (2001). "Body image" drugs: a growing psychosomatic problem. *Psychotherapy and Psychosomatics, 7,* 61–65.

Kanayama, G., Pope, H. G., Cohane, G., & Hudson, J. I. (2003). Risk factors for anabolic-androgenic steroid use among weightlifters: A case-control study. *Drug and Alcohol Dependence, 71*, 77–86.

Kindlundh, A. M., Isacson, D. G., Berglund, L., & Nyberg, F. (1999). Factors associated with adolescent use of doping agents: Anabolic-androgenic steroids. *Addiction, 94*, 543–553.

Koepp, M. J., Gunn, R. N., Lawrence, A. D., Cunningham, V. J., Dagher, A. & Jones, T. (1998). Evidence for striatal dopamine release during a video game. *Nature, 383* (6682), 266–268.

Kohlberg, L. (1976). Moral stages and moralization: Cognitive-developmental approach. In R. Lickona (Ed.), *Moral development and behaviour: Theory, research and social issues* (pp. 31–53). Chicago: Rand McNally.

Kroger, J. (2000). *Identity development: adolescence through adulthood.* Thousand Oaks, CA: Sage.

Larose, S., & Bernier, A. (2001). Social support processes: Mediators of attachment state of mind and adjustment in late adolescence. *Attachment and Human Development, 3*, 96–120.

Larson, R., & Ham, M. (1993). Stress and "storm and stress" in early adolescence: The relationship of negative events with dysphoric affect. *Developmental Psychology, 29*, 130–140.

Larson, R., & Richards, M. H. (1994). *Divergent realities: The emotional lives of mothers, fathers and adolescents.* New York: Basic Books.

Laursen, B., Coy, K. C., & Collins, W. A. (1998). Reconsidering changes in parent–child conflict across adolescence: A meta-analysis. *Child Development, 69*, 817–832.

Lee, A., & Hankin, B. L. (2009). Insecure attachment, dysfunctional attitudes and low self-esteem predicting prospective symptoms of depression and anxiety during adolescence. *Journal of Clinical Child and Adolescent Psychology, 38*(2), 219–231.

Marcia, J. E. (1980). Identity in adolescence. In J. Adelson (Ed.), *Handbook of adolescent psychology* (pp. 159–187). New York: John Wiley & Sons, Ltd.

Markiewicz, D., Lawford, H., Doyle, A. B., & Haggart, N. (2006). Developmental differences in adolescents' and young adults' use of mothers, fathers, best friends and romantic partners to fulfill attachment needs. *Journal of Youth and Adolescence, 35*, 127–140.

Markovits, H., Benenson, J., & Dolensky, E. (2001). Evidence that children and adolescents have internal models of peer interactions that are gender differentiated. *Child Development, 72*, 879–886.

Matsumoto, D., & Juang, L. (2008). *Culture and psychology* (4th ed.). Belmont, CA: Wadsworth.

McGivern, R. F., Andersen, J., Byrd, D., Mutter, K., & Reilly, J. (2002). Cognitive efficiency on a match to sample task decreases at the onset of puberty in children. *Brain and Cognition, 50*(1), 73–89.

Mendle, J., Turkheimer, E., & Emery, R. E. (2007). Detrimental psychological outcomes associated with early pubertal timing in adolescent girls. *Developmental Review, 27*, 151–171.

Mikulincer, M. (1995). Attachment style and mental representations of the self. *Journal of Personality and Social Psychology, 69*, 1203–1215.

Mikulincer, M., Gillath, O., Sapir-Lavid, Y., Yaakobi, E., Artas, K & Tal-Aloni, L. (2003). Attachment theory and concern for others' welfare: evidence that activation of the sense of secure base promotes endorsement of self-transcendence values. *Basic and Applied Social Psychology, 25*, 299–312.

Miller, J. G. (1997). Culture and self: Uncovering the cultural grounding of psychological theory. In J. D. Snodgrass & R. L. Thompson (Eds.), *Morality in everyday life: Developmental perspectives* (pp. 259–282). Cambridge: Cambridge University Press.

Moss, E., Cyr, C., & Dubois-Comtois, K. (2004). Attachment at early school age and developmental risk: Examining family contexts and behavior problems of controlling-caregiving, controlling-punitive and behaviorally disorganized children. *Developmental Psychology, 40,* 519–532.

Mulholland, A. M., & Mintz, L. B. (2001). Prevalence of eating disorders among African American women. *Journal of Counseling Psychology, 48*(1), 111–116.

Newman, B. M., & Newman, P. R. (2001). Group identity and alienation. Giving the we its due. *Journal of Youth and Adolescence, 30,* 515–538.

Nowak, M. (1998). The weight-conscious adolescent: Body image, food intake, and weight related behavior. *Journal of Adolescent Health, 23*(6), 389–398.

Parker, S., Nichter, M., Vuckovic, N., Sims, C., & Ritenbaugh, C. (1995). Body image and weight concerns among African American and white adolescent females: Differences that make a difference. *Human Organization, 54*(2), 103–114.

Patock-Peckham, J. A., King, K., Morgan-Lopez, A. A., Ulloa, E. C., & Filson Moses, J. M. (2011). Gender-specific meditational links between parenting styles, parental monitoring, impulsiveness, drinking control, and alcohol-related problems. *Journal of Studies on Alcohol and Drugs, 72*(2), 247–258.

Paus, T., Keshavan, M., & Giedd, J. N. (2008). Why do many psychiatric disorders emerge during adolescence? *Nature Reviews Neuroscience, 9*(12), 947–957.

Phillips, K. A. (1996). *The broken mirror: Understanding and treating body dysmorphic disorder.* New York: Oxford University Press.

Phillips, K. A., McElroy, S. L., Keck, P. E., Jr., Pope, H. G., Jr., & Hudson, J. I. (1993). Body dysmorphic disorder: 30 cases of imagined ugliness. *American Journal of Psychiatry, 150,* 302–308.

Pope, H. G., Gruber, A. J., Choi, P., Olivardia, R., & Phillips, K. A. (1997). Muscle dysmorphia: An underrecognized form of body dysmorphic disorder. *Psychosomatics, 38,* 548–557.

Pope, H. G., Gruber, A. J., Mangweth, B., Bureau, B., deCol, C., Jouvent, R., & Hudson, J. I. (2000a). Body image perception among men in three countries. *American Journal of Psychiatry, 157,* 1297–1301.

Pope, H. G., Olivardia, R., Borowiecki, J. J., & Cohane, G. H. (2001). The growing commercial value of the male body: A longitudinal survey of advertising in women's magazines. *Psychotherapy and Psychosomatics, 70,* 189–192.

Pope, H. G., Phillips, K. A., & Olivardia, R. (2000b). *The Adonis complex: The secret crisis of male body obsession.* New York: Free Press.

Reyna, V., & Farley, F. (2008). Risk and rationality in adolescent decision-making: Implications for theory, practice and public policy. *Psychological Science in the Public Interest, 7,* 1–44.

Rubin, K., Dwyer, K., Booth-LaForce, C., Kim, A., Burgess, K., & Rose-Krasnor, L. (2004). Attachment, friendship and psychosocial functioning in early adolescence. *Journal of Early Adolescence, 24,* 326–356.

Saraswathi, T. S. (1999). Adult–child continuity in India: is adolescence a myth or an emerging reality? In T. S. Saraswathi (Ed.), *Culture, socialization and human development: Theory, research and applications in India* (pp. 213–232). Thousand Oaks, CA: Sage.

Sarracino, D., Presaghi, F., Degni, S., & Innamorati, M. (2011). Sex-specific relationships among attachment security, social values, and sensation seeking in early adolescence: Implications for adolescents' externalizing problem behavior. *Journal of Adolescence, 34,* 541–554.

Schindler, A., Thomasius, P. S., Gemeinhardt, B., Kustner, U., & Eckert, J. (2005). Attachment and substance use disorders: a review of the literature and a study in drug dependent adolescents. *Attachment and Human Development, 7,* 207–228.

Schlegel, A., & Barry, H. (1991). *Adolescence: An anthropological inquiry.* New York: Free Press.

Schwartz, S. J., Cote, J. E., & Arnett, J. J. (2005). Identity and agency in emerging adulthood: Two developmental routes in the individuation process. *Youth and Society, 37,* 201–229.

Selman, R. (1980). *The growth of interpersonal understanding*. New York: Academic Press.

Simmons, R. G., Burgeson, R., Carlton-Ford, S., & Blyth, D. A. (1987). The impact of cumulative change in early adolescence. *Child Development, 58,* 1220–1234.

Simons, K., Paternite, C. E., & Shore, C. (2001). Quality of parent/adolescent attachment and aggression in young adolescents. *Journal of Early Adolescence, 21,* 182–203.

Simons, L. G., & Conger, R. D. (2011). Linking mother–father differences in parenting to a typology of family parenting styles and adolescent outcomes. *Journal of Family Issues, 28*(2), 212–241.

Skrandies, W., Reik, P., & Kunze, C. (1999). Topography of evoked brain activity during mental arithmetic and language tasks: Sex differences. *Neuropsychologia, 37,* 421–430.

Smetana, J. G. (1995). Parenting styles and conceptions of parental authority. *Child Development, 66*(2), 299–316.

Smith, E. (1997, November 24). Bodybuilders face "flip side" of anorexia. *USA Today,* p. 1.

Snarey, J. R. (1995). In a communitarian voice: The sociological expansion of Kohlbergian theory research and practice. In W. M. Kurtines & J. L. Gewirtz (Eds.), *Moral development; An introduction* (pp. 109–134). Boston: Allyn and Bacon.

Snarey, J. R., & Bell, D. (2003). Distinguishing structural and functional models of human development: A response to "what transits in an identity status transition?" *Identity, 3,* 221–230.

Snarey, J. R., Reimer, J., & Kohlberg, L. (1985). The development of social-moral reasoning among kibbutz adolescents: A longitudinal cross-cultural study. *Developmental Psychology, 21,* 3–17.

Sroufe, L. A. (2005). Attachment and development: A prospective longitudinal study from birth to adulthood. *Attachment and Human Development, 7,* 349–367.

Steinberg, L., Albert, D., Cauffman, E., Banich, M., Graham, S., & Wollard, J. (2008). Age differences in sensation seeking and impulsivity as indexed by behavior and self report: Evidence for a dual systems model. *Developmental Psychology, 44,* 1764–1778.

Steinberg, L., Graham, S., O'Brien, L., Woolard, J., Cauffman, E., & Banich, M. (2009). Age differences in future orientation and delay discounting. *Child Development, 80,* 28–44.

Stice, E., & Whitenton, K. (2002). Risk factors for body dissatisfaction in adolescent girls: A longitudinal investigation. *Developmental Psychology, 38,* 669–678.

Tanner, J. M. (1990). *Foetus into man: Physical growth from conception to maturity* (revised and enlarged ed.). Cambridge, MA. Harvard University Press.

Tiggemann, M., & Pickering, A. S. (1996). Role of television in adolescent women's body dissatisfaction and drive for thinness. *International Journal of Eating Disorders, 20,* 199–203.

Tunbridge, E. M., Weickert, C. S., Kleinman, J. E., Herman, M. M., Chen, J., & Kolachana, B. S. (2007). Catechol-o-methyltransferase enzyme activity and protein expression in human prefrontal cortex across the postnatal lifespan. *Cerebral Cortex, 17*(5), 1206–1212.

Walcott, D. D., Pratt, H. D., & Patel, D. R. (2003). Adolescents and eating disorders: Gender, racial, ethnic, sociocultural and socioeconomic issues. *Journal of Adolescent Research, 18,* 223–243.

Wark, G. R., & Krebs, D. L. (2000). The construction of moral dilemmas in everyday life. *Journal of Moral Education, 29*(1), 5–17.

Williams, S. K., & Kelly, F. D. (2005). Relationships among involvement, attachment and behavioural problems in adolescence: Examining father's influence. *Journal of Early Adolescence, 25,* 168–196.

Windle, M., Spear, L. P., Fuligni, A. J., Angold, A., Brown, J. D., Pine, D., ... Dahl, R. E. (2008). Transitions into underage and problem drinking: Developmental processes and mechanisms between 10 and 15 years of age. *Pediatrics, 121,* S273–S289.

Yang, C. J., Gray, P., & Pope, H. G. (2005). Male body image in Taiwan versus the West: *Yanggang Zhiqi* meets the Adonis complex. *American Journal of Psychiatry, 162,* 263–269.

5

Development from a Clinical and Educational Perspective

Chapter preview and learning objectives

One of the major challenges facing psychologists working with children and adolescents is distinguishing normal behavior from behavior that is atypical or maladaptive. In *Chapter 1*, readers were introduced to Pat, a 12-year-old boy who had a history of academic difficulties and who was responding to academic frustrations with increased emotional reactivity. Within the context of that case study, readers were briefly introduced to a discussion of clinical and educational approaches to diagnosis and treatment/intervention for Pat. In this chapter, the discussion will focus on the decision-making process involved in the assessment, diagnosis, and treatment/intervention programs for child and adolescent problems. The chapter closes with a discussion of ethical challenges facing practitioners who work with children and adolescents in their practice and research settings.

After completing this chapter, readers will have an increased understanding of:

- clinical and educational perspectives concerning the nature and severity of child problems;
- assessment as an on-going process of generating hypotheses about behavior;
- various methods used by psychologists to assess child and adolescent behavior;
- data gathering, problem solving, and developing interventions;
- the different systems used to classify child problems (dimensional and categorical classification systems);
- global issues in the use of different categorical classification systems (the *Diagnostic and Statistical Manual of Mental Disorders* (DSM) and the *International Classification of Diseases* (ICD));
- the strengths and limitations of the different classification systems;
- descriptive and experimental research methods in child psychology;
- strengths and limitations of the different research approaches;
- ethical concerns and considerations in working with children and adolescents.

Developmental deviations: clinical and educational perspectives

Developmental milestones provide benchmarks for evaluating deviations from the norm. Although a three-year-old child might frequently engage in tantrum behaviors, the same behaviors in an eight-year-old would be cause for concern. Not all behavioral deviations will be that obvious, hence the question: ***When is a behavioral deviation from the norm considered serious enough to warrant intervention?***

It is likely time to intervene when the behavior is . . .

- developmentally inappropriate;
- occurring with greater frequency than anticipated;
- occurring with greater severity than expected;
- causing concern for the safety of the child or others;
- causing significant dysfunction (school, home, peers);
- causing significant distress to the child or caregiver.

Steps in the decision-making process

In order to make decisions about the nature and severity of dysfunctional behavior, practitioners need to have a plan of action that will inform the decision-making process. In the case of child and adolescent development, the practitioner will need to assess the behavior(s) carefully, taking into consideration developmental expectations, and known risks and protective factors given the child's age, gender, and culture.

Step 1 – assessment The first step in the decision-making process is assessment. Assessment is a term that has come to be associated with "testing," although on a broader level, assessment can also be seen as a process that involves the on-going evaluation of behaviors and situations/events, or monitoring of treatment outcomes. In the latter sense, the goal of assessment could be to develop a **diagnosis** concerning the dynamics of the problem; for example, what caused the problem (**precipitating cause**) and what is maintaining the problem (**maintaining cause**). Assessments can measure development in broad areas of functioning, such as cognitive, behavioral, or emotional assessments, or they can pinpoint specific areas, such as determining one's level of depression (syndrome specific test) or self-esteem.

Step 2 – diagnosis and classification In addition to conceptualizing diagnosis as a process of inquiry, the term diagnosis can also refer to *taxonomy* and specific nomenclature, or how disorders are classified. The goal is to define the problem in a way that is diagnostically relevant, by classifying symptoms or characteristics within a specific diagnostic category (learning disability, anxiety disorder, and so on). Once the "problem" is diagnosed, then the psychologist can access empirically supported methods that are available to treat the disorder.

Initially, this form of information gathering may produce a number of *provisional diagnoses* (hypotheses) that will be confirmed or rejected during the course of the evaluation.

Ultimately, on the basis of information derived from interviews, observations, and responses to different types of assessment instruments, the problem becomes more clearly defined and a specific intervention or treatment can now be recommended.

Step 3 – treatments and interventions Throughout this book, interventions and treatment alternatives will be discussed as they relate to specific child and adolescent problems. There has been increasing emphasis on the "end usability" of developmental research to inform child intervention and treatment:

> Within developmental studies, there has been increased focus on the connection between normative development, atypical development and intervention, including the importance of understanding atypical development through a normative lens that can guide interventions.
>
> (Guerra, Graham, & Tolan, 2011, p. 7)

To this end, Cicchetti and Toth (2006) have emphasized the need for research to investigate and improve our "understanding of the mechanisms and processes that initiate and maintain the developmental pathway to disease" (p. 621).

As will become evident throughout these chapters, treatments and interventions can be delivered in a number of different settings (clinics, schools, home) and can be based on a number of different theoretical perspectives (behavioral, cognitive, psychodynamic, family systems). In addition, treatments and interventions can target outcomes in a number of different areas, including child outcomes (enhanced child functioning in academic, social, emotional, and behavioral areas) and family outcomes (improved quality of life, stress reduction, and reduced level of family chaos).

Assessment and evaluation

Three primary goals of assessment and case formulation include:

1. problem identification, clarification, and classification;
2. problem interpretation and problem evaluation;
3. treatment formulation. (Wilmshurst, 2008, p. 149)

Mash and Hunsley (2005) outline a number of forms that assessments can take, including: diagnosis (case formulation), screening (at-risk populations), prognosis (charting the course of a disorder), and the monitoring and evaluation of treatment.

Assessment methods

There are many assessment instruments available to evaluate functioning in broad areas of learning and achievement, neuropsychological development, emotional and behavioral concerns, as well as measures to evaluate syndrome-specific concerns (such as depression, anxiety, and so on). The purpose of this section is not to provide an exhaustive review of assessment instruments but to provide information about how these methods assist psychologists to arrive at decisions about diagnosis and treatment or intervention.

In their survey of school psychologists in the United States, Shapiro and Heick (2004) found that intelligence testing (84%) was the most common form of assessment, followed by the use of interviews, behavioral rating scales, and observations (67–75%).

Interviews   Interviews provide an opportunity to obtain significant information about a child's medical, developmental, and educational history; family history; parental expectations; and parent and teacher perceptions of the problem. Interviews can take a variety of forms and can be highly structured, semistructured, or unstructured.

Depending on the nature of the problem, practitioners often want to obtain information from parents and teachers prior to seeing the child or adolescent. When interviewing a child, it is important to engage the child at a developmentally appropriate level, and establish rapport prior to asking more difficult questions. **Unstructured interviews** allow for considerable flexibility and are useful for obtaining initial impressions about the problem, or parent/teacher expectations about potential outcomes. **Semistructured interviews** provide opportunities for obtaining specific information, but also have built-in flexibility to allow deviation from the structure along the way. The *Semistructured Clinical Interview for Children and Adolescents* (SCICA;

McConaughy & Achenbach, 2001) is an example of a semistructured interview. The SCICA contains specific questions (which can later be ranked and scored), in addition to some open-ended questions. Children can also participate in semistructured interviews depending on their age, as part of the interview process. For example, the initial part of the Achenbach System of Empirically Based Assessment (ASEBA; Achenbach & Rescorla, 2001) contains a number of specific questions for youth which can later be scored, as well as a number of open-ended questions (such as "*Please describe the best things about yourself*"). These initial questions become part of the overall evaluation of adaptive functioning on the ASEBA. The **mental status exam** is a specific type of semistructured interview designed as a quick check to determine an individual's orientation in time and space. For example, an adolescent who appears somewhat dazed and confused might be asked questions about current events (day and time), math calculations, and questions requiring insight and judgment (Sattler & Hodge, 2006, p. 638).

The most rigid form of interview is the **structured interview** which asks very specific questions with a goal of obtaining information to confirm or rule out a potential diagnosis. This type of interview is also helpful in obtaining information about demographics or historical background when retaining the sequence of information is important.

Strengths and limitations of the interview   While interviews can provide a wealth of information, it is not always possible to determine whether an individual is completely truthful about the information (wanting to project a socially desirable image), whether information is recalled accurately, or the extent to which personal bias alters recall.

Observations   There are several methods of observation that can be used to assist in the development of a functional behavioral assessment, or to monitor behaviors once a plan is set in place. The observational methods discussed below are summarized in Table 5.1.

Narrative recording   This procedure involves keeping an anecdotal record of behaviors and events as they occur. Often this can represent the first stage of observation where the psychologist obtains a general impression of the nature and types of behaviors that are occurring. Although this form of observation provides an opportunity to see cause and effect connections, information may be subject to **observer drift** (losing focus, becoming distracted, or missing key elements).

Event recording   Recording of **discrete** events is helpful in measuring low frequency behaviors (e.g., the number of times a child raises his or her hand to ask a question) or the amount of lapsed time between a request and a response. For example, it may be important to determine the length of time between when a teacher or parent makes a request and the child initiates a response. Recording can often take the form of a tally sheet with pre-recorded responses. This is the preferred method for low frequency behaviors. However, the disadvantage is that information is not obtained about why the behavior occurred.

Table 5.1   Methods of recording observed behaviors

Observation type	Appropriate use	Description
Event recording	Discrete, low frequency behaviors, e.g., the child asks a question, raises his/her hand, or talks out of turn	Record the number of times a behavior occurs during an observational period.
Interval recording	Continuous behaviors, e.g., on-task behavior, remaining seated, etc.	Measurement is contingent on pre-determined time intervals. The observer creates a time schedule (e.g., observe behavior for 15 seconds at the top of each minute). Recording behaviors at one-minute intervals provides a high yield of behavioral observations (i.e., it is possible to record 30 observations in 30 minutes).
Template matching child	Record alternate observations of the target child's behavior and that of another "model" student	This method can be adapted to either event or interval recording depending on the nature of the behavior to be observed. Information about the frequency of the model child's behaviors can be used to set goals for the target child.

Interval recording   Interval observations are best used for **continuous** behaviors (e.g., on-task behavior) which are best recorded through timed intervals (e.g., observing every 60 seconds to determine whether on-task performance is evident for the next 20-second interval and recording a "yes or no" on a tally sheet). The process would be repeated each minute and would allow for 30 (20-second) observations within a half-hour period. If more than one observer is present, it is also possible to obtain an estimate of inter-rater agreement for the behavior observed.

Template matching child   In addition to the target child, the observer also observes an exemplary child to determine the optimum ratio of on-task behavior in a 30-minute period (using the event recording procedure above, with the first 20 seconds viewing the exemplary child and the second 20-second period observing the target child). This provides the advantage of having a benchmark to compare the behavior to, rather than selecting an arbitrary ideal.

Rating scales   Behavioral rating scales are an effective and efficient method of obtaining information from multiple informants about a child's behavior in a number of important areas. Behavioral rating scales such as the Achenbach System of Empirically Based Assessment (ASEBA; Achenbach & Rescorla, 2001), the Devereux Behavior Rating Scale – School Form (DSMD; Naglieri, LeBuffe, & Pfeiffer, 1994), and the Conners' Rating Scales (CRS-R; Conners, 1998) provide parallel forms that can be completed by parents, teachers, and children (of certain ages) regarding behaviors

Table 5.2   Examples of the types of question that might be found in a behavior rating scale

Please complete the following statements regarding the child's behaviors during the last six months	Not true (0)	Somewhat true (1)	Always true (2)
1. Fails to finish assignments, tests			
2. Argues			
3. Prefers to be alone			
4. Enjoys playing sports			
5. Restless			
6. Complains of headaches			
7. Has a friend stay over			
8. Has destroyed an article of personal or family value			
9. Gets into fights			
10. Complains of stomach aches			

in a number of areas (self-concept, social skills, aggression, attention and concentration, learning style). Syndrome scales can also be helpful in having parents, teachers, and youth rate levels of emotional distress (such as depression, anxiety) relative to similar-aged peers.

Behavioral rating scales, such as the ASEBA and Devereux scales, are popular for several reasons, including the following:

- They are in a multi-rater format (parents, teachers, and older children can complete the questionnaires).
- Behaviors are surveyed across a variety of areas.
- The responses are hand-scored or computer-scored and generate a behavioral profile.
- The profile allows for a comparison of a child's behaviors with normative data available for similar-aged peers.
- Rating scales are empirically supported and derived.

The statements contained in Table 5.2 are similar to those found in many of the rating scales used to evaluate behaviors.

We will revisit the topic of behavioral rating scales later in this chapter, when discussing the dimensional classification system. An example of a behavioral profile generated by a behavioral rating scale is available in Figure 5.1.

Functional behavioral assessment (FBA)   Derived from applied behavioral analysis and the behavioral model, a functional behavioral assessment (FBA) is a tool that allows psychologists to develop a behavioral intervention plan, based on systematic observation and analysis of the problem behavior as it relates to events/situations that precipitate the behavior (**antecedent condition**) and the possible environmental factors that reinforce and perpetuate the problem (**consequence**). Unlike the psychoanalytic perspective which attributes behavior to internal and unconscious origins, the behavioral perspective conceptualizes patterns of behavior as learned responses that are

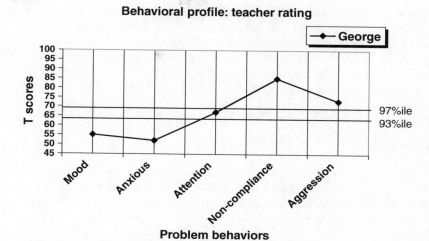

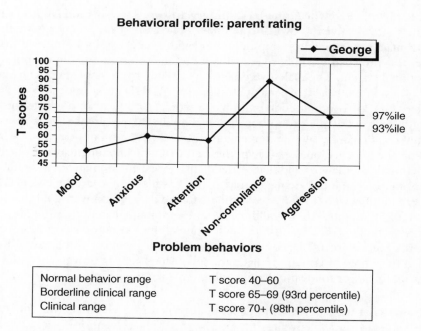

Normal behavior range	T score 40–60
Borderline clinical range	T score 65–69 (93rd percentile)
Clinical range	T score 70+ (98th percentile)

Figure 5.1 Example of a behavioral profile based on teacher and parent ratings.

based on external conditions of reinforcement and punishment (i.e., we are motivated to increase behaviors that are rewarded and decrease those that are punished).

FBA is a "multimethod, multisource approach to identify relationships between specific individual characteristics and contextual variables that trigger and maintain behaviour" (Hawkins & Axelrod, 2008, p. 841). In the United States, the reauthorization of the Individuals with Disabilities Education Act (IDEA, 2004) and the focus on early intervention have drawn considerable attention to FBA and its potential role in developing intervention plans. As a result, FBA has been the focus of significant empirical investigations in an attempt to "bridge the gap between research and practice" (Hoff, Ervin, & Friman, 2005, p. 46). Recent investigations have applied FBA methods to interventions and treatment plans for a host of child and adolescent behavior problems, in the classroom (Hoff et al., 2005; Moore, Anderson, & Kumar, 2005) and home environments (Hawkins & Axelrod, 2008).

Target the deficit or the excess?

In developing a behavior management program, it is always best to select a **behavioral deficit** (such as non-compliance, or off-task behavior) rather than a **behavioral excess** (such as aggressive behaviors, or getting out of seat), since this provides the opportunity for increasing positive outcomes.

An example of a FBA for home-based intervention   Hawkins and Axelrod (2008) examined the effectiveness of FBA methods applied to on-task homework behavior for four male residents in a group home under the supervision of a trained married couple who provided a family-style living arrangement using a token economy as a motivational system. The males were between 12 and 16 years of age and had diagnoses of attention deficit hyperactivity disorder (ADHD) and oppositional defiant disorder (ODD). Youth attended an on-site school, and were responsible for completing homework at the group home after school. The researchers interviewed the staff, reviewed records, and conducted a narrative observation of homework periods. Based on the information, it was hypothesized that all four students were capable of completing the homework and that off-task behavior during homework was motivated by wanting to escape task demands, rather than an inability to do the task (Hawkins & Axelrod, 2008, p. 845). After collecting baseline data, youth were told that if they worked for 10 minutes, they would receive a reward immediately after the 10-minute period was completed. Rewards represented one of three conditions: break alone (five minutes); break with preferred activities (five minutes); or an edible treat. Results revealed that three of the youth made the most significant improvements in on-task homework behavior following the five-minute break (alone) conditions.

An example of a FBA for school-based intervention   Hoff, Ervin, and Friman (2005) assessed the effectiveness of applying a FBA intervention for a 12-year-old boy who was diagnosed with ADHD/ODD and who was disruptive in the regular classroom. Interviews, a review of records, and observations (with partial interval recording) revealed a number of disruptive verbal behaviors (talking to peers, making noises) and intrusive behaviors (making faces, taking others' possessions, getting out of his seat). The analysis revealed that during the structured portion of the lessons, the boy's behaviors were very similar to his peers. However, when the teacher assigned a task to the class, and then walked around to check their homework and answer questions, his disruptive behavior increased dramatically. Two potential hypotheses were generated: disruptive behavior was motivated by trying to attract peer attention; or it was motivated by escape from a task of little interest to him. Teacher comments

Table 5.3 Examples of functional behavioral analysis

Antecedent condition	Behavior	Consequence	What happened
Teacher asks the child to read out loud to the class	Child acts out in class	Child is removed from class	Reinforcement: reading is removed, avoidance is reinforced
Mother requests clean-up time	Child refuses to clean up his toys	Mother cleans up	Reinforcement: clean-up is removed, avoidance is reinforced
Child calls himself "stupid"	Child feels depressed	Feelings of low self-esteem	Reinforcement: child feels worse
Child is ignored by peers	Child tries to get peers' attention	Child is rejected by peers	Punishment: child withdraws

during the interview referred to his acting "silly" and being the "class clown," which gave more credence to the "attention-getting" hypothesis. Further observation confirmed that his behavior was rewarded by peer laughter and attention more than half the time, but also that his behavior was more disruptive when the task assigned was silent reading (escape).

Further examples of FBA can be found in Table 5.3.

Recall that in *Chapter 2*, when discussing different reinforcement and punishment paradigms, reinforcement always resulted in an increase in behavior (in Table 5.3, avoidance is reinforced), while punishment resulted in decreased behaviors (social interaction declines). The psychologist can use this information to develop an intervention plan to reinforce replacement behaviors that are adaptive as opposed to maladaptive. An example of this will be presented in the case of George Nash, to be discussed shortly.

Clinical and psychometric instruments   In addition to rating scales and observation, an **assessment battery** (a group of instruments) can be selected to conduct an assessment. Information concerning the **validity** (the degree to which the tests measure what they purport to measure), **reliability** (the likelihood of obtaining the same score on test/retest and between raters), and the **population** upon which the tests were standardized are available in the instruments' technical manuals.

Reliability and validity

Reliability is a measure of a test's consistency across administrations (an individual takes the same test at Time 1 and Time 2 (**test-retest reliability**)), or the extent of agreement between two test administrators or observers evaluating the same individual (**inter-rater, or inter-observer reliability**). The term validity refers to the extent that a test measures what it intends to measure, including:

the degree to which test items represent the entire range of possible items (**content validity**) and the extent to which the test can predict the construct that is being measured (**criterion validity**).

Individual psychometric instruments   There are many possible explanations for a child's academic and behavioral difficulties, including the fact that behaviors may be a response to frustrations resulting from problems in information processing, memory, or cognitive ability. An **intelligence test** or a measure of **cognitive functioning** might provide valuable information about strengths and weaknesses that a child brings to the learning task, while **neuropsychological tests** can provide information about executive processing, memory, and attention. Standardized achievement tests can provide an index of academic functioning relative to standard intelligence scores to allow direct comparison of these two levels (an approach called the discrepancy formula or **discrepancy criterion**, which will be discussed at length in *Chapter 8*).

A practitioner who is concerned about a child's emotional status may conduct a **personality assessment** or administer **response inventories** aimed at more specific emotional difficulties (such as anxiety, depression, somatic concerns, disruptive behaviors).

Projective assessments   Asking children to draw a picture of a person or their family, or to tell a story in response to pictures, are forms of **projective assessment**. Information can be analyzed for content of recurring themes such as feelings of powerlessness, feelings of isolation, family cohesion, and sibling rivalry.

Diagnosis and classification

After assessment and evaluation, the next step is to identify how the problem is classified, relative to other problems. Practitioners are guided in the decision-making process through the use of systems of classification that clarify the nature of the problem, its causes, course, and treatment alternatives. The classification system provides professionals with a "common" language for accessing and discussing relevant information about the disorder. There are two main systems of classification for child and adolescent disorders: the **categorical classification system**, and the **dimensional** or **empirical classification system**.

Categorical classification systems

The two most widely used categorical systems for the classification of mental diseases or disorders are the *International Classification of Diseases* (ICD-10; WHO, 1992), and the *Diagnostic and Statistical Manual of Mental Disorders* (DSM-IV-TR; APA, 2000). Both systems are currently in the process of revision and historically there has been a concentrated effort to align the two systems, although some differences exist in how the disorders are conceptualized and in the terminology used.

Although the two systems share the same goal, the DSM provides more explicit rules and criteria to guide the decision-making process. The ICD is most frequently found in Europe, while the DSM is predominantly used in North America. The ICD is the most frequently used system, worldwide, for clinical diagnoses and training, while the DSM is the source that is most often used for research (Mezzich, 2002).

Comorbidity and classification

Children tend to experience a significantly higher number of comorbid (co-occurring) disorders compared to adults. A major difference between the ICD and the DSM, which has important implications regarding the diagnosis of child psychopathology, is that while the ICD seeks to determine a predominant diagnosis, the DSM allows for comorbidity for as many diagnoses that meet the criteria (Kolvin & Trowell, 2002).

Despite the differences in these two diagnostic systems, they share a categorical decision-making format; namely, a disorder is considered to be present or absent based on the degree of "fit" between the symptom presentation and the defining criteria. What follows is a brief description of each of the categorical systems.

DSM   The DSM contains classification criteria for over 400 mental disorders. Child and adolescent disorders occur throughout the manual but are primarily concentrated in sections devoted to **neurodevelopmental disorders** (intellectual developmental disabilities (IDD), autism spectrum disorders (ASD), specific learning disabilities (SLD), motor skills impairments and specific language impairments (SLI), disruptive behavior disorders (ODD, CD), and disorders of attention, overactivity, and impulsivity (ADHD)).

Child symptoms versus adult symptoms

While adults with depression may often appear "sad," this is not always the case with children. The DSM cautions that depression in children may appear as "**irritability**." Furthermore, while adults with post-traumatic stress disorder (PTSD) may experience flashbacks, young children are more likely to engage in repetitive play about the trauma.

ICD   The ICD provides an international standard for diagnosis and classification for general epidemiological purposes. Disorders that specifically relate to mental and behavioral concerns are contained in **Chapter V**, including disorders with onset usually occurring in childhood and adolescence. Currently, categories which relate most specifically to child and adolescent concerns can be found in the following sections: Mental Retardation (**F70–F79**), Disorders of Psychological Development

Table 5.4   DSM-IV-TR and ICD-10: a multiaxial comparison

DSM-IV-TR	
Axis I	Name of disorder; if more than one, principal one is listed first
Axis II	Mental retardation and personality disorders
Axis III	Any relevant general medical conditions
Axis IV	Psychosocial and environmental problems: e.g., family situation (divorce, separation, custody arrangements), school or occupational problems, financial problems, etc.
Axis V	Global Assessment of Functioning (GAF). Rating on GAF scale from 0 (incapacitated) to 100 (superior functioning). Often rated at intake and discharge
ICD-10	
Axis One	Clinical psychiatric syndrome. Main diagnosis
Axis Two	Specific disorders of development (speech, language, academic, motor)
Axis Three	Intellectual level (rated on an eight-point scale from highly intelligent to profound retardation)
Axis Four	Any relevant general medical conditions
Axis Five	Associated abnormal psychosocial situations; two-point rating scale from most (2) to least (0) severe. Nine categories are available, each with specific subcategories: 00: No significant difficulty

1. Abnormal intrafamilial relationships	6. Acute life events
2. Mental disorder, deviance, or handicap in child's primary support	7. Societal stressors
3. Inadequate/distorted intrafamilial communication	8. Chronic interpersonal stress associated with school/work
4. Abnormal qualities of parenting	9. Stressful events/situations resulting from child's own disorder/disability

(**F80–F89**), and Behavioral and Emotional Disorders with Onset Usually in Child-hood and Adolescence (**F90–F98**).

DSM and ICD: a comparative view   Although there are many similarities in the number and nature of disorders represented by each system, differences in classification are still evident. As will be discussed in *Chapter 8*, the DSM differs from the ICD-10 in criteria for attention deficit hyperactivity disorder (ADHD; DSM) and hyperkinetic disorder of childhood (HKD; ICD-10). There are other differences, some subtle and others not so subtle, that can cause confusion when individuals communicate from different sides of these classification systems. As each of the disorders is discussed, similarities and differences in the two systems will be addressed, as well as proposed changes for future revisions of both systems.

Multi-axial systems   Clinicians using the DSM report the client's problems on each of five axes, while the ICD uses a six-axis system for reporting child and adolescent problems (WHO, 1996). A comparison of the two multiaxial systems is available in Table 5.4.

The six-axis system of the ICD-10, especially Axis Five, provides significant information and draws attention to the many aspects of the child's psycho-social world that may impact on functioning, above and beyond the specific disorder with which

Table 5.5 Empirical and categorical systems: strengths and limitations.

Classification system	How disorders are classified/conceptualized	Strengths	Limitations
Categorical classification system (DSM, ICD)	Observation, clinical judgment Structured and semistructured interviews (e.g., NIMH DISC-IV, K-Sads) Matching symptoms to criteria (medical model) Disorder present or absent Qualitative and mutually exclusive	Widely adopted in clinical practice and research Acceptance by third-party payers DSM: multiaxial presentation and documentation of associated features, nature, and course	Clinical judgment may vary Disorders as present/absent (yes/no) Mutually exclusive; may pose problems for comorbid disorders Issues of reliability and validity
Empirical/ dimensional classification system (ASEBA, BASC2, Conners)	Behavioral rating scales Empirically derived (factor analysis) Symptoms present by degree Multirater, parallel forms Syndromes are on continuum Age-based norms Degree of variance from the norm Internalizing and externalizing Quantitative and continuous	Provides a range of deviation from norm Developmental norms Multiple informants Syndromes can be comorbid Can chart progress of interventions Quantitative	Not as widely accepted by third-party payers Multiple informants may result in discrepant information Issues of reliability and validity

the child may be diagnosed. For each of the nine situations referred to on Axis Five, there are several subcategories. For example, "1. Abnormal intrafamilial relationships" lists five possibilities: 1.0 lack of warmth in parent–child relationships; 1.1 intrafamilial discord among adults; 1.2 hostility toward or scapegoating of the child; 1.3 physical child abuse; 1.4 sexual abuse (within the family).

Strengths and limitations of the categorical systems

Strengths   The widespread use of the categorical system by clinical professionals assures its continued use, and dissemination of information about disorders using prescribed criteria. The all-or-nothing paradigm brings greater clarity to the diagnosis and the clinical decision-making process. The manuals are often comprehensive and based on significant field research.

Weaknesses   The DSM has been criticized concerning the appropriateness of the symptoms for child populations, since many of the field trials did not include child samples. Also, the categorical (all-or-nothing) nature of the symptoms does not support the continuum of symptoms that occurs in childhood. Neither of the categorical systems can accommodate a continuum, at present, which would be appropriate for developmental concerns. The strengths and weaknesses of the dimensional and categorical systems are presented in Table 5.5.

Clinical and Educational Child Psychology

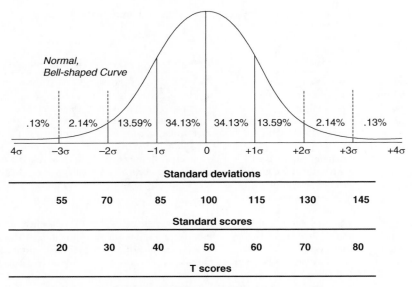

Figure 5.2 Standard normal distribution and T scores.

Dimensional classification system

The **dimensional classification system** conceptualizes problem behaviors along a continuum of severity. The Achenbach System of Empirically Based Assessment (ASEBA; Achenbach & Rescorla, 2001) is an example of a dimensional classification system. Since this system is used on a worldwide basis, it will provide the template for the following discussion.

Achenbach System of Empirically Based Assessment (ASEBA) The ASEBA has been translated into 80 languages and has been reported in over 5000 research studies (Achenbach, 2008; Berube & Achenbach, 2004). Although the entire scale contains 112 (youth self-report form) to 113 (parent and teacher reports) items, factor analysis has revealed that items cluster into eight **syndromes**: *anxious/depressed, withdrawn/depressed, somatic complaints, social problems, thought problems, attention problems, rule-breaking behaviors, and aggressive behaviors*. The ASEBA syndrome scales were derived based on samples of children from Australia, England, and 40 states in the United States of America.

Behavioral rating scales and the T score distribution

In a T score distribution, the average T score is 50 and the standard deviation is 10. Children and youth who score within one standard deviation of the mean (range of scores between 40 and 60) are considered to score within average limits. As the scores increase, the cause for concern also increases. The normal distribution and T score distribution are available in Figure 5.2.

The ASEBA reports behaviors in terms of **T scores** that provide an index of the severity of the behavior relative to normative functioning based on the child's age and gender. Scores between 65 and 69 are considered to fall within the **Borderline Clinical Range** and in need of monitoring and potential intervention. Scores of 70 or above represent behaviors that are two standard deviations above the mean, at the ninety-eighth percentile, and are considered to be **Clinically Significant**. Children and youth who score in the top 2% of the population are considered to have significant problems in need of intervention. (See Figure 5.1 for an example of a behavioral profile and T score distribution.)

Internalizing problems and externalizing problems In addition to the syndrome scales, there are two broad groupings of syndromes: **internalizing problems** (**behavioral deficits** representing a lack of some quality) and **externalizing problems** (representing **behavioral excesses**). Symptoms of withdrawal, anxiety, and somatic complaints all fall within the realm of internalizing problems, while rule-breaking behaviors and aggressive behaviors are considered to be externalizing behaviors. There are high rates of **comorbidity** (co-occurring disorders) among the internalizing disorders (anxiety, depression, somatic complaints), and the externalizing disorders (rule-breaking and aggressive behaviors). It is not uncommon to find a child who is anxious and depressed, or a child who is aggressive and engages in rule-breaking behaviors. Internalizing and externalizing behaviors may also co-exist (a child may be anxious and aggressive).

Strengths and limitations of the dimensional classification system

Strengths The strengths of the system lie in its ability to provide:

- a continuum of severity from mild to severe;
- empirically supported benchmarks;
- data that are both quantitative and continuous;
- two broad-band behavioral dimensions (internalizing and externalizing);
- a multi-rater format;
- test and retest data for an index of clinical change before and after intervention;
- data that allow for a comparison with ratings for peers of the same age and gender.

Weaknesses Despite a number of strengths, one of the major weaknesses is that the dimensional system has not been endorsed by some third-party payers (such as insurance companies), and poses difficulties, at times, when multiple informants present very different profiles concerning the same child. However, different perspectives can also demonstrate consistency or inconsistency of symptoms across a variety of different situations (e.g., at home and at school).

Issues in classification: clinical and educational perspectives

While the DSM and ICD provide diagnostic guidelines, there are several limitations to the usefulness of these diagnoses when working with children, due to the ambiguity and reliance on clinical judgment inherent in these systems. This is especially true for children who have "*hidden disabilities*" which often have common symptom presentations, and are difficult to diagnose, such as: attention deficit hyperactivity disorder (ADHD), dyslexia, dyspraxia/developmental coordination disorder (DCD), autism spectrum disorder, or speech and language difficulties (McKay & Neal, 2009). Hidden disabilities can be misdiagnosed or can evade a diagnosis altogether.

Global initiatives have targeted early intervention, often by tiered systems of screenings and graduated interventions, such as Response to Intervention (RTI) in the United States and the All-Wales Strategy for Child and Adolescent Mental Health (NAW, 2001) in the United Kingdom. However, these systems are not without their problems and have been criticized for delaying formal assessment and the fact that more elusive disabilities are less likely to be detected early, and more likely to be misclassified as "delays" rather than disabilities. In their critique of the system in Wales, McKay and Neal (2009) suggest that "tier 1 frontline services including teaching staff, school nurses, health visitors, foster carers and other non-specialist key staff" may not have the necessary training to detect these hard-to-diagnose conditions (p. 167). As a result, because the student has not been correctly identified, appropriate intervention is not provided and instead the child begins the long journey to more punitive types of interventions (disciplinary activities, detentions) and eventual involvement in the criminal justice system. Rather than effective engagement, the student becomes progressively disengaged from the system, in a "continuum of disengagement" (McKay & Neal, 2009, p. 170).

Another area where diagnosis is flawed with respect to the recognition of special needs is in the category of social, emotional, and behavioral disorders (SEBD), also referred to as emotional and behavioral disorders (EBD). The Special Education Needs: Code of Practice (DfES, 2001) reports there is "a lack of clarity about which particular groups of children and which behaviours constitute EBD" and where "behavior problems" and the strategies to contain them differ from more general discipline problems. At the other extreme, there is lack of clarity as to whether behavior difficulties in school indicate some underlying mental health problems that need medical or psychiatric intervention. In general, there is a distinction made between emotional and behavioral difficulties and more deep-seated mental health problems which require psychiatric interventions; however, the British government has acknowledged that there is some overlap between the group of children with EBD and those who have mental health problems (DfES, 2001).

Based on their survey of mental health concerns in children and adolescents in the United Kingdom, using ICD and DSM criteria, Meltzer, Gatward, Goodman, and Ford (2003) found that 10% of children between five and 15 years of age had a mental disorder, with 5% meeting criteria for conduct disorder. Within the United States, 21% of children aged nine to 17 were estimated to have a diagnosable mental or addictive disorder, with at least minimal impairment, while 11% were considered to meet criteria for significant functional impairment. Of this sample, approximately 10% met criteria for disruptive disorders (Shaffer et al., 1996).

While the Code of Practice (DfES, 2001) provides a list of general areas that may be associated with lower academic performance and special education needs (SEN), such as communication and interaction, cognition and learning, behavior, emotional and social development, and sensory and/or physical problems, however, it does not specify criteria, stating instead that it does not assume that there are hard and fast categories of special educational need. In this way, the Code of Practice differs

Table 5.6 Summary of quantitative research methods.

Research method/type of data collection	Data analysis	Strengths and weaknesses

Descriptive research
Survey
Questionnaires
Case studies
Observation (naturalistic)
	Frequency distribution
	Measures of central tendency
	  (mean, median, mode,
	  standard deviation)
		Strengths
		Allows for easy access to data
		Ecological validity (naturalistic settings)
		Case study provides in-depth analysis
		Weaknesses
		Limited statistical power, rigor, and
		  control
		Limited ability to generalize

Correlational research
Compare pre-existing data
Descriptive data collection
	Correlation coefficient
	  (Pearson's r)
	Measures of strength (-1 to
	  + 1) and direction
	  (positive or negative) of
	  association between
	  variables
		Strengths
		Can access large data sources of
		  pre-existing data
		High external validity (generalizability)
		Weaknesses
		Limited statistical power; cannot imply
		  causation

Epidemiological
  information
	Prevalence, incidence, and
	  lifetime prevalence rates
		Low internal validity (low rigor and
		  control)

Experimental research
Scientific method, control
  group and experimental
  group
	Statistical methods designed
	  to test hypotheses with
	  goal to reject the null
	  hypothesis
	Manipulate variables under
	  controlled conditions
		Strengths
		High statistical power; can determine
		  causes
		High internal validity (rigor and control)
		Weaknesses
		Limited external validity (narrow band
		  results may not generalize)
		Low ecological validity (controlled or
		  analogue studies)

significantly from the Individuals with Disabilities Education Act (IDEA, 2004) in the United States, which outlines 13 categories of disability that are eligible for special education services and the requirements needed to meet those criteria.

Research methods in child psychopathology

Guided by the scientific method, research goals are to describe, predict, control (prevent), and understand the nature of clinical problems. As a result, research questions are designed to explore (descriptive methods); to test hypotheses about the relationships among a set of variables (correlational research); or to determine a cause and effect relationship between two or more variables (experimental research). While correlational research evaluates the association among existing variables, experimental research involves the actual manipulation of variables under controlled conditions. A summary of the different types of research methods, their strengths, and their weaknesses can be found in Table 5.6.

More recently, there has been an increased emphasis on "translational" research in child development in an attempt to develop innovative research programs and designs that can inform policy and practices, using a blend of basic and applied research (Guerra, Graham, & Tolan, 2011). For example, using a qualitative and mixed methods research approach, Guerra, Williams, and Sadek (2011) interviewed students about the nature and the causes of bullying and determined that bullying takes on more sexualized connotations in middle school and high school. Other research programs have found that certain variables, such as poor literacy, can act as **mediating variable** between early poverty and later depression (Kellam, Rebok, Mayer, Ialongo, & Kalonder, 1994), while other variables can act as **moderating variables**, such as a calm and soothing parent who can over-ride the fearful and heightened physiological reactions of a child with a wary temperament (Kagan & Fox, 2006).

Descriptive research and methods

Descriptive methods increase our knowledge about the relative frequency and distribution of variables in the environment (e.g., do children spend more time studying or watching television?). Data can be obtained from a variety of methods, including: **naturalistic observation**, **laboratory observation**, **case studies**, or **surveys** and **questionnaires** (paper and pencil, or individual interviews conducted face to face or by telephone or e-mail).

Naturalistic observation and laboratory observation   A researcher may observe a child playing in a laboratory setting under controlled conditions, or in a natural setting like the playground.

Strengths and limitations of naturalistic versus laboratory observation   Collecting data in a laboratory setting has the advantage of increased control, while the strength of naturalistic observation exists in the **ecological validity** of observations obtained in naturally occurring settings. However, observation is not without its challenges and limitations due to a number of potential biases, including: **observer bias**, **observer drift** (difficulties sustaining attention), **central tendency bias** (tendencies to pick the middle category more frequently when rating behaviors), and **observer effect** (the fact that individuals tend to alter their behavior when observed). Because of the lack of control over competing factors and variables, the success of recording behaviors in the natural setting depends to a great extent on which behaviors are selected and how objectively they are defined. Recall that different observational methods were discussed earlier in this chapter.

Correlational research and methods   Researchers who conduct correlational studies are interested in how characteristics "co-vary" (e.g., hours of studying and academic grades).

What is a correlation?

The co-relationship between two variables is defined by a continuum that ranges from −1 to +1, with +1 indicating a perfect **positive correlation** and −1 indicating a perfect **negative correlation**. Characteristics at zero are unrelated.

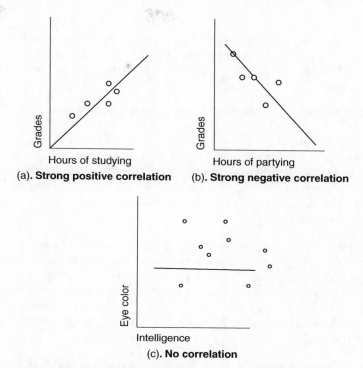

Figure 5.3   Graphic examples of positive, negative, and zero correlation.

A researcher finds that as hours of studying increase, grades increase, and as television viewing increases, grades decrease. Results indicate a strong positive correlation (+0.70) between studying and academic performance, and a modest negative correlation (−0.30) between television viewing and grades. In all cases of correlation, the **number indicates the strength** of the association, while the **positive or negative sign indicates the direction** of the association. Examples of positive and negative correlations are presented in Figure 5.3.

Based on this hypothetical study, can the researcher claim that either (a) increased studying increases grades, or (b) television viewing decreases grades? The correct answer is that neither of the statements is true. The important point to remember is that **correlation does not imply causation**, because we have not controlled for a possible third factor that may be operating to influence the strength and direction of the association.

Association versus causation

In the hypothetical correlational study discussed here, there may be several "other" factors that have influenced grade reduction or increases for these students, including:

a. students can spend a number of hours studying the wrong material or using ineffective study methods which would not increase their academic scores;
b. some television viewing might enhance understanding of some academic material (e.g., documentaries).

Strengths and limitations of the correlational method Correlational research affords **high external validity** (it is possible to generalize across a wide variety of variables, and replicate results to include greater sample variance) and data can be readily available from pre-existing data bases. However, although one is able to cast a wide net, the method does not allow for cause and effect inferences, thereby resulting in **low internal validity**.

Epidemiological studies Correlational studies that provide information about the rates of occurrence of different disorders are called **epidemiological studies**. These studies inform clinicians about disorder **incidence rates** (*number of new cases of a disorder within a given period of time; for example, new cases in a given year*), **prevalence rates** (*total number of cases of a disorder within a given time frame*), and **lifetime prevalence rates** (*number of cases of a disorder which might be expected to occur over the course of one's lifespan*).

Case study The **case study** is an intense and on-going observation of a single subject over the course of time. While it has the advantage of providing rich detailed information, its weakness is the limited ability to generalize the information.

Survey method Surveys can be completed in person, on the telephone, or via the internet. An obvious strength of the survey method is the fact that it can be an efficient and effective method of collecting information, in a relatively short period of time. Weaknesses of the method can include response biases (only those willing to participate are surveyed; the responses may reflect what is socially acceptable, rather than reality).

Descriptive methods and statistical measurement The descriptive methods discussed above can provide information regarding the **frequency distribution** of the responses measured, in terms of: **percentages**, **cumulative percentages** and **percentiles**, as well as the **mean** (average), **median** (mid-point), and **mode** (most frequent response) for the distribution.

Mean, median, and mode

A student takes a series of exams and produces the following scores out of a possible 50 points: 35, 48, 20, 50, 35, 42, 40.

In this distribution, the **mean** (average) score would be 38.5, the **median** (mid-point) would be 40, and the **mode** (most frequent score) would be 35.

The experimental method

The experimental method is the most rigorous method and allows the researcher to manipulate variables to determine **cause and effect** relationships. For example, a researcher hypothesizes that viewing television violence increases aggressive behavior in children. To test this hypothesis, the researcher must disprove (or reject) the **null hypothesis** which states there is "no difference" in the level of aggressive behavior in children who watch violent versus non-violent television programs. The researcher **randomly assigns** children (say, boys aged four to five years) to one of two groups: a **control group** (not exposed to television violence) and an **experimental group** (exposed to a violent television program). The variable that is manipulated (television program, violent versus non-violent) is the **independent variable** and the outcome (aggressive behavior) is the **dependent variable**.

A possible research design might be to randomly assign 50 boys, matched for ages (four to five years) and socio-economic status (SES) to one of two groups:

Experimental Group: watch violent television show (Kung Fu Bears);
Control Group: watch non-violent television show (Cuddle Bears).

For 15 minutes prior to watching the shows, the children are observed playing in a laboratory play room (**baseline** record of play before exposure to television program), and again for 15 minutes after viewing the shows. Toys have been pre-selected for their violent (guns, punching bag) and non-violent content (blocks, stuffed animals, building materials). Researchers who are recording play behaviors are **blinded** (have no knowledge) as to whether the child is from the control group or experimental group.

Internal validity The experimental method provides **high internal validity**, since controls limit external variability (e.g., the sample has been matched for gender, age, and SES to limit the extraneous confounds). Play data were collected pre- and post-viewing and long-term effects were monitored by having subjects return to the play laboratory two weeks after the experiment and observing them play again. The researcher has attempted to limit **observer/experimenter bias effects** by insuring that the rater was **blind to/unaware of** group affiliation. If more than one observer was used, the researcher would have included training periods to establish high rates of **inter-rater reliability** (e.g., raters agree on the amount of violent versus non-violent play within 80% accuracy).

External validity The rigorous and controlled nature of the experimental method limits the generalizability of the findings. Therefore, while the experimental method yields high internal validity (experimental control), the "artificial" or "contrived" nature of the "experimental situation" may result in a lack of **ecological validity** (**validity of context**). In fact, in the example, if the results demonstrate a significant increase in aggressive behaviors, researchers are bound to limit the nature of these findings to low SES boys, between the ages of four and five, who watched the program Kung Fu Bears. To increase generalizability, studies are often **replicated** to see if results are similar for different populations (older boys, females, and so on).

Ethical standards   In the above experiment, the researcher has the boys who were exposed to Kung Fu Bears return for a 15-minute play session two weeks later to measure any long-term effects. If the children who originally viewed Kung Fu Bears (the experimental group) continued to demonstrate elevated levels of aggressive play relative to controls, it could be argued that the study violates the ethical principle of **beneficence and non-maleficence**, or the clinician's duty to "do no harm," since exposure to the study created long-term violent behaviors in the subjects.

Quasi-experimental design   In some situations, random placement is not possible and might even be construed as unethical. For example, arbitrarily withholding treatment from one group might be considered unethical. In a **wait-list control** situation, the group not receiving treatment can still be used to measure the effects between the two groups after group one finishes treatment, and then receive treatment in the next phase. Researchers can also use a **matched control group** (i.e., compare children that have been matched for all relevant variables other than the experimental variable).

Empirically based treatments   In order to study the effects of specific treatments for specific problems, studies use **replication** to determine whether treatment effects can generalize to different age groups, populations, or the wait-list control. Recall that in the wait-list control condition, children are not deprived of treatment; treatment is merely delayed until the experimental group completes their treatment phase.

Single subject experiment   In this design, the subject acts as their own control. In this case, the variable to be manipulated (the **independent variable**) would be a clinical intervention and the subject would be observed prior to intervention (**baseline data**) and again after the intervention was introduced. This is also referred to as an ABA design. Many clinicians prefer to add another level of analysis to rule out any potential confound. For example, George's on-task behavior has increased after the introduction of a token economy in his classroom (George can gain 10 minutes of free play, if he works for three 10-minute sessions on his seatwork). However, the school psychologist wants to insure that the intervention is responsible for the change in behavior by ruling out any other source of influence (e.g., George's desire to impress a new little red-headed girl who is sitting beside him).

The ABAB or reversal design

The psychologist uses an ABAB design and observes if there is a difference between behaviors at Time 2, Time 3, and Time 4. If the behavior deteriorates at Time 3, and improves again at Time 4, then there is strong support for the claim that behavior improved because of the intervention.

No intervention	Token economy	Remove intervention	Token economy
Condition A	Condition B	Condition A	Condition B
Time 1	Time 2	Time 3	Time 4

Developmental considerations in child research

The study of behavior over time Studies of **developmental pathways** or **trajectories** examine **protective factors** that serve to buffer the child from harm, or **risk factors** that place the child at increased risk. Researchers also investigate how symptoms present at various developmental stages (e.g., depression in a two-year-old may appear as "acting out," whereas depression in adolescence may be evident in social withdrawal). Some children may be more **vulnerable** to negative influences due to other risk factors (low self-esteem, poor social skills, learning problems) while others may be more **resilient** due to protective factors (family support system, mentors, peer support, and so on).

Developmental pathways: equifinality and multifinality

Equifinality emphasizes that different pathways can lead to the same outcome. For example, two children may share symptoms of depression; however, one is reacting to peer rejection, while the other is in the midst of a custody battle.

Multifinality relates to the fact that very similar paths can produce very different outcomes. For example, one child whose parents are divorcing may spend increasing time engaged in athletic competitions, while another child in similar circumstances may engage in delinquent activity.

Longitudinal, cross-sectional, and accelerated longitudinal designs The **longitudinal study** (such as a study that follows the course of development of the same group of children from the age of five to 20 years) has the advantage of measuring differences in the same population. However, weaknesses of the method include: time, cost, and loss of subjects over time (**subject attrition**). A **cross-sectional** approach studies change over time in different populations; for example: comparing three groups of children at three different ages: Group A, five years of age; Group B, 12 years of age; and Group C, 20 years of age. The design allows for data collection in a relatively short period of time; however, there is a loss of information about developmental pathways that might have been evident longitudinally. Another limitation is the possibility of **cohort effects** (the three groups of children actually represent different generations and have been exposed to different environmental factors). One alternative method that allows for a reduction in time, while protecting against cohort effects, is the **accelerated longitudinal design**. Using this method, the researcher might study one group of children aged five to 12 and a second group of children aged 13 to 20, thereby effectively reducing his research time commitment by half.

Qualitative research and mixed methods

Historically, the primary research method has focused on quantitative methods (statistical analysis of data); however, there has been an increase in the collection of more subjective data (such as information from interviews). As a result, more recently there has been a focus on combining the best of both worlds, in what is referred to as "mixed methods."

Advantages and disadvantages   Quantitative methods use statistical analyses of variables to test hypotheses, while qualitative methods focus on information about the underlying processes or experiences, often obtained through such activities as: focus groups, observations, or transcripts of interviews. While the goal in quantitative analysis is to find a significant mathematical difference between variables, in qualitative analysis the focus is on finding the underlying patterns and themes. Strengths of the quantitative approach include the ability to test hypotheses mathematically, while the strength of qualitative research lies in the rich information on individual differences that would be lost mathematically. While the quantitative approach loses information about "individual differences," the qualitative approach lacks the ability to prove or disprove a hypothesis, and may have limited generalizability.

Ethical concerns and challenges in practice and research

Clinicians working with children face many unique challenges. Very young children may not have adequate insight into their problems or lack the necessary language to articulate their feelings or concerns. Licensed practitioners are guided by ethical principles and standards that are monitored by their professional organizations. Some of the challenges facing psychologists in practice or conducting research with children and adolescents may include:

- the need to obtain the child's assent (consent) for participation;
- issues of confidentiality when working with adolescents;
- the need to determine who is the custodial parent in divided families;
- ensuring that the child understands that participation is "voluntary."

Although different cultures vary in whether practices favor a more individualistic or collectivistic orientation, there is a universal code, the Universal Declaration of Ethical Principles for Psychologists (2008), that has been developed to guide psychological services, globally, which is supported by the International Union of Psychologists, the International Association of Applied Psychology, and the International Association for Cross-Cultural Psychology. The Universal Declaration recognizes four aspirational principles, which are found in most ethical codes, namely: respect for the dignity of others; provision of competent care; integrity; and professional responsibility to society.

Do young children understand the concept of voluntariness?

When Abramovitch, Freedman, Henry, and Van Brunschot (1995) asked 121 children (five to 10 years of age) if they would like to stop participating in the study, only seven children withdrew. However, when the examiner added "and I won't be angry with you if you do stop," twice as many children terminated their involvement. The researchers concluded that children may not have an understanding of the right to "voluntariness" (e.g., that they can withdraw from participation).

However, there are a number of issues that are unique to working with children and adolescents that may fluctuate widely based on local laws, including the rights bestowed to the adolescent once they reach the age of majority, and what that age represents in that location. This is crucial to granting permission for involvement in research or therapy, and issues of confidentiality regarding information which may take place in therapy sessions, or the access to/and dissemination of reports concerning the adolescent. In the United States and Canada, the age of majority ranges from 18 to 21 years, depending on the state or province in which one resides.

Furthermore, the American Psychological Association (2010, Standard 3.10b) states that it is a violation of ethics if a psychologist obtains "passive permission" from a guardian (e.g., asking a parent to return a form only if they desire that their child not be included in a research study, or therapy program).

References

Abramovitch, R., Freedman, J., Henry, K., & Van Brunschot, M. (1995). Children's capacity to agree to psychological research: Knowledge of risks and benefits and voluntariness. *Ethics and Behavior, 5*, 25–48.

Achenbach, T. M. (2008). Assessment, diagnosis, nosology and taxonomy of child and adolescent psychopathology. In M. Hersen & A. Gross (Eds.), *Handbook of clinical psychology, Volume 2: Children and adolescence* (pp. 429–457). Hoboken, NJ: John Wiley & Sons, Ltd.

Achenbach, T. M., & Rescorla, L. A. (2001). *Manual for the ASEBA school-age forms and profiles.* Burlington, VT: University of Vermont, Research Center for Children, Youth and Families.

American Psychiatric Association (APA). (2000). *Diagnostic and statistical manual of mental disorders* (4th ed., text revision). Washington, DC: Author.

American Psychological Association (APA). (2010). Ethical principles of psychologists and code of conduct. Retrieved from http://www.apa.org/ethics/code/index.aspx

Berube, R. L., & Achenbach, T. M. (2004). *Bibliography of published studies using ASEBA instruments: 2004 edition.* Burlington, VT: University of Vermont, Department of Psychiatry.

Cicchetti, D., & Toth, S. L. (2006). Building bridges and crossing them: Translational research in developmental psychopathology. *Development and Psychopathology, 18*, 619–622.

Conners, C. K. (1998). *Conners Rating Scales – revised technical manual.* North Tonawanda, NY: Multi-Health Systems.

Department for Education and Skills (DfES). (2001). Inclusive schooling. Retrieved from https://www.education.gov.uk/publications/eOrderingDownload/DfES-0774-2001.pdf

Guerra, N. G., Graham, S., & Tolan, P. H. (2011). Raising healthy children: Translating child development research into practice. *Child Development, 82*(1), 7–16.

Guerra, N. G., Williams, K. R., & Sadek, S. (2011). Understanding bullying and victimization during childhood and adolescence: A mixed methods study. *Child Development, 82*(1), 295–310.

Hawkins, R. O., & Axelrod, M. I. (2008). Increasing the on-task homework behavior of youth with behavior disorders using functional behavioral assessment. *Behavior Modification, 32*(6), 840–859.

Hoff, K. E., Ervin, R. A., & Friman, P. C. (2005). Refining functional behavioral assessment: Analyzing the separate and combined effects of hypothesized controlling variables during ongoing classroom routines. *School Psychology Review, 34*(1), 45–57.

Individuals with Disabilities Education Act (IDEA). (2004). Retrieved from http://idea.ed. gov/download/finalregulations.pdf

Kagan, J., & Fox, N. A. (2006). Biology, culture and temperamental biases. In N. Eisenberg (Ed.), *Handbook of child psychology: Vol. 3. Social, emotional, and personality development* (6th ed.) (pp. 167–225). Hoboken, NJ: John Wiley & Sons, Ltd.

Kellam, S. G., Rebok, G. W., Mayer, L. S., Ialongo, N. & Kalonder, C. R. (1994). Depressive symptoms over first grade and their responsiveness to a preventative trial aimed at improving achievement. *Development and Psychopathology, 6*, 463–489.

Kolvin, I., & Trowell, J. (2002). Diagnosis and classification in child and adolescent psychiatry: The case of unipolar disorder. *Psychopathology, 35*, 117–121.

Mash, E. J., & Hunsley, J. (2005). Evidence-based assessment of child and adolescent disorders: Issues and challenges. *Journal of Clinical Child and Adolescent Psychology, 34*(3), 362–379.

McConaughy, S. H., & Achenbach, T. M. (2001). *Manual for the semistructured clinical interview for children and adolescents* (2nd ed.). Burlington, VT: University of Vermont, Research Center for Children, Youth and Families.

McKay, J., & Neal, J. (2009). Diagnosis and disengagement: Exploring the disjuncture between SEN policy and practice. *Journal of Research in Special Education Needs, 9*, 164–172.

Meltzer, H., Gatward, R., Goodman, R., & Ford, T. (2003). Mental health of children and adolescents in Great Britain. *International Review of Psychiatry, 15*, 185–187.

Mezzich, J. E. (2002). International surveys on the use of ICD-10 and related diagnostic systems. *Psychopathology, 35*, 2–3.

Moore, D. W., Anderson, A., & Kumar, K. (2005). Instructional adaptation in the management of escape-maintained behavior in a classroom. *Journal of Positive Behavior Interventions, 7*, 216–223.

Naglieri, J. A., LeBuffe, P. A., & Pfeiffer, S. I. (1994). *The Devereux Scales of Mental Disorders: DSMD manual.* San Antonio, TX: Psychological Corporation.

National Assembly for Wales (NAW). (2001). *Everybody's business: All Wales CAMHS strategy document.* Cardiff: Author.

Sattler, J. M., & Hodge, R. D. (2006). *Assessment of children: Behavioral, social and clinical foundations* (5th ed.). San Diego, CA: Jerome M. Sattler Inc.

Shaffer, D., Fisher, P., Dulcan, M. K., Davies, M., Piacentini, J., Schwab-Stone, M. E., . . . Regier, D. A. (1996). The NIMH Diagnostic Interview Schedule for Children Version 2.3 (DISC-2.3): description, acceptability, prevalence rates and performance in the MECA Study. *Journal of the American Academy of Child and Adolescent Psychiatry, 35*, 865–877.

Shapiro, E. S., & Heick, P. (2004). School psychologist assessment practices in the evaluation of students referred for social/behavioural/emotional problems. *Psychology in the Schools, 41*(5), 551–561.

Universal Declaration of Ethical Principles for Psychologists. (2008). Retrieved from http://www.am.org/iupsys/resources/ethics/univdecl2008.pdf

Wilmshurst, L. (2008). *Abnormal child psychology; A developmental perspective.* New York: Routledge, Taylor and Francis Group.

World Health Organization (WHO). (1992). *The ICD-10 classification of mental and behavioral disorders. Clinical descriptions and diagnostic guidelines.* Geneva: WHO.

World Health Organization (WHO). (1996). *Multiaxial classification of child and adolescent psychiatric disorders: The ICD-10 classification of mental and behavioural disorders in children and adolescents.* Cambridge: Cambridge University Press.

Part Two

Child and Adolescent Problems and Disorders

6

Adjustment Problems and Disorders in Childhood and Adolescence

Clinical and Educational Child Psychology, First Edition. Linda Wilmshurst.
© 2013 John Wiley & Sons, Ltd. Published 2013 by John Wiley & Sons, Ltd.

Chapter preview and learning objectives

The first five chapters have provided foundation skills for understanding typical and atypical behaviors that may be evident at different stages of development. At this point, the reader has accumulated the necessary tools to address:

- how and why problems may develop in some children from a variety of perspectives (Chapter 2);
- developmental differences and difficulties based on normal expectations, given the child's chronological and mental age (Chapters 3 and 4); clinical and educational perspectives on the nature of diagnosis; different systems of classification; and how to evaluate problems using several empirical procedures and methods (Chapter 5).

In the previous chapters, we discussed six important questions that can serve as guidelines for evaluating the need for intervention. The questions are repeated in the text box below for review.

In keeping with the major themes of this book, developmental problems will be explored along a continuum of severity. In this chapter, the focus is on mild variations in behavior patterns that occur in children and adolescents in response to specific stressors in their environment (school, family, neighborhood, or peers).

Difficulties coping with stressors may result in the development of an **adjustment disorder** which can be accompanied by *anxiety* (fears, doubts, restlessness, separation anxiety), *depression* (irritability, moodiness, sadness, withdrawal) or *disruptive behaviors* (aggression, rule violations, truancy). Awareness of these typical adjustment problems can provide an increased understanding of more serious disorders that will be discussed in later chapters.

Six important questions to ask about the behavior pattern

1. Is it developmentally inappropriate?
2. Does it occur with greater frequency than anticipated?
3. Does it occur with greater severity than expected?
4. Is it causing concern for the safety of the child or others?
5. Is it causing significant dysfunction (school, home, peers)?
6. It is causing significant distress to the child or caregiver?

Although a transactional-bio-psycho-social approach recognizes that a child's problems result from the interaction between all aspects of the child's world, in some cases environmental factors may play a more prominent role (family, peers), while child characteristics may play a greater role in the development of other problems (genetics and heritability).

Introduction to adjustment problems

Adjustment problems represent emotional or behavioral symptoms of distress in response to a known stressor. The stressor can be a stressful event or situation, or involve a life change. The *Diagnostic and Statistical Manual of Mental Disorders* (DSM) and the *International Classification of Diseases* (ICD) define **adjustment disorders** as clinically significant behaviors indicating either "marked distress" in excess of what one would normally anticipate, or "significant impairment" in social or occupational (academic) functioning. Onset can manifest as early as one month after exposure to the stressor, but must be evident within three months, and terminate within six months. Adjustment disorders are considered to represent a temporary period of adaptation to the condition which caused the distress. Response to an acute event, such as a change of schools, is usually more immediate and subsides within a few months. However, if the stressor persists, and if there are other comorbid problems, then the response may progress to other more severe disorders. According to the ICD, if symptoms persist beyond six months, then the diagnosis should be changed to reflect the current clinical picture. The ICD includes culture shock, grief reaction, and hospitalization as possible sources of adjustment disorders. Although the current DSM distinguishes between **bereavement** (an expected response to the loss of a loved one) and adjustment disorder, the recommendation is that in the revision, a subtype, "related to bereavement," be included as a special type of adjustment disorder with symptoms enduring for at least 12 months following the death of a relative or close friend.

ICD and DSM: adjustment disorders and reactions to stress

The DSM considers adjustment disorders as a separate category of disorders, while the ICD clusters adjustment disorders under the major classification of neurotic, stress-related, and somatoform disorders (F40–F48). Currently, the DSM includes the stress disorders as part of the 10 anxiety disorders; however, it has been proposed that the revision contain a separate category for trauma and stress-related disorders.

Symptoms and prevalence of adjustment disorders

The nature of the response to the stressor may vary according to an individual's cultural background, developmental stage, temperament, and gender. Women are diagnosed twice as frequently as men; however, boys and girls have an equal likelihood of being diagnosed. Between 2% and 8% of children and adolescents will experience an adjustment disorder, and those living in high stress environments are vulnerable to increased risk. For children, headache and stomachache are the most common somatic symptoms (Alfven, 2001), while feeling "mad" is the most common cognitive/emotional response to a stressor (Sharrer & Ryan-Wenger, 1995). Compas, Connor-Smith, Saltzman, Thomsen, and Wadsworth (2001) reviewed 63 studies concerning coping with stress in childhood and adolescence. Results yielded four potential coping styles, namely: two styles of **engaged coping**, such as active coping (cognitive decision making, problem solving), and seeking social support (emotion-focused support), and two types of **disengaged coping**, such as distraction and avoidance (avoidance of negative emotions). Compas et al. (2001) concluded that children who use problem-focused and engaged coping tend to be better adjusted than those who use patterns of disengaged coping.

Temperament, emotional reactivity, and response to stressors

In *Chapter 2*, temperament was described as a genetic trait that emerges early in childhood and is characterized as an individual's "*general behavioral style that is relatively constant across situations.*" Initially, Thomas and Chess (1977) described nine traits, which were later consolidated into six traits by Rothbart and colleagues (Rothbart, Ahadi, & Evans, 2000; Rothbart & Bates, 2006), namely: **general activity level** (intensity of responsiveness); **fearful distress** (attempts to withdraw from stimulation); **irritable distress** (negative emotionality; frustrating events produce restless, fussy, and irritable responses); **positive affect** (positive disposition); **attention span persistence** (focus on the task and avoidance of distractions); and **rhythmicity** or adherence to routines (Rothbart, Ahadi, & Evans, 2000; Rothbart & Bates, 2006). Rothbart's model of temperament provides a unique distinction between *fearful distress* (triggered by fear) and *irritable distress* (triggered by frustration) based on the nature of the stressor. Ultimately, Rothbart's model clusters the traits into three major components: *emotion* (fearful distress, irritable distress, positive affect), *attention* persistence and general *activity* level (Rothbart, 2003; Rothbart & Bates, 2006). These characteristics of temperament have been found to be relatively stable from early childhood to adulthood (Buss & Plomin, 1984).

Theorists have argued whether temperament is more "state-like" (certain types of situations will evoke certain types of characteristics) or more "trait-like" (individuals' response patterns are stable across different situations) (Kenny & Zautra, 2001). However, although a case can be made for the influences of maturation and experience on temperament (Henderson & Wachs, 2007; Rothbart & Bates, 2006), researchers who have focused on **differential consistency** have found that individual differences in patterns of responses become more pronounced with age, as responses influence the trajectory of experience and patterns become more engrained over time (Rothbart & Bates, 2006, pp. 124–127).

Differential consistency

In their discussion of differential consistency, Neppl et al. (2010) suggest that with increased autonomy comes the ability to selectively choose social contexts that are the best fit for one's disposition (the cumulative continuity principle of development). Over the course of time, these "person–environment transactions," in which temperament influences social responses as well as social responses influencing temperament, "reinforce and accentuate those very aspects of temperament" (p. 387). As an example, Neppl et al. (2010) suggest that if a toddler is outgoing and cheerful, responses in kind will likely reinforce similar behaviors in the future (positive affectivity); however, if a toddler is angry and upset, the likely responses that this toddler will receive will reinforce negative affectivity.

Five- and three-factor models of personality

What we think of as temperament in children, in its mature form is "personality" in adulthood. There have been many theories of personality; however, trait theory is closest to what we would relate to temperament traits. Historically, Cattell (1957) was renowned for reducing a list of 18,000 words of traits into a 16-factor theory of personality (including such traits as warm, suspicious, tense, cheerful, and so on). Since that time, researchers have continued to use more sophisticated types of factor analysis to reduce the list even further into five superordinate personality traits which have come to be known as the "Big Five Factor" or the "Five-Factor Model" (Goldberg, 1993). Although the labels differ somewhat between the different variations on the model, the most popular is the version by Costa and McCrae (1990) which includes five traits (each on a continuum from most to least) represented by the acronym *OCEAN:* openness to experience, conscientiousness, extroversion, agreeableness, and neuroticism.

Recently, many researchers have found that Tellegan's (1985) three-factor model, or the "Big Three," is a better fit for research because it has fewer factors and contains much of the same information. The three factors are: **positive emotionality** (*extroverted: energized and active*); **negative emotionality** (*threatened and distressed*); and **constraint** (*high control, risk aversion, planning*). Tellegan's model, although constructed for adults, has many of the same features evident in the discussion of temperament, namely *positive emotionality* (surgency, approach, and pleasure), *negative reactivity* (negative affect response to fearful distress or irritable distress), and *effortful control* (behavioral inhibition and attentional control).

Recently, Neppl et al. (2010) reported results of their longitudinal investigation of the stability of temperament (using the three factors above: positive emotionality, negative emotionality, and constraint) for 273 families over the course of three developmental periods: toddlerhood (two years), early childhood (three to five years), and middle childhood (six to 10 years). Results revealed that there is stability and continuity of temperament measured by all three factors of the "Big Three," from toddlerhood to middle childhood, despite the use of multiple raters, multiple instruments, and obvious differences in social contexts evident at different developmental stages. Furthermore, not only were the dimensions of temperament consistent, stability increased with age for all three dimensions, such that stability quotients from early childhood to middle childhood were higher than those measured from toddlerhood to early childhood. Similar results achieved by Tackett, Krueger, Iacono, and McGue (2008), comparing measures of the "Big Three" collected at middle childhood with those obtained in late adolescence, provide comprehensive evidence of the stability of the "Big Three" dimension across the lifespan from toddlerhood to late adolescence.

Effortful control (constraint)

According to Rothbart, the self-regulatory system of **effortful control** is one of the most important aspects of temperament that influences a child's ability to cope with stressors. Effortful control is the voluntary ability to manage emotional (emotion regulation) and behavioral responses (behavioral inhibition) to stressors by suppressing a dominant (prepotent) response in favor of a more adaptive response. **Behavioral inhibition** will be revisited in *Chapter 8* in discussions of problems of attention persistence and executive functioning deficits in children with attention deficit hyperactivity disorder (ADHD). Children who have better effortful control are more successful than peers with less effortful control, in areas of: task persistence, academic achievement, social competency, social relatedness (give and take, sharing and cooperativeness), and moral maturity (Eisenberg, 2010; Kochanska & Aksan, 2006; Posner & Rothbart, 2007).

Behavioral inhibition in high and low reactive temperaments

Kagan's work with infants (Kagan & Snidman, 2004; Kagan & Fox, 2006) has demonstrated how infant reactivity at a very early age (four months) can predict later responses to such stressful situations as stranger anxiety (seven to nine months of age). Kagan and colleagues have determined that there are brain-based differences in how arousal of the amygdale takes place in individuals who experience novel stimuli. Shy and inhibited toddlers respond to stimulation with increased activation in the right frontal lobe (associated with negative emotions, such as fear), while more outgoing and social toddlers have less activation in the right, but more activation in the left frontal cortex (associated with more pleasurable emotions). Researchers suggest that increased activity in the brains of inhibited children is associated with other physiological reactions such as increases in heart rate, cortisol level, pupil dilation, and increased skin surface temperature, which are all responses associated with sympathetic nervous system arousal and preparation for a fight or flight response (Kagan, 2007; Schmidt, Santesso, Schulkin, & Segalowitz, 2007; Zimmerman & Stansbury, 2004).

How the brain registers emotions

Contrary to early speculation that all brain activity was filtered through the cortex (the brain's executive function) LeDoux (1996; Cain & LeDoux, 2008) suggests that separate systems in the brain handle cognition versus emotional responding, and that the fear circuit actually bypasses the cortex as messages go directly from the sensory receptors to the thalamus which sends the message to the amygdale. This would explain why our initial responses to fear can be so powerful and lacking in logic.

Adjustment problems in early and middle childhood

Adjustment to school stressors

Does involvement in preschool programs place children at greater risk than children who are reared in the home environment? This is a highly controversial question, but one that needs to factor in the quality of preschool care versus the quality of home care and any enrichment that the preschool program can provide that may be instrumental in increasing the child's exposure to positive learning experiences and peer relationships. For children growing up in a high poverty and highly stressed environment, an enriched and quality child care experience can have a protective effect, while for children living in an adequate environment, this experience can expand opportunities for stimulating educational and social engagement with peers.

Transition to school   Transition to school can be a stressful life event for some children (Garmezy, Masten, & Tellegen, 1984). Schor (1986) found that access to public health services for complaints of headaches, stomachaches, and body pains peaked for children and youth during two key periods: transition to elementary school (six years of age) and entry into junior high school (12 years of age). Recently, Turner-Cobb, Rixon, and Jessop (2008) studied stress resulting from the transition to school for 105 four-year-old children who were about to enter primary school for the first time in the United Kingdom. Parents collected morning and evening saliva samples: four to six months before the children were to begin attending school; two weeks into the first term; and at six and 12 months follow-up. Assessment of the anticipation, transition, and adaptation to school revealed that **cortisol** levels were considerably higher in the anticipatory stage than levels collected at transition or six-month follow-up. Furthermore, children with poor **effortful control** exhibited higher cortisol levels at transition, while those who experienced social isolation in the first six months exhibited higher cortisol levels at follow-up.

The hypothalamic–pituitary–adrenal (HPA) pathway

Recall that under stress, the hypothalamus activates the pituitary gland which in turn causes the adrenal glands to release corticosteroids, a group of stress hormones, such as **cortisol**, into the system. Cortisol mobilizes vital organs to respond to increased stress or pending threat. Cortisol levels can be analyzed through saliva samples.

Role of temperament

Overcontrolled behaviors   There is increasing interest in the adjustment problems of overly shy and inhibited children (Kagan, 1997; Kagan & Fox, 2006). Extremely shy children have a lower threshold for arousal of the **amygdale** (which regulates emotions and the fear response), and evidence higher cortisol levels, increased heart rate, and greater right frontal activation (Fox, Henderson, Rubin, Calkins, & Schmidt, 2001). Shy and reticent children are more likely to be exposed to peer rejection, exclusion, loneliness, and victimization in the early school years (Coplan, Closson, & Arbeau, 2007; Gazelle & Ladd, 2003). At least one study reported that some teachers believe shyness to have as much of a negative impact on social and school adjustment as aggression (Arbeau & Coplan, 2007).

Children who respond to situations with high emotional reactivity, and have low effortful control or low attentional control, have fewer strategies for adapting to anxiety-provoking situations and are at increased risk for developing internalizing disorders (Eisenberg et al., 1997; Anthony, Lonigan, Hooe, & Phillips, 2002). Children high in **negative emotionality**, or **trait negative affect** (Watson & Clark, 1984), demonstrate characteristics of nervousness, guilt, self-dissatisfaction, sense of rejection and sadness, tension, anger, and frustration resulting from high levels of arousal of their motor, affective, and sensory systems. As a result, preschoolers can feel overwhelmed, fearful, and distressed, which can predict the development of internalizing behaviors in later childhood and adolescence (Mun, Fitzgerald, Von Eye, Puttler, & Zucker, 2001; Rothbart, Ahadi, Hersey, & Fisher, 2001). Preschoolers who are overly shy and inhibited have higher cortisol levels, and poorer peer relations (Eisenberg et al., 1993; Gunnar, Tout, de Haan, Pierce, & Stansbury, 1997). Researchers have found that very shy preschoolers who develop effortful or attentional control as they mature are less likely to remain shy and inhibited over the course of time (Henderson, Fox, & Rubin, 2001). However, if these children are in high-risk environments (negative parent traits; low family cohesion) and do not develop increased ability for attentional control and effortful control, then internalizing symptoms can remain stable into later childhood and adolescence.

Undercontrolled behaviors   Aggressive behaviors contribute significantly to school adjustment problems. The ability to detect aggressive behaviors in infants as young as five months of age has prompted researchers to suggest that aggression can be innate (Tremblay, LeMarquand, & Vitaro, 1999). The nature, severity, and intensity of aggressive responses can vary widely, with some children demonstrating aggression at an earlier age (**early starters**).

Hot- or cold-blooded?

Aggressive responses can be **proactive or cold-blooded** (planned and premeditated), or they can be **reactive and hot-blooded** (Dodge, Lochman, Harnish, Bates, & Pettit, 1997).

In *Chapter 9*, the focus will be on the more serious and stable patterns of aggressive and defiant behaviors that can develop in children (oppositional defiant disorder; ODD) and youth (conduct disorder; CD) and the nature of interventions to assist in treating these disorders.

Children who exhibit undercontrolled behaviors (difficult temperament, with hyperactivity and poor ability to inhibit responses) are at the greatest risk for negative outcomes, including school adjustment problems. Preschoolers who demonstrate "exuberance" or **surgency** (Ahadi, Rothbart, & Ye, 1993) often demonstrate high activity levels and traits of impulsivity, and seek out novel and sensational (pleasurable) experiences. Because these exuberant children's behaviors can escalate out of control, they are at increased risk for peer rejection, and for developing more serious externalizing problems, such as disruptive behavior disorders (Rimm-Kaufman et al., 2002). However, similar to their peers who are at risk for developing internalizing problems, researchers have found that if exuberant children develop greater effortful control, then the risk of developing externalizing problems dissipates (Rubin, Coplan, Fox, & Calkins, 1995).

Other school-related factors   Other problems that can cause school adjustment difficulties include: comorbid problems (learning disabilities, emotional and social difficulties), child perceptions of teacher support, and a chaotic school environment.

Comorbid problems   Children who have pre-existing learning, emotional, or social problems are at increased risk for school adjustment problems. Adding additional risks can have a **multiplier effect** (Sameroff & Fiese, 2000). Rutter (1979) found that children exposed to two risk factors predicted a fourfold increase in psychopathology, while exposure to four risk factors increased the chances tenfold. Although children with the inattentive type of ADHD are less severely impaired than those with both inattentive and hyperactive-impulsive symptoms, they demonstrate more comorbid internalizing disorders, learning disabilities, and academic problems, and are two to five times more likely to be referred for speech and language problems (Weiss, Worling, & Wasdell, 2003).

Teacher support   At least one study found that two of the most powerful stressors for school children are assessments and teacher psychological abuse. Piekarska (2000) investigated the causes of stress for 271 children enrolled in the Polish public school system. The researcher concluded that teachers' psychological abuse caused stress and anxiety in the children, who developed survival-coping strategies that were not only destructive to their school achievements but also to their psychological well-being.

On a more positive note!

Gruman, Harachi, Abbott, Catalano, and Fleming (2008) found that teacher support had a positive influence on children who had mobility issues (multiple school moves).

Gruman et al. (2008) studied the potential risk from multiple school moves in second-through fifth-grade children (N = 1,003). School changes predicted declines in academic performance and classroom participation; however, these effects were moderated by peer acceptance and teacher support, which increased positive attitudes toward school among children who had experienced the most school changes.

Chaos in the school environment   Chaos in the school environment, which can contribute to the development of stress and interfere with learning in children, can take many forms, including "high levels of noise, crowding, confusion, instability of school or residence, changes in adult caregivers or friends, and low level of structure and regularity of routines" (Maxwell, 2010, p. 83). Although there are individual differences in children's sensitivity to external noise, the majority of children attending schools located in high traffic areas (near flight paths, subways, or train stations) report the noise as "annoying" (Hygge, Evans, & Bullinger, 2002), and interfering with their ability to do their work or concentrate (Haines & Stansfeld, 2000; Simon, 2005). Classroom crowding has been related to increases in disruptive behaviors (Maxwell, 2003) and lower academic achievement (Evans, Lepore, Shejwal, & Palsane, 1998). Ehrenberg, Brewer, Gamoran, and Willms (2001) demonstrated positive academic outcomes for elementary school children who were randomly assigned to smaller classes with 13 to 17 children, compared to peers assigned to larger classrooms containing 22 to 25 children. Classrooms are visually complex settings and can become very "busy" with visual displays (such as posters or art) that can be distracting to young learners, although this is an area that has not received much research interest to date (Maxwell, 2003). Since studies have demonstrated how noise and crowding can impede the learning process for children in general, it would not be surprising to find that a chaotic classroom would interfere with learning and add to the challenges that children with disabilities and special needs face in the learning environment.

Adjustment to family stressors

Parental stress and family conflict   Essex, Klein, and Lakin (2002) found that maternal stress beginning in infancy was the most potent predictor of elevated cortisol levels in children. Furthermore, preschoolers with high cortisol levels exhibited more mental health symptoms in first grade than their peers. In their sample of seven- to 10-year-old children, Stocker and Youngblade (1999) found that increased marital conflict was related to more hostile parent–child interactions (with both mothers and fathers), more conflicted sibling relationships, and difficulties relating to peers. Persistent marital conflict has been associated with a number of negative child outcomes, including conduct problems, anxiety, and aggression (Grych & Fincham, 1990). High levels of stress or marital conflict may be evident in preschool children's negative play with peers, anxiety concerning parent welfare, and increased risk for behavioral problems (Frosch & Mangelsdorf, 2001).

Can the termination of marriage have benefits?

Morrison and Coiro (1999) found that living in a two-parent family with a high degree of marital conflict can be more problematic for children than the actual termination of the marriage following high degrees of conflict.

Recently, Crawford, Schrock, and Woodruff-Borden (2011) investigated the interaction between child temperament (negative affect and effortful control) and environmental factors (maternal negative affect and family functioning) in the prediction of internalizing symptoms in young children. The results of their study revealed a direct and indirect pathway to internalizing disorders. In the direct model, child negative affect and family functioning predicted childhood internalizing symptoms. In the indirect model, effortful control is linked to internalizing by way of the impact that it has on family functioning. Children high in negative affect often respond to stressful situations by withdrawal and avoidance; a pattern that only serves to reinforce the maintenance of their anxiety symptoms. Crawford et al. (2011) propose that "maternal negative affect plays a meditational role with child effortful control contributing to the overall tenor of the family environment" (p. 60). Since mothers with negative affect are less positive and sensitive in their parenting practices, it is possible that they exacerbate their child's symptoms of negative affect (anxiety, fears, depression, withdrawal, somatic complaints, and social problems).

Chaos in the home Ackerman and Brown (2010) discuss several aspects of *physical* (noise, crowding, order, predictability of family routines) and *psychosocial* (family stability, parental mental illness or well-being, employment schedules) chaos in the home that can impact cognitive and social outcomes for early and middle childhood. Although family income (socio-economic status; SES) can influence chaos, some studies suggest that some factors like family relocations, when controlled for SES, still can have a negative influence on academic achievement (Adam, 2004). Unpredictability and lack of structure in the home can influence children's motivation and their feelings of self-worth, and can be associated with negative outcomes for children in a number of areas, including: behavior regulation (attention, working memory), reading, and parent–child communication (Evans, Gonnella, Marcynyszyn, Gentile, & Salpekar, 2005).

The ramifications of family instability can be far-reaching, and can impact development in a number of ways, including teacher ratings of popularity and social competency, as well as child self-ratings of loneliness (Hertzman, 2010). According to results from the Canadian National Longitudinal Survey of Children and Youth (NLSCY) conducted in the late 1990s, 41% of preschool children had experienced a residential move, and "behavioural and receptive language delays in development by age 4 or 5 rose consistently with the number of residential moves experienced by the child" (Hertzman, 2010, p. 114).

Divorce and separation Divorce may be harder on younger children compared to older children, since they are unable to cognitively process the fact that the marital breakup was not their fault (Hetherington & Stanley-Hagan, 1999). Feelings of self-blame are the most common responses that young children experience (three-and-a-half to six years of age) in response to a marital split (Wallerstein & Kelly, 1982). Divorce can be preceded by a history of conflict, and often the conflict continues throughout the process, as issues of custody and access enter into the fray. For school-age children, the outcome will be moderated by the severity of the conflict and how disputes are managed (Hetherington & Kelly, 2002). Parenting practices may also be inconsistent during a tumultuous divorce and parents may vacillate between being controlling and intrusive, or lacking in discipline (Madden-Derdich & Leonard, 2001). When parents are cooperative and peaceful, children have much better outcomes, regardless of whether the custody arrangement involves joint or sole custody (Parke & Buriel, 1998).

Gender effects when security is threatened by a divorce

Boys respond to the perceived threat inherent in a divorce with increased aggressive and assertive responses, while girls become engaged in futile attempts to reunite the parents, resulting in feelings of anxiety and depression (Davies & Lindsay, 2001).

Siblings: allies or rivals

Sibling conflict Siblings can experience elements of positive as well as negative feelings towards each other. However, compared to peers, emotions surrounding siblings tend to have a more intense and enduring impact (Buhrmester & Furman, 1990). Studies suggest less *perceived* sibling conflict among children under the age of eight, since social comparisons are outside the realm of their cognitive capacity, and on the surface, primary school children *seem* to have less conflict with siblings than peers. Yet when the amount of time spent together is taken into consideration, the rate of conflict is higher for siblings (DeHart, 1999).

Although conflict and disagreements can be a normal part of sibling relationships (Shantz & Hobart, 1989), persistent and severe hostility between siblings can contribute to internalizing problems in elementary school children, such as depressed mood, loneliness, and low self-esteem (Stocker, 1994), or externalizing problems and deviant behaviors (Stocker, Burwell, & Briggs, 2002), especially if parental rejection is also evident (Garcia, Shaw, Winslow, & Yaggi, 2000). With respect to externalizing problems, sibling conflict at an early age has been linked to hostility and aggression in five-year-olds (Garcia et al., 2000), and later on in adolescence (Kim, Hetherington, & Reiss, 1999).

Sibling rivalry increases in middle childhood, especially if parents compare accomplishments or characteristics among children resulting in the "lesser" child feeling resentful, which can impact future adjustment (Dunn, 2004). Sibling rivalry is often most intense when the goal is to obtain parental attention and approval, and siblings are both males, close in age, or if the elder sibling is a male; the situation intensifies if there is marital conflict, or family stress due to financial problems (Dunn, Slomkowski, & Beardsall, 1994; Jenkins, Rasbash, & O'Connor, 2003).

Siblings and the ICD

Although it is not uncommon for siblings to have conflict, the ICD recognizes **sibling rivalry disorder** (F93.3), under the category of *emotional disorders with onset specific to childhood*. The disorder is characterized by a combination of:

a. evidence of sibling rivalry and/or jealousy;
b. onset following the birth of a younger sibling (usually the child next in age is affected);
c. marked emotional disturbance associated with psychosocial problems.

Associated features may include: competitiveness for parental attention, high degree of negative feelings, and possible malicious intent to undermine the sibling, as well as lack of positive regard and unwillingness to share. Frequently, the child may demonstrate regressive behaviors, such as reverting to bottle feeding, and baby talk. There is no comparable disorder in the DSM.

Sibling support Despite the possibility of intense negative emotions, siblings can also provide a sense of mutual support to each other in times of family difficulties, such as parental conflict or divorce (Jenkins, 1992), or when there is a lack of peer support; in these times children will treat older siblings as surrogate attachment figures in the absence of the parent, seeking comfort when distressed (Seibert & Kerns, 2009). Older siblings can gain confidence in their leadership skills or responsibility when caring for younger siblings (Marvinney, 1988) or gain experience in teaching and nurturing others (Eisenberg & Fabes, 1998).

Sisters report more intimacy at all age levels, while maternal acceptance has been identified as a significant correlate of peer intimacy, regardless of gender, at all ages (Kim, McHale, Osgood, & Crouter, 2006). Regardless of the nature of the sibling relationship, it tends to remain stable from early to middle childhood (Buhrmester & Furman, 1990).

Adjustment to environmental stressors

In Bronfenbrenner's bioecological model (1979, 2001), there are four primary influences that can be found in the child's immediate environment: family (including the home, parents, and siblings), schools (including preschool and elementary or primary school settings, teachers, classrooms); the neighborhood (safe versus violent; access to leisure activities, playgrounds), and peers (friends and playmates). In this section, the focus is on stressors existing in the young child's neighborhood or peer relationships.

Neighborhood disadvantage   All children who grow up in impoverished environments do not develop problem behaviors; however, low SES at an early age can be a predictor of delinquency in adolescence (Brooks-Gunn & Duncan, 1997). The earlier the onset of risk factors, such as poor peer relationships, neighborhood ecology, or academic achievement, the stronger the predictor of problem behaviors in the future (Appleyard, Egeland, van Dulmen, & Sroufe, 2005). At-risk toddlers who do not have the benefit of quality child care are at increased risk for school drop-out and committing juvenile offences as adolescents (Harlow, 2002; Schweinhart, Barnes, & Weikart, 1993). Duncan, Brooks-Gunn, and Klebanov (1994) found that having more low-income neighbors put five-year-olds at increased risk for externalizing behaviors (temper tantrums, destructive behaviors), even when controlling for family income, SES, and other family variables. Exposure to negative peer group influences, and attending schools and preschools of lower quality (e.g., those with lower quality resources, or higher pupil–teacher ratios), may also predispose young children to these risks, contributing to an overall negative neighborhood effect (McLoyd, 1998). Children living in impoverished neighborhoods often experience barriers to involvement in organized recreation due to lack of financial support and neighborhood resources (Jones & Offord, 1989). Life transitions, stressful life events, and exposure to neighborhood violence at a young age can predispose a child to aggressive behavior in later years (Attar, Guerra, & Tolan, 1994).

Peer relationships   Children's peer relations can be instrumental in shaping the course of social and emotional development (Asher & Coie, 1990). However, children can experience the stress of poor peer relationships due to a number of different reasons, including the development of inadequate social skills as a result of externalizing problems (aggression), internalizing problems (shyness, anxiety, and social withdrawal), impulsivity (attention deficit disorder), or other comorbid disorders (such as learning disabilities). Children who are aggressive and are prone to interpret ambiguous behaviors of peers as having hostile intent (**hostile attribution bias**) are often rejected by peers (Dodge, Price, Bachorowski, & Newman, 1990). Children who are shy demonstrate a wariness and anxiety concerning social situations due to their fear of being evaluated negatively by peers (Coplan & Armer, 2007). As a result, although these children often desire to interact with peers, they are simultaneously inhibited by their social fear and anxiety (Coplan, Prakash, O'Neil, & Armer, 2004). As previously discussed, shyness and being inhibited can result from underlying biological factors (Kagan, 1997), or overprotective (or over-involved) parenting (Rubin, Burgess, & Hastings, 2002). Children who have attention deficit hyperactivity disorder (ADHD) often experience problems with social adaptation, and approximately 50% of children diagnosed with ADHD will experience difficulties in their relationships with peers (Pelham & Bender, 1982).

Social difficulties are so prominent among individuals with specific learning disabilities that it has been argued that social disability should be included in the definition proper (Rourke, Young, & Leenaars, 1989). Stone and La Greca (1990) conducted a **sociometric survey** in a sample of children in the fourth through sixth grades. Based on the responses, children were classified into categories of popular, rejected, and neglected. Children with specific learning disabilities were overly represented in the rejected (28%) and neglected (26%) categories, relative to their peers.

Sociometric surveys of peer status

Since the 1950s, researchers have used sociometric surveys to categorize children's peer relationships. A study by Vasa, Maag, Torrey, and Kramer (1994) indicated that 41% of teachers used the surveys to better understand classroom dynamics. Initially, only social acceptance (peer nomination as a friend or preferred play-mate) was indexed due to ethical concerns about having children label disliked peers. Since that time, the sociometric survey has evolved into a two-dimensional survey that classifies **peer status** (social likability) and **social impact** and has been found to have virtually no negative influence on peer responders (Bell-Dolan & Wessler, 1994; Mayeux, Underwood, & Risser, 2007).

Newcomb, Bukowski, and Pattee (1993) conducted a meta-analysis of 41 studies that employed sociometric techniques to obtain evaluations of peer status and found the following traits associated with each status:

Popular status When compared to their "average" peers, popular children evidence higher levels of sociability and cognitive abilities, greater problem-solving skills, more social traits. and lower levels of aggression and withdrawal. They also have the ability to maintain friendships over time and are often sought after as preferred play-mates by their peers.

Rejected status Aggressive children who are less skilled cognitively and socially are often rejected by peers. Furthermore, rejected children often express aggression physically and in negative behaviors that are disruptive. Rejected children may also experience depression and anxiety resulting from their stressful peer relations.

Neglected status   Neglected children have low social impact and are less aggressive and social than average children. Although they may share traits of their "average" peers, their low visibility may result in them not being selected in favor of the more popular peers.

Controversial status   Children in this group have a mix of traits from the popular and rejected categories. Controversial children share elevated levels of aggression similar to their rejected peers (in fact, in some studies they demonstrate more aggression than rejected children), but have better-developed cognitive and social skills and are more socially aware than the rejected children.

Adjustment problems in adolescence

Adjustment to school stressors

School transitions   Although students begin secondary school with moderate interest, there is a significant decline in interest, motivation, and academic performance across adolescence (Barber & Olsen, 2004). Declines may be related to changes in the school setting and expectations that accompany the transition from primary school to secondary school, as smaller settings with close teacher contact and direct supervision are replaced by larger classes, multiple teachers, higher expectations, and less guidance and supervision (Seidman, Aber, & French, 2004). By secondary school, it has been reported that half of students (between 40% and 60%) become increasingly and chronically disengaged from school (Klem & Connell, 2004), and 30% of students engage in behaviors that are high-risk, and not conducive to academic performance (Eaton et al., 2008). Furthermore, as the number of *life changes* increase (school transition, pubertal development, onset of dating, residential moves, family conflict), academic performance decreases accordingly (de Bruyn, 2005; Seidman, Lambert, Allen, & Aber, 2003).

Academic interest and gender

Although Dotterer, McHale, and Crouter (2009) found an overall decline in interest from late school age (10–11 years) to secondary school (13–14 years), girls reported significantly higher levels of interest at the beginning and end of secondary school. This finding is interesting, given the significant decreases in male college enrolment figures from the 1970s (55%) to recent times (45%) (King, 2006).

While transitions to secondary school can be stressful, Rothon et al. (2009) found that graduation can be equally stressful, especially for those with poor academic performance. Rothon and colleagues found that students attending East London secondary schools who scored high on a distress measure at 13 to 14 years of age performed the worst on the General Certificate of Secondary Education (GCSE), administered at the end of compulsory education (16 years of age).

In the United States, transition from high school has taken on greater significance in federal education law, improving services for students transitioning from public education to vocational programs or the community work force. In 1997, it became mandatory to have a student's Individualized Educational Program (IEP) include such transition plans, with respect to adult living objectives. Transition plans are now an integral part of the IEP (IDEA, 2004).

The transition to secondary school may also represent a transition to a larger school. Studies have shown that student absenteeism is lower in smaller versus larger secondary schools (Finn & Voelkl, 1993) where there is more engagement in prosocial behaviors and extracurricular activities (Moore & Lackney, 1993). Youth with close and positive friendships often will sustain these friendships in times of transition, which may ease their adjustment to the new school both socially and academically (Aikins, Bierman, & Parker, 2005).

Role of affect regulation and comorbidity   Faced with a stressful event, arousal can be seen as a two-stage process involving: *reactivity* (increased physiological arousal) and *recovery* (post-stress response of decreased arousal) (Linden, Earle, Gerin, & Christenfeld, 1997). Different parts of the **autonomic nervous system** (**ANS**) are involved in the reactivity phase (**sympathetic nervous system**) and the recovery phase (**parasympathetic nervous system**). The sympathetic nervous system appraises the level of stress and mobilizes the internal arousal system (**"fight or flight"** response), while the parasympathetic system returns responses to normal (Porges, 2003). Weak recovery by the parasympathetic system and an overly sensitive or overactive sympathetic system can result in strong emotions of anger and avoidance (Beauchaine, Gatzke-Kopp, & Mead, 2007). Developmentally, as affect regulation becomes more controlled, individuals acquire positive skills to cope with stressful circumstances. However, youth with externalizing problems or internalizing problems often experience more problems with affect regulation in difficult circumstances.

In their study of students enrolled in two secondary schools in the US mid-west, Martyn-Nemeth, Penckofer, Gulanick, Velsosr-Friedrich, and Bryant (2009) found that stress and low self-esteem were related to both avoidant coping patterns and depressed mood. Furthermore, the combined effect of low self-esteem and avoidant coping were also related to unhealthy eating behaviors (dietary restraint, or overconsumption).

Parenting and affect regulation

Having a secure parent relationship facilitated emotion regulation and recovery after exposure to a stressful task for youth with externalizing problems, but not for those with internalizing problems. Willemen, Schuengel, and Koot (2009) suggest that "frustration and irritability" demonstrated by youth with externalizing problems was a much easier response for parents to recognize than less obvious responses (such as guilt or shame) that youth with internalizing problems may be experiencing.

Emotion regulation and the adolescent brain   Recall that in situations of heightened emotionality, adolescents are more likely to make impulsive decisions and engage in risky behaviors. According to Casey, Jones, and Somerville (2011), during adolescence increased production of cortical dopamine levels, and an imbalance between heightened awareness of emotional cues (overactivation of the subcortical regions of the brain), in the presence of immaturity in cognitive control (the prefrontal cortex responsible for planning ability and logical problem solving) place the adolescent at increased risk for sensation seeking, impulsivity, and risky decisions.

Adjustment to family stressors

Parenting practices and family cohesion   There is increased risk for negative mental health outcomes for **cumulative risks** rather than any single risk factor (Gutman, Sameroff, & Eccles, 2002; Prelow & Loukas, 2003). In a large community sample of adolescents, Roberts, Roberts, and Chan (2009) found that 7.5% of their population developed the first episode of a psychiatric disorder during adolescence. Experiencing two or more stressors was a significant predictor of a clinical diagnosis, while adverse family circumstances (poor family satisfaction, high maternal stress, and stressful relations with mother, father, or both parents) predicted the incidence of being diagnosed with a disorder for every disorder examined in the study, including: anxiety, mood, attention deficit hyperactivity disorder (ADHD), disruptive, and substance abuse/dependence disorders. Adolescents who live with the stress of family conflict are prone to chronic emotional arousal and increased reactivity to other stressful events (Repetti, Taylor, & Seeman, 2002), and are at increased risk of feeling helpless to control their environment (Chorpita & Barlow, 1998).

Family instability can cause stress due to disruptions of normal family routines, alteration of the family constellation, or frequent family relocations. Adam and Chase-Lonsdale (2002) found that adolescent adjustment problems increased in proportion to the number of residential moves experienced, even after controlling for demographic variables, such as SES. Researchers suggest that feelings of insecurity, disconnection from social relationships, and stress reactivity may contribute to adjustment problems (Cummings, Davies, & Campbell, 2000; Pribesh & Downey, 1999).

Studies have also examined the role of attachment and parenting style as moderators of stress in adolescents. In a recent longitudinal study of community-based adolescents, Dick et al. (2011) investigated gene–environment interaction and the biological and environmental contributors to adolescent externalizing behaviors. The results revealed that the association between genotype (CHRM2; cholinergic muscarinic 2 receptor) and externalizing behavior was the strongest in environments with low parent monitoring and weakest in environments with high parent monitoring. In another study, Lee and Hankin (2009) found that anxious and avoidant attachment patterns predicted anxiety and depression in youth, while anxious attachment mediated by low self-esteem and dysfunctional attitudes also predicted internalizing symptoms for this group.

Siblings   Sibling support, intimacy, and companionship are lower in adolescence, compared with middle childhood, due to the increasing significance of peer group support (Buhrmester & Furman, 1990). In a longitudinal prospective design, Stocker, Burwell, and Briggs (2002) monitored sibling conflict from middle childhood (seven to nine years of age) to early adolescence (11 to 12 years of age) and found sibling conflict was predictive of anxiety, depressed mood, and delinquent behaviors in early adolescence. In their study of sibling relationships between younger and older sisters, Slomkowski, Rende, Conger, Simons, and Conger (2001) found older sisters' hostility was predictive of the younger sister developing subsequent delinquent behaviors. Bank, Patterson, and Reid (1996) found sibling conflict predicted later adjustment problems in adolescence and adulthood. Siblings who have a warm, supportive relationship in adolescence also tend to have more gratifying friendships with peers (Yeh & Lempers, 2004).

Sibling conflict and adjustment problems

Stocker, Burwell, and Briggs (2002) suggest several explanations for the negative influence of sibling conflict, including **social learning theory** (observation and imitation of externalizing behaviors), **negative attribution style** (inescapable conflict and feelings of self-blame resulting in internalizing behaviors), and **social cognition** (living in a conflicted environment providing little opportunity to interpret normative social cues, resulting in the **hostile attribution bias**). Younger children may be more strongly influenced by conflict with older siblings, since the older siblings may dominate the relationship and engage the younger siblings in **deviancy training**, introducing them to their deviant peers (Rowe & Gully, 1992).

Adjustment to environmental stressors

Peer relationships   A supportive network of peers can provide a protective influence against negative outcomes (Criss, Pettit, Bates, Dodge, & Lapp, 2002). A failure to meet socio-developmental milestones in forming healthy peer relationships can lead to externalizing or internalizing problems based on one of two possible trajectories. Oland and Shaw (2005) suggest that children may develop *internalizing symptoms* (highly anxious and inhibited responses) leading to avoidance of involvement with peers and lack of healthy peer relationships; or develop *externalizing symptoms* (impulsivity, poor emotional control, idealized self-concept, callous unemotional traits) leading to a failure to develop normal reciprocal and empathic relationships.

Youth with internalizing symptoms who eventually establish positive peer relationships have far better outcomes than those who cannot (Gazelle & Ladd, 2003), since social avoidance leads to progressive social impairment and reduced social acceptance (Ginsburg, La Greca, & Silverman, 1998). Youth with externalizing problems lack the emotion regulation and self-monitoring necessary to establish successful social interactions and are often rejected by peers (Keiley, Lofthouse, Bates, Dodge, & Petit, 2003), placing them at increased risk for linking up with similar peers (Lahey, Waldman, & McBurnett, 1999). Deviant peer affiliations have been linked to increased risk for suicide (Fergusson, Beautrais, & Horwood, 2003), substance use, and antisocial behaviors (Beautrais, 1999).

Adolescent girls who feel friendless and isolated are at twice the risk for suicide ideation (Pfeffer, 2000), while support group cohesion serves as a protective factor for depression and suicide. For boys, protection from suicide risk was found in activity-based groups rather than peer friendships (Bearman & Moody, 2004).

Can you be a stress magnet?

The **stress-generation hypothesis** suggests that stressful interpersonal life events can be generated by dysfunctional behaviors and attitudes (Hammen, 2006).

Other environmental stressors   A negative cognitive style (Safford, Alloy, Abramson, & Crossfield, 2007), poor interpersonal problem solving (Davila, Hammen, Burge, Paley, & Daley, 1995), excessive reassurance seeking (Potthoff, Holahan, & Joiner, 1995), and avoidant coping (Holahan, Moos, Holahan, Brennan, & Schutte, 2005) are all mechanisms that can increase the risk for generating stressful interpersonal life events. Harkness and Stewart (2009) found that adolescents' scores on a depression inventory collected at Time 1 predicted higher rates of stressful interpersonal events experienced within the next 12-month period.

McLaughlin and Hatzenbuehler (2009) examined the role of stressful life events in the development of anxiety sensitivity in 1065 adolescents in a community sample. Anxiety sensitivity is a "fear of symptoms, including bodily sensations, which results from beliefs about the harmful, social, psychological, or physiological consequences of such symptoms" (McLaughlin & Hatzenbuehler, 2009, p. 659). This lowered threshold for anxious responding has been linked to panic attacks, trait anxiety, and anxiety disorders in children and adolescents (Pollock et al., 2002). Stress and experiencing of stressful life events has been shown to impact child and adolescent mental health in negative ways (Grant, Compas, Thurm, & McMahon, 2004). Stressful life events can contribute to increases in anxiety sensitivity, especially if the stressors are health-related (fear of disease) or related to family discord; however, anxiety sensitivity predicted anxiety but not depressive symptoms seven months later (McLaughlin & Hatzenbuehler, 2009).

References

Ackerman, B. P., & Brown, E. D. (2010). Physical and psychosocial turmoil in the home and cognitive development. In G. W. Evans and T. D. Wachs (Eds.), *Chaos and its influence on children's development: An ecological perspective* (pp. 35–47). Washington, DC: APA.

Adam, E. K. (2004). Beyond quality: Parental and residential stability and children's achievement. *Current Directions in Psychological Science, 13*, 210–213.

Adam, E. K., & Chase-Lonsdale, P. L. (2002). Home sweet home(s): Parental separations, residential moves and adjustment in low-income adolescent girls. *Developmental Psychology, 38*, 792–805.

Ahadi, S., Rothbart, M., & Ye, R. (1993). Children's temperament in the US and China: Similarities and differences. *European Journal of Personality, 7*, 359–377.

Aikins, J., Bierman, K., & Parker, J. (2005). Navigating the transition to junior high school: The influence of pre-transition friendship and self-system characteristics. *Social Development*, *14*(1), 42–60.

Alfven, G. (2001). Understanding the nature of multiple pains in children. *Journal of Pediatrics*, *138*(2), 156–158.

Anthony, J. L., Lonigan, C. J., Hooe, E. S., & Phillips, B. M. (2002). An affect-based, hierarchical model of temperament and its relations with internalizing symptomatology. *Journal of Clinical Child and Adolescent Psychology*, *31*, 480–490.

Appleyard, K., Egeland, B., van Dulmen, M. H. M., & Sroufe, L. A. (2005). When more is not better: The role of cumulative risk in child behaviour outcomes. *Journal of Child Psychology and Psychiatry*, *46*, 235–245.

Arbeau, A., & Coplan, R. J. (2007). Kindergarten teachers' beliefs and responses to hypothetical prosocial, asocial and antisocial children. *Merrill-Palmer Quarterly*, *53*, 291–318.

Asher, S. R., & Coie, J. D. (1990). *Peer rejection in childhood*. New York: Cambridge University Press.

Attar, B. K., Guerra, N. G., & Tolan, P. H. (1994). Neighborhood disadvantage, stressful life events and adjustments in urban elementary-school children. *Journal of Clinical Child and Adolescent Psychology*, *23*, 391–400.

Bank, L., Patterson, G., & Reid, J. (1996). Negative sibling interaction patterns as predictors of later adjustment problems in adolescent and youth adult males. In G. H. Brody (Ed.), *Sibling relationships: Their causes and consequences* (pp. 197–229). New York: Ablex.

Barber, B. K., & Olsen, J. A. (2004). Assessing the transitions to middle and high school. *Journal of Adolescent Research*, *19*, 3–30.

Bearman, P. S., & Moody, J. (2004). Suicide and friendships among American adolescents. *American Journal of Public Health*, *94*, 89–95.

Beauchaine, T. P., Gatzke-Kopp, L., & Mead, H. K. (2007). Polyvagal theory and developmental psychopathology: Emotion dysregulation and conduct problems from preschool to adolescence. *Biological Psychology*, *74*, 174–184.

Beautrais, A. L. (1999). Risk factors for suicide and attempted suicide and among young people, in *Commonwealth Department of Health and Aged Care, national youth suicide prevention strategy – Setting the evidence-based research agenda for Australia (a literature review)* (pp. 113–278). Canberra: Commonwealth of Australia.

Bell-Dolan, D., & Wessler, A. E. (1994). Ethical administration of sociometric measures: Procedures to use and suggestions for improvement. *Professional Psychology: Research and Practice*, *25*, 23–32.

Bronfenbrenner, U. (1979). *The ecology of human development*. Cambridge, MA: Harvard University Press.

Bronfenbrenner, U. (2001). The bioecologial theory of human development. In U. Bronfenbrenner (Ed.), *Making human beings human: Bioecological perspectives on human development* (pp. 3–15). Thousand Oaks, CA, Sage Publications.

Brooks-Gunn, J., & Duncan, G. J. (1997). The effects of poverty on children. *Future of Children*, *7*, 55–71.

Buhrmester, D., & Furman, W. (1990). Perceptions of sibling relationships during middle childhood and adolescence. *Child Development*, *61*, 1387–1398.

Buss, A. H., & Plomin, R. (1984). *Temperament: Early developing personality traits*. Hillsdale, NJ: Erlbaum.

Cain, C. K., & LeDoux, J. E. (2008). Emotional processing and motivation: In search of brain mechanisms. In A. J. Elliott (Ed.), *Handbook of approach and avoidance motivation* (pp. 17–34). New York: Psychology Press.

Casey, B. J., Jones, R. M., & Somerville, L. H. (2011). Braking and accelerating of the adolescent brain. *Journal of Research on Adolescence*, *21*(1), 21–33.

Cattell, R. B. (1957). *Personality and motivation: Structure and measurement*. Yonkers-on-Hudson, NY: World Book Co.

Chorpita, B. F., & Barlow, D. H. (1998). The development of anxiety: The role of control in the early environment. *Psychological Bulletin, 124,* 3–21.

Compas, B. E., Connor-Smith, J. K., Saltzman, H., Thomsen, A., & Wadsworth, M. E. (2001). Coping with stress during childhood and adolescence: Problems, progress and potential in theory and research. *Psychological Bulletin, 127,* 87–127.

Coplan, R. J., & Armer, M. (2007). A "multitude" of solitude: A closer look at social withdrawal and nonsocial play in early childhood. *Child Development Perspectives, 1,* 26–32.

Coplan, R. J., Closson, L., & Arbeau, K. (2007). Gender differences in the behavioural associates of loneliness and social dissatisfaction in kindergarten. *Journal of Child Psychology and Psychiatry (Special Issue on Preschool Mental Health), 48,* 988–995.

Coplan, R. J., Prakash, K., O'Neil, K., & Armer, M. (2004). Do you "want" to play? Distinguishing between conflicted-shyness and social disinterest in early childhood. *Developmental Psychology, 40,* 244–258.

Costa, P. T., Jr., & McCrae, R. R. (1990). Personality: another "hidden factor" in stress research. *Psychological Inquiry, 1,* 22–24.

Crawford, M. A., Schrock, M., & Woodruff-Borden, J. (2011). Child internalizing symptoms: contributions of child temperament, maternal negative affect, and family functioning. *Child Psychiatry and Human Development, 42,* 53–64.

Criss, M., Pettit, G. S., Bates, J. D., Dodge, K. A., & Lapp, A. L. (2002). Family adversity, positive peer relationships and children's externalizing behavior: A longitudinal perspective on risk and resilience. *Child Development, 73*(4), 1220–1237.

Davies, P., & Lindsay, L. (2001). Does gender moderate the effects of marital conflict on children? In J. Grych & F. Fincham (Eds.), *Interpersonal conflict and child development; Theory, research and applications* (pp. 64–97). New York: Cambridge University Press.

Davila, J., Hammen, C., Burge, D., Paley, B., & Daley, S. E. (1995). Poor interpersonal problem solving as a mechanism of stress generation in depression among adolescent women. *Journal of Abnormal Psychology, 104,* 592–600.

de Bruyn, E. H. (2005). Role strain engagement and academic achievement in early adolescence. *Educational Studies, 31,* 15–27.

DeHart, G. B. (1999). Conflict and averted conflict in preschoolers' interactions with siblings and friends. In W. A. Collins & B. Laursen (Eds.), *Minnesota Symposia on Child Psychology: Vol. 30. Relationships as developmental contexts: Festschrift in honor of Williard W. Hartup* (pp. 281–303). Mahwah, NJ: Erlbaum.

Dick, D. M., Meyers, J., Latendresse, S. J., Creemers, H., Lansford, J. E., Pettit, G. S., . . . Muizink, A. C. (2011). CHRM2, parental monitoring and adolescent externalizing behavior: Evidence for gene-environment interaction. *Psychological Science, 22*(4), 481–489.

Dodge, K. A., Lochman, J. E., Harnish, J. D., Bates, J., & Pettit, G. (1997). Reactive and proactive aggression in school children and psychiatrically impaired chronically assaultive youth. *Journal of Abnormal Psychology, 106,* 37–51.

Dodge, K. A., Price, J. M., Bachorowski, J., & Newman, J. P. (1990). Hostile attribution albiases in severely aggressive adolescents. *Journal of Abnormal Psychology, 99,* 385–392.

Dotterer, A. M., McHale, S. M., & Crouter, A. C. (2009). The development and correlates of academic interests from childhood through adolescence. *Journal of Educational Psychology, 101,* 509–519.

Duncan, G., Brooks-Gunn, J., & Klebanov, P. (1994). Economic deprivation and early childhood development. *Child Development, 65,* 296–318.

Dunn, J. (2004). Sibling relationships. In P. K. Smith & C. H. Hart (Eds.), *Handbook of childhood social development* (pp. 223–237). Oxford: Blackwell.

Dunn, J., Slomkowski, C. L., & Beardsall, L. (1994). Sibling relationships from the preschool period through middle childhood and early adolescence. *Developmental Psychology, 30,* 315–324.

Eaton, D. K., Kann, L., Kinchen, S., Shanklin, S., Ross, J., Hawkins, J., . . . Wechsler, H. (2008). *Youth Risk Behavior Surveillance – United States, 2007. MMWR Surveillance*

Summaries, *57*(SS04), 1–131. Retrieved from http://www.cdc.gov/mmwr/preview/mmwrhtml/ss5704a1.htm?s_cid=ss5704a1_e

Ehrenberg, R. G., Brewer, D. J., Gamoran, A., & Willms, J. D. (2001). Class size and student achievement. *Psychological Science in the Public Interest*, *2*(1), 1–30.

Eisenberg, N. (2010). Empathy-related responding: Links with self-regulation, moral judgment, and moral behaviors. In M. Mikulincer & P. R. Shaver (Eds.), *Prosocial motives, emotions, and behavior: The better angels of our nature* (pp. 129–148). Washington, DC: APA.

Eisenberg, N., Fabes, R., Bernzweig, J., et al. (1993). The relations of emotionality and regulation to preschoolers' social skills and sociometric status. *Child Development*, *64*(5), 1418–1438.

Eisenberg, N., Guthrie, I. K., Fabes, R. A., Reiser, M., Murphy, B. C., Holgren, R., Maszk, P., & Losoya, S. (1997). The relations of regulation and emotionality to resiliency and competent social functioning in elementary school children. *Child Development*, *68*, 295–311.

Eisenberg, N., & Fabes, R. (1998). Prosocial development. In N. Eisenberg (Ed.), *Handbook of child psychology: Vol. 3. Social, emotional, and personality development* (5th ed., series Ed. W. Damon) (pp. 701–778). New York: John Wiley & Sons, Ltd.

Essex, M. J., Klein, M. H., & Lakin, N. H. (2002). Maternal stress beginning in infancy may sensitize children to later stress exposure: effects on cortisol and behavior. *Biological Psychiatry*, *52*(8), 776–784.

Evans, G. W., Gonnella, C., Marcynyszyn, L. A., Gentile, L., & Salpekar, N. (2005). The role of chaos in poverty and children's socioemotional adjustment. *Psychological Science*, *16*, 560–565.

Evans, G. W., Lepore, S. J., Shejwal, B. R., & Palsane, M. N. (1998). Chronic residential crowding and children's well-being: An ecological perspective. *Child Development*, *69*(6), 1514–1523.

Fergusson, D. M., Beautrais, A. L., & Horwood, L. J. (2003). Vulnerability and resiliency to suicidal behaviors in young people. *Psychological Medicine*, *33*, 61–73.

Finn, J. D., & Voelkl, K. E. (1993). School characteristics related to student engagement. *Journal of Negro Education*, *62*(3), 249–268.

Fox, N. A., Henderson, H. A., Rubin, K. H., Calkins, S. D., & Schmidt, L. A. (2001). Continuity and discontinuity of behavioral inhibition and exuberance: Psychophysiological and behavioral influences across the first four years of life. *Child Development*, *72*, 1–21.

Frosch, C., & Mangelsdorf, S. (2001). Marital behavior, parenting behavior, and multiple reports of preschoolers' behavior problems: Mediation or moderation? *Developmental Psychology*, *37*, 502–519.

Garcia, M., Shaw, D., Winslow, E., & Yaggi, K. (2000). Destructive sibling conflict and the development of conduct problems in young boys. *Developmental Psychology*, *36*, 44–53.

Garmezy, N., Masten, A., & Tellegen, A. (1984). The study of stress and competence in children: A building block for developmental psychopathology. *Child Development*, *55*(1), 97–111.

Gazelle, H., & Ladd, G. (2003). Anxious solitude and peer exclusion: A diathesis-stress model of internalizing trajectories in childhood. *Child Development*, *74*, 257–279.

Ginsburg, G., La Greca, A., & Silverman, W. (1998). Social anxiety and in children with anxiety disorders: Relation with social and emotional functioning. *Journal of Abnormal Child Psychology*, *26*, 175–186.

Goldberg, L. R. (1993). The structure of phenotypic personality traits. *American Psychologist*, *48*, 26–34.

Grant, K. E., Compas, B. E., Thurm, A. E., & McMahon, S. D. (2004). Stressors and child and adolescent psychopathology: Measurement issues and prospective effects. *Journal of Clinical Child and Adolescent Psychology*, *33*, 412–425.

Gruman, D., Harachi, T., Abbott, R. D., Catalano, R. F. & Fleming, C. B. (2008). Longitudinal effects of student mobility on three dimensions of elementary school engagement. *Child Development, 79*(6), 1833–1852.

Grych, J. H., & Fincham, F. D. (1990). Marital conflict and children's adjustment: A cognitive-contextual framework. *Psychological Bulletin, 108,* 267–290.

Gunnar, M., Tout, K., de Haan, M., Pierce, S., & Stansbury, K. (1997). Temperament, social competence, and adrenocortical activity in preschoolers. *Developmental Psychobiology, 31*(1), 65–85.

Gutman, L. M., Sameroff, A. J., & Eccles, J. S. (2002). The academic achievement of African American students during early adolescence: An examination of multiple risk, promotive, and protective factors. *American Journal of Community Psychology, 30,* 367–399.

Haines, M. M., & Stansfeld, S. A. (2000). Measuring annoyance and health in child social surveys. In D. Cassereau (Ed.), *Proceedings of Inter-Noise 2000,* vol. 3 (pp. 1609–1614). Indianapolis, IN: Institute of Noise Control Engineering of the USA.

Hammen, C. (2006). Stress generation in depression: Reflections on origins, research and future directions. *Journal of Clinical Psychology, 62,* 1065–1082.

Harkness, K. I., & Stewart, J. G. (2009). Symptom specificity and the prospective generation of life events in adolescence. *Journal of Abnormal Psychology, 118,* 278–287.

Harlow, C. W. (2002). *Educational and correctional populations.* Washington, DC: Bureau of Justice Statistics, Office of Justice Programs.

Henderson, H. A., Fox, N. A., & Rubin, K. A. (2001). Temperamental contributions to social behavior. The moderating roles of frontal EEG asymmetry and gender. *Journal of the American Academy of Child and Adolescent Psychiatry, 40,* 68–74.

Henderson, H. A., & Wachs, T. D. (2007). Temperament theory and the study of cognition–emotion interactions across development. *Developmental Review, 27,* 396–427.

Hertzman, C. (2010). Framework for the social determinants of early child development. In *Encyclopedia on Early Childhood Development.* Retrieved from http://child-encyclopedia.com/pages/PDF/HertzmanANGxp.pdf

Hetherington, E. M., & Kelly, J. (2002). *For better or for worse: Divorce reconsidered.* New York: W.W. Norton.

Hetherington, E. M., & Stanley-Hagan, M. (1999). The adjustment of children with divorced parents. A risk and resiliency perspective. *Journal of Child Psychology and Psychiatry and Allied Disciplines, 40,* 129–140.

Holahan, C. J., Moos, R. H., Holahan, C. K., Brennan, P. L., & Schutte, K. K. (2005). Stress generation, avoidance coping, and depressive symptoms: A 10-year model. *Journal of Consulting and Clinical Psychology, 73,* 658–666.

Hygge, S., Evans, G. W., & Bullinger, M. (2002). A prospective study of some effects of aircraft noise on cognitive performance in school children. *Psychological Science, 13,* 469–474.

Individuals with Disabilities Education Act (IDEA). (2004). Retrieved from http://idea.ed.gov/download/finalregulations.pdf

Jenkins, J. (1992). Sibling relationships in disharmonious homes: Potential difficulties and protective effects. In F. Boer & J. Dunn (Eds.), *Children's sibling relationships* (pp. 125–138). Hillsdale, NJ: Erlbaum.

Jenkins, J., Rasbash, J., & O'Connor, T. G. (2003). The role of the shared family context in differential parenting. *Developmental Psychology, 39,* 99–113.

Jones, M. B., & Offord, D. R. (1989). Reduction of antisocial behavior in poor children in nonschool skill development. *Journal of Child Psychology and Psychiatry, 30,* 737–750.

Kagan, J. (1997). Temperament and the reactions to unfamiliarity. *Child Development, 68,* 139–143.

Kagan, J. (2007). A trio of concerns. *Perspectives on Psychological Science, 2*(4), 361–376.

Kagan, J., & Fox, N. A. (2006). Biology, culture and temperamental biases. In N. Eisenberg (Ed.), *Handbook of child psychology: Vol. 3. Social, emotional, and personality development* (6th ed.) (pp. 167–225). Hoboken, NJ: John Wiley & Sons, Ltd.

Kagan, J., & Sniderman, N. (2004). *The long shadow of temperament.* Cambridge, MA: Belknap Press.

Keiley, M., Lofthouse, N., Bates, J., Dodge, K., & Petit, G. (2003). Differential risks of covarying and pure components in mother and teacher reports of externalizing and internalizing behaviour across ages 5 to 145. *Journal of Abnormal Child Psychology, 31,* 267–283.

Kenny, D. A., & Zautra, A. (2001). New methods for the analysis of change. In L. M. Collins & A. G. Sayers (Eds.), *New methods for the analysis of change (decade of behavior)* (pp. 243–263). Washington, DC: APA.

Kim, J. E., Hetherington, E. M., & Reiss, D. (1999). Associations among family relationships, antisocial peers, and adolescents' externalizing behaviors: Gender and family type differences. *Child Development, 70,* 1209–1230.

Kim, J-Y., McHale, S. M., Osgood, D. W., & Crouter, A. C. (2006). Longitudinal course and family correlates of sibling relationships from childhood through adolescence. *Child Development, 77*(6), 1746–1761.

King, J. (2006). *Gender equity in higher education: 2006.* Washington, DC: American Council on Education.

Klem, A. M., & Connell, J. P. (2004). Relationships matter: Linking teacher support to student engagement and achievement. *Journal of School Health, 74,* 262–273.

Kochanska, G., & Aksan, N. (2006). Children's conscience and self-regulation. *Journal of Personality, 74,* 1587–1617.

Lahey, B., Waldman, I., & McBurnett, K. (1999). The development of antisocial behavior: An integrative causal model. *Journal of Child Psychology and Psychiatry and Allied Disciplines, 40,* 669–682.

LeDoux, J. (1996). *The emotional brain: The mysterious underpinnings of emotional life.* New York: Simon and Schuster.

Lee, A., & Hankin, B. L. (2009). Insecure attachment, dysfunctional attitudes, and low self-esteem predicting prospective symptoms of depression and anxiety during adolescence. *Journal of Clinical Child and Adolescent Psychology, 38*(2), 219–231.

Linden, W., Earle, T. L., Gerin, W., & Christenfeld, N. (1997). Physiological stress reactivity and recovery: Conceptual siblings separated at birth? *Journal of Psychosomatic Research, 42,* 117–135.

Madden-Derdich, D., & Leonard, S. (2001). Parent–child relationships: The moderating influence between interparental conflict and child adjustment. Poster presented at the biennial meeting of the Society for Research in Child Development, April, Minneapolis, MN.

Martyn-Nemeth, P., Penckofer, S., Gulanick, M., Velsosr-Friedrich, B., & Bryant, F. S. (2009). The relationship among self-esteem, stress, coping, eating behavior, and depressive mood in adolescence. *Research in Nursing and Health, 32*(1), 96–109.

Marvinney, D. (1988). *Sibling relationships in middle childhood: Implications for social-emotional development* (PhD thesis). University of Minnesota, Minneapolis.

Maxwell, L. E. (2003). Home and school density effects on elementary school children: The role of spatial density. *Environment and Behavior, 35,* 566–578.

Maxwell, L. E. (2010). Chaos outside the home. The school environment. In G. W. Evans & T. D. Wachs (Eds.), *Chaos and its influence on children's development: An ecological perspective* (pp. 83–95). Washington, DC: APA.

Mayeux, L., Underwood, M. K., & Risser, S. D. (2007). Perspectives on the ethics of sociometric research with children: How children, peers, and teachers help to inform the debate. *Merrill-Palmer Quarterly, 53*(1), 53–78.

McLaughlin, K. A., & Hatzenbuehler, M. L. (2009). Stressful life events, anxiety sensitivity, and internalizing symptoms in adolescents. *Journal of Abnormal Psychology, 118*(3), 659–669.

McLoyd, V. (1998). Socioeconomic disadvantage and child development. *American Psychologist, 53,* 185–201.

Moore, G. T., & Lackney, J. A. (1993). School design: Crisis, educational performance and design applications. *Children's Environments, 10*(2), 1–22.

Morrison, D. R., & Coiro, M. J. (1999). Parental conflict and marital disruption: Do children benefit when high-conflict marriages are dissolved? *Journal of Marriage and the Family, 61,* 626–637.

Mun, E. Y., Fitzgerald, H. E., Von Eye, A., Puttler, L. I., & Zucker, R. A. (2001). Temperament characteristics as predictors of externalizing and internalizing child behavior problems in the contexts of high and low parent psychopathology. *Infant Mental Health Journal, 22,* 393–415.

Neppl, T. K., Donnellan, M. B., Scaramella, L. V., Widaman, K. F., Spilman, S. K., Ontai, L. L., & Conger, R. D. (2010). Differential stability of temperament and personality from toddlerhood to middle childhood. *Journal of Research in Personality, 44,* 386–396.

Newcomb, A. F., Bukowski, W. M., & Pattee, L. (1993). Children's peer relations: A meta-analytic review of popular, rejected, neglected, controversial, and average sociometric status. *Psychological Bulletin, 113,* 99–128.

Oland, A. A., & Shaw, D. S. (2005). Pure versus co-occurring externalizing and internalizing symptoms in children: The potential role of socio-developmental milestones. *Clinical Child and Family Psychology Review, 8,* 247–270.

Parke, R. D., & Buriel, R. (1998). Socialization in the family: Ethnic and ecological perspectives. In N. Eisenberg (Ed.), *Handbook of child psychology: Vol. 3. Social, emotional, and personality development* (5th ed., series Ed. W. Damon) (pp. 463–552). New York: John Wiley & Sons, Ltd.

Pelham, W. E., & Bender, M. E. (1982). Peer relationships in hyperactive children: Description and treatment. In K. D. Gadow & I. Bialer (Eds.), *Advances in learning and behavioral disabilities,* vol. 1 (pp. 365–436). Greenwich, CT: JAI Press.

Pfeffer, C. R. (2000). Suicidal behavior in prepubertal children: From 1980s to the new millennium. In R. W. Maris, S. S. Canetto, J. L. McIntosh, & M. M. Silverman (Eds.), *Review of Suicidology, 2000* (pp. 159–169). New York: Guilford.

Piekarska, A. (2000). School stress, teachers' abusive behaviors, and children's coping strategies. *Child Abuse and Neglect, 24*(11), 1443–1449.

Pollock, R. A., Carter, A. S., Avenevoli, S., Dierker, L. C., Chazan-Cohen, R., & Merikangas, K. R. (2002). Anxiety sensitivity in adolescents at risk for psychopathology. *Journal of Clinical Child and Adolescent Psychology, 31,* 343–353.

Porges, S. W. (2003). Social engagement and attachment: A phylogenic perspective. *Roots of Mental Illness in Children, 1008,* 31–47.

Posner, M. I., & Rothbart, M. K. (2007). Temperament and learning. In M. I. Posner & M. K. Rothbart (Eds.), *Educating the human brain* (pp. 121–146). Washington, DC: APA.

Potthoff, J. G., Holahan, C. J., & Joiner, T. D. (1995). Reassurance seeking, stress generation and depressive symptoms: An integrative model. *Journal of Personality and Social Psychology, 68,* 664–670.

Prelow, H. M., & Loukas, A. (2003). The role of resource, protective, and risk factors on academic achievement-related outcomes of economically disadvantaged Latino youth. *Journal of Community Psychology, 31,* 513–529.

Pribesh, S., & Downey, D. B. (1999). Why are residential and school moves associated with poor school performance? *Demography, 36,* 521–534.

Repetti, R. L., Taylor, S. E., & Seeman, T. E. (2002). Risky families: Family social environments and the mental and physical health of offspring. *Psychological Bulletin, 128,* 330–336.

Rimm-Kaufman, S., Early, D. B., Cox, M. J., Saluja, G., Pianta, R. C., Bradley, R. H., & Payne, C. (2002). Early behavioral attributes and teacher sensitivity as predictors of competent behavior in the kindergarten classroom. *Journal of Applied Developmental Psychology, 23,* 451–470.

Roberts, R. E., Roberts, C. R., & Chan, W. (2009). One-year incidence of psychiatric disorders and associated risk factors among adolescents in the community. *Child Psychology and Psychiatry, 50,* 405–415.

Rothbart, M. K. (2003). Temperament and the pursuit of an integrated developmental psychology. *Merrill-Palmer Quarterly, 50,* 492–505.

Rothbart, M. K., Ahadi, S. A., & Evans, D. E. (2000). Temperament and personality: Origins and outcomes. *Journal of Personality and Social Psychology, 78*(1), 122–135.

Rothbart, M. K., Ahadi, S. A., Hersey, K. I., & Fisher, P. (2001). Investigations of temperament at three to seven years: The children's behavior questionnaire. *Child Development, 72,* 1394–1408.

Rothbart, M. K., & Bates, J. E. (2006). Temperament. In N. Eisenberg (Ed.), *Handbook of child psychology: Vol. 3. Social, emotional, and personality development* (6th ed.) (pp. 99–166). Hoboken, NJ: John Wiley & Sons, Ltd.

Rothon, C., Head, J., Clark, C. M., Klineberg, E., Cattell, V., & Stansfeld, S. (2009). The impact of psychological distress on the educational achievement of adolescents at the end of compulsory education. *Social Psychiatry and Psychiatric Epidemiology, 44,* 421–427.

Rourke, B. P., Young, G. C., & Leenaars, A. A. (1989). A childhood learning disability that predisposes those afflicted to adolescent and adult depression and suicide risk. *Journal of Learning Disabilities, 22,* 169–175.

Rowe, D., & Gully, B. (1992). Sibling effects on substance abuse and delinquency. *Criminology, 30,* 217–233.

Rubin, K. H., Coplan, R. J., Fox, N. A., & Calkins, S. D. (1995). Emotionality, emotion regulation, and preschoolers' social adaptation. *Development and Psychopathology, 7,* 49–62.

Rubin, K. H., Burgess, K. B., & Hastings, P. D. (2002). Stability and social-behavioral consequences of toddlers' inhibited temperament and parenting behaviors. *Child Development, 73,* 483–495.

Rutter, M. (1979). Protective factors in children's responses to stress and disadvantage. In M. Whalen & J. E. Rolf (Eds.), *Primary prevention of psychopathology: Vol. 3. Social competence in children* (pp. 49–79). Hanover, NH: University Press of New England.

Safford, S. M., Alloy, L. B., Abramson, L. Y., & Crossfield, A. G. (2007). Negative cognitive style as a predictor of negative life events in depression-prone individuals. A test of the stress generation hypothesis. *Journal of Affective Disorders, 99,* 147–154.

Sameroff, A., & Fiese, B. H. (2000). Transactional regulation: The developmental ecology of early intervention. In J. P. Shonkoff & S. J. Meisels (Eds.), *Handbook of early childhood intervention* (2nd ed.) (pp. 135–159). New York: Cambridge University Press.

Schmidt, L. A., Santesso, D. L., Schulkin, J., & Segalowitz, S. J. (2007). Shyness is a necessary but not sufficient condition for high salivary cortisol in typically developing 10-year-old children. *Personality and Individual Differences, 43,* 1541–1551.

Schor, E. (1986). Use of health care services by children and diagnoses received during presumably stressful life transitions. *Pediatrics, 77,* 834–841.

Schweinhart, L. J., Barnes, H. V., & Weikart, D. P. (1993). *Significant benefits: The High/Scope Perry Preschool Study through age 27. Monographs of the High/Scope Educational Research Foundation,* no. 10. Ypsilanti, MI: High/Scope Press.

Seibert, A. C., & Kerns, K. A. (2009). Attachment figures in middle childhood. *International Journal of Behavioral Development, 33,* 347–355.

Seidman, E., Aber, J. L., & French, S. (2004). The organization of schooling and adolescent development. In K. Maton, C. Schellenbach, B. Leadbeater, & A. Solarz (Eds.), *Investing in child, youth, families, and communities: Strengths-based research and policy* (pp. 233–250). Washington, DC: APA.

Seidman, E., Lambert, L. E., Allen, L., & Aber, J. (2003). Urban adolescents' transition to junior high school and protective family transactions. *Journal of Early Adolescence, 23,* 166–193.

Sharrer, V. W., & Ryan-Wenger, M. (1995). A longitudinal study of age and gender differences of stressors and coping strategies in school-aged children. *Journal of Pediatric Health Care, 9*, 123–130.

Shantz, C. U., & Hobart, C. J. (1989). Social conflict and development: Peers and siblings. In T. J. Berdt & G. W. Ladd (Eds.), *Peer relationships in child development. Wiley Series on Personality Processes* (pp. 71–94). New York: John Wiley & Sons, Ltd.

Simon, N. S. (2005). *Building quality, academic achievement, and self-competency in New York City Schools* (Master's thesis). Cornell University, Ithaca, NY.

Slomkowski, C., Rende, R., Conger, K. J., Simons, R., & Conger, R. D. (2001). Sisters, brothers, and delinquency: Evaluating social influence during early and middle adolescence. *Child Development, 72*, 271–283.

Stocker, C. M. (1994). Children's perceptions of relationships with siblings, friends, and mothers: Compensatory processes and links with adjustment. *Journal of Child Psychology and Psychiatry, 35*, 1447–1459.

Stocker, C. M., Burwell, R., & Briggs, M. (2002). Sibling conflict in middle childhood predicts children's adjustment in early adolescence. *Journal of Family Psychology, 16*, 50–57.

Stocker, C. M., & Youngblade, L. (1999). Marital conflict and parental hostility: Links with children's sibling and peer relationships. *Journal of Family Psychology, 13*, 598–609.

Stone, W. L., & La Greca, A. M. (1990). The social status of children with learning disabilities: A reexamination. *Journal of Learning Disabilities, 23*, 32–37.

Tackett, J. L., Krueger, R. F., Iacono, W. G., & McGue, M. (2008). Personality in middle childhood: A hierarchical structure and longitudinal connections with personality in late adolescence. *Journal of Research in Personality, 42*, 1456–1462.

Tellegen, A. (1985). Structures of mood and personality and their relevance to assessing anxiety, with an emphasis on self-report. In A. H. Tuma & J. D. Maser (Eds.), *Anxiety and the anxiety disorders* (pp. 681–706). Hillsdale, NJ: Erlbaum.

Thomas, A., & Chess, S. (1977). *Temperament and development.* New York: Brunner/Mazel.

Tremblay, R. E., LeMarquand, D., & Vitaro, F. (1999). The prevention of oppositional defiant disorder and conduct disorder. In H. C. Quay & A. E. Hogan (Eds.), *Handbook of disruptive behavior disorders* (pp. 525–558). New York: Kluwer Academic.

Turner-Cobb, J., Rixon, L., & Jessop, D. (2008). A prospective study of diurnal cortisol responses to the social experience of school transition in four-year-old children: Anticipation, exposure, and adaptation. *Developmental Psychobiology, 50*(4), 377–389.

Vasa, S. F., Maag, J. W., Torrey, G. K., & Kramer, J. J. (1994). Teachers' use and perceptions of sociometric techniques. *Journal of Psychoeducational Assessment, 12*(2), 135–141.

Wallerstein, J. S., & Kelly, J. B. (1982). *Surviving the breakup: How children and parents cope with divorce.* New York: Basic Books.

Watson, D., & Clark, L. A. (1984). Negative affectivity: The disposition to experience aversive emotional states. *Psychological Bulletin, 96*, 465–490.

Weiss, M., Worling, D., & Wasdell, M. (2003). A chart review study of the inattentive and combined types of ADHD. *Journal of Attention Disorders, 7*, 1–9.

Willemen, A. M., Schuengel, C., & Koot, H. M. (2009). Physiological regulation of stress in referred adolescents: The role of the parent-adolescent relationship. *Journal of Child Psychology and Psychiatry, 50*, 482–490.

Yeh, H., & Lempers, J. D. (2004). Perceived sibling relationships and adolescent development. *Journal of Youth and Adolescence, 33*, 133–147.

Zimmerman, K. K., & Stansbury, K. K. (2004). The influence of emotion regulation, level of shyness, and habituation on the neuroendocrine response of three-year-old children. *Psychoneuroendocrinology, 29*, 973–982.

7

Early Onset Problems: Preschool and Primary School

Clinical and Educational Child Psychology, First Edition. Linda Wilmshurst.
© 2013 John Wiley & Sons, Ltd. Published 2013 by John Wiley & Sons, Ltd.

Chapter preview and learning objectives

In this chapter, three neurodevelopmental disorders will be discussed, including intellectual developmental disabilities (IDD), autism spectrum disorders (ASD, formerly known as pervasive developmental disorders (PDD)), and communication disorders. Our notion of IDD (formerly mental retardation) has evolved over time, and is currently conceptualized as a condition of subnormal intellectual capacity manifesting during the developmental period, accompanied by impairments in adaptive functioning. The change in terminology from mental retardation to IDD is in keeping with how the disability is currently conceptualized. The American Association of Mental Retardation (AAMR) recently changed its name to the American Association of Intellectual and Developmental Disability (AAIDD; www.aamr.org) in keeping with this movement.

Children with ASD evidence qualitative impairments in social reciprocity and communication skills, and engage in a restricted range of activities often involving non-functional and stereotypical routines. Many with ASD also have comorbid intellectual disabilities.

While not all children with language impairments are diagnosed with IDD or ASD, many children with these developmental disorders also evidence some degree of language impairment. Within this chapter, the essential features of developmental language impairments will be discussed, as they relate to difficulties with expressive, receptive, and social communication.

In addition to the neurodevelopmental disorders mentioned above, the chapter will also focus on two other disorders that have early onset: feeding disorders and selective mutism. While some children are "fussy" eaters, other children demonstrate food refusal, a predominant symptom of a condition known as "failure to thrive" which can result in significant health risks. Children who are diagnosed with selective mutism refuse to speak in public, although their speech is often otherwise unimpaired. Currently, there is much controversy regarding how best to conceptualize selective mutism.

This chapter will provide increased understanding of:

- the role of intellectual and adaptive functioning in meeting criteria for intellectual disabilities;
- the difference between developmental delay and developmental deficit;
- the difference between a general learning disability and a specific learning disability;
- the nature and range of autism spectrum disorders;
- the multi-faceted nature of language impairments, and how these are related to other developmental disorders;
- the nature and characteristics of other early onset problems, such as feeding disorders and selective mutism.

Neurodevelopmental disorders and disabilities

This chapter reviews three neurodevelopmental disorders: intellectual developmental disability, autism spectrum disorders, and communication disorders. Two other neurodevelopmental disorders, attention deficit hyperactivity disorder (ADHD) and the specific learning disabilities, will be discussed in the next chapter.

Intellectual developmental disorder/disability (IDD)

Clinical description: nature and course

Introduction   Understanding (IDD) requires an appreciation of how intelligence relates to mental age and an awareness of differences between specific or global delays in development (**developmental delay**) versus **life-long deficits** in the ability to reason and learn, resulting in limitations in adaptive functioning.

Idiocy versus madness

In 1838, Jean Esquirol (1772–1840) devoted a large section of his book on mental health to the topic of **"idiocy."** Esquirol was the first to articulate the difference between *"idiots"* who never developed their mental capacity and the "mentally deranged" who once had mental capacity, but lost it (Sattler, 2001, p. 129).

Global developmental delay   The term **global developmental delay** captures the concept of development as a continuum, and individual differences in the rate of acquiring expected skills in areas such as language, motor, or cognitive and adaptive functioning. Children suspected of having significant delays in these areas are often assessed using standardized, norm-referenced measures to determine the extent and nature of the delay and to provide guidelines for early intervention programs that will target skills that require remediation. Repeated assessments are essential to chart progress and any "changes in the rate of development in order to arrive at a valid diagnosis" (Sattler & Hoge, 2006, p. 440).

Intellectual developmental disability (formerly mental retardation)   Currently, IDD refers to significantly subnormal intellectual functioning in the presence of impairment in adaptive functioning (life skills, such as communication, self-help, leisure activities) that manifest during the developmental period. Cognitive deficits are considered significant if an IQ (intelligence quotient) score on a standardized measure of intelligence is two standard deviations (sd) below the norm (IQ of approximately 70, when the average IQ is 100). Standardized measures of adaptive functioning are often obtained through questionnaires completed by parents and teachers. While developmental delays are likely to remit with appropriate intervention, children who have IDD will experience life-long difficulties in areas requiring "higher order cognitive processes (such as efficient problem-solving strategies, generalization and abstraction)" compared to "subordinate processes (such as attention, rehearsal, ability to inhibit responses, and discrimination of the elements of a problem)" (Sattler & Hoge, 2006, p. 438).

Learning disability: general versus specific   The general public can be confused since the term **"learning disability"** has been used interchangeably to refer to IDD on various websites, and in various publications, especially in the United Kingdom. The

Royal College of Psychiatrists (2004, p. 1) has attempted to clarify the distinction between a **general learning disability** and a **specific learning disability**, stating that a child with a general disability "finds it more difficult to learn, understand and do things compared to other children of the same age." Therefore, while a *general learning disability* (IDD) refers to reduced overall capacity to learn due to lowered cognitive ability/intelligence quotient (an IQ of approximately 70 or below), the term specific learning disability is used to refer to a learning difficulty in a specific area, such as reading (dyslexia), writing, or understanding what is said to them, despite having general learning ability at least within the average range (an IQ range of at least 85–115). Specific learning disabilities will be addressed in *Chapter 8*.

A major communication gap

In North America, the term learning disability is synonymous with specific learning disability, which refers to a significant discrepancy between intelligence (usually average or above) and academic performance (well below average). Specific learning disabilities can occur in reading (dyslexia), writing, or mathematics. However, in the United Kingdom, the term learning disability can also be used as a generic term to refer to intellectual disability, a generalized impairment in learning capacity and adaptive functioning due to subnormal intelligence.

The nature of IDD IDD is defined as a condition of subnormal intellectual functioning (DSM) or arrested/incomplete development of the mind (ICD) with accompanying impairments in adaptive functioning. IDD manifests within the developmental period, prior to 18 years of age.

Intelligence (IQ) Historically, intellectual deficit has traditionally been classified by degree of severity (mild, moderate, severe, or profound) based on IQ scores obtained from individually administered intelligence tests. These tests have a mean (average) of 100 and a standard deviation (sd) of 15. Functioning levels of those diagnosed with IDD can vary depending on the IQ scores. Those with mild impairment (IQ range 50 to 70) can be expected to achieve academic levels as high as the sixth grade, and be gainfully employed with minimal supervision, while those with moderate levels (IQ range 35 to 49) may achieve more modest education levels and work in sheltered workshops. Those with severe (IQ range 20 to 24) and profound (IQ range below 20) levels of IDD will experience more pronounced impairments due to increased neurological dysfunction. Approximately 85% of all those classified with IDD will have a mild level of disability, while 10% will experience moderate levels of impairment (APA, 2000).

   The way in which intellectual disabilities are conceptualized has continued to evolve, with the AAIDD shifting its emphasis from classifications based on IQ range to more practical applications based on levels of service needed. This model is based on the **intensity of intervention** required, ranging across intermittent, limited, extensive, and pervasive service needs.

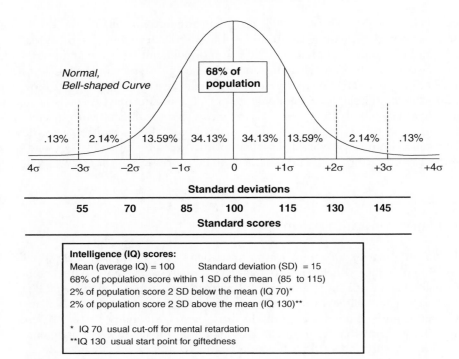

Figure 7.1   Standard normal distribution and IQ scores.

The measurement of intelligence   Recall that the normal distribution was previously discussed when the T score distribution was introduced (Figure 5.1). The relationship of IQ scores (standard scores) to the normal distribution is presented in Figure 7.1.

The majority of individuals (68%) will score within 1 sd of the mean (IQ range 85–115). Note that as scores move away from the center, the population under the curve shrinks on either side of the midpoint. An IQ score of 70 is 2 sd below the mean and is the cut point for a diagnosis of IDD. Approximately 2% of the population can be expected to obtain an IQ score below 70. On the other hand, individuals who obtain an IQ score of 130 (2 sd above the mean) are functioning at the ninety-eighth percentile, which is often seen as the cut point for "gifted" classifications which include the top 2% of the population.

With the introduction of mandatory education, the French government commissioned Alfred Binet (1857–1911) and Théodore Simon (1873–1961) to develop a measure of mental ability to identify children at risk for academic difficulties. The original **Binet–Simon Scales** (1905) consisted of 30 questions of increasing difficulty based on age-related cognitive probes (Sattler, 2001). In 1916, Terman devised the **intelligence quotient** (**IQ**) to provide a **ratio IQ** of a child's mental age (MA) relative to chronological age (CA). Although the ratio IQ has since been replaced by the deviation IQ derived from more sophisticated statistical procedures, the ratio IQ can be a helpful heuristic in understanding the relationship between mental age (MA) and chronological age (CA), as is evident in the following example: Robby is five years old (CA), but has the mental age of a three-year-old (MA). His ratio IQ would be 60 which would likely place him in the mild range of mental retardation.

Ratio IQ:

$$IQ = \frac{MA}{CA} \times 100$$

Example (Robby):

$$IQ = \frac{3}{5} \times 100 = 60$$

Adaptive functioning Impairment in **adaptive functioning** (ability to function independently) is a criterion for IDD. Deficits are measured using standardized scales of social maturity and adaptation, which will be discussed shortly. Neither the DSM nor the ICD provides guidelines regarding the extent of "deficit" required in adaptive functioning to meet the criteria for IDD; however, the DSM does indicate that deficits must exist in at least two of these 10 adaptive areas: *communication skills, self-care, home living, social/interpersonal skills, use of community resources, self-direction, functional academic skills, work, leisure*, or *health and safety.*

Developmental and associated features The majority of children with IDD have mild deficits and will benefit from special education resources available in their own communities, although those with greater needs may require more comprehensive services. Early identification is essential, since brain development is rapid in the first two years of life. Delays or deficits may be evident in the following global areas:

- gross motor skills (*sitting, walking*);
- fine motor skills (*drawing, letters, coloring*)
- communication skills (*speech, articulation, vocabulary*);
- cognitive skills (*problems solving, transferring information from one situation to another*);
- social skills.

Behavior problems can add to academic or social difficulties and those with comorbid communication problems, self-injurious behaviors, stereotypical movements, and overactivity are at increased risk for negative outcomes (Aman, Hammer, & Rohahn, 1993).

Comorbidity Children with IDD are four times more likely to have comorbid disorders than peers without IDD (APA, 2000).

IDD and comorbidity

The most common disorders associated with IDD include: ADHD, mood disorders, PDD, and stereotypical movement disorder (APA, 2000). Specific types of IDD may exhibit certain patterns of comorbidity.

Subtypes and prevalence: etiology of chromosomal abnormalities/genetic origins

Down syndrome   Children with **Down syndrome (DS)** are born with a defect on chromosome 21; either an extra number 21 chromosome (**trisomy 21**) or damage to the chromosome. Children with DS have unique physical characteristics (short stature, almond-shaped eyes, short broad hands, low muscle tone) and may experience problems with motor skills (awkwardness, lack of coordination) and speech (grammar, expressive language, and articulation). They have strong imitative skills. The average IQ range is between 30 and 70, with the average IQ score around 50 (Chapman & Hesketh, 2000; Vicari, 2006). IQ scores tend to decrease with age (Pennington, Moon, Edgin, Stedron, & Nadel, 2003). Those with **upper level Down syndrome** (IQ in the lower average range: 80–90) do not meet criteria for a diagnosis of IDD.

DS and child-bearing age

The prevalence rate for DS is usually one in 800 births; however, for women over 45 years of age, the risk increases to one in 25 births.

Prader–Willi syndrome   Individuals with **Prader–Willi syndrome** have a defect on chromosome 15, inherited from the father, causing mild intellectual impairment (IQ range 60–80) (Milner et al., 2005). Low muscle tone and weak reflex responses are evident at birth. School-age children have short stature (small hands and feet), poor emotion regulation (impulsivity, temper tantrums, mood swings), compulsive eating, aggression, and stubbornness (Dykens & Cassidy, 1995). Obsessive compulsive behaviors and picking at their skin can be problematic (Wigren & Hansen, 2005). Compulsive eating can result in obesity.

Angelman syndrome   A defect on chromosome 15, inherited from the mother, results in **Angelman syndrome**, once called "happy puppet" syndrome, due to frequent and inappropriate laughing/smiling that accompanies the disorder (Horsler & Oliver, 2006). Developmental delay, speech impairment, and movement disorder are associated characteristics. The syndrome is rare (one in 10,000 births), and **microcephaly** (small head size), seizures, and a flat-shaped head may be evident (Horsler & Oliver, 2006).

Williams syndrome (WS)   J.C.P. Williams, a New Zealand cardiologist, identified **Williams syndrome** (WS) in a number of cardiovascular patients. Although caused by a random mutation on chromosome 7 (ELN, a gene responsible for maintaining heart valves and blood tissue, is missing), recipients have a 50% risk of passing on the mutation to offspring. Children with WS are hypersensitive to sound and have distinct facial features including puffiness around the eyes, a wide mouth, and a short nose. Infants can be colicky and irritable, while adolescents are prone to diabetes (Bellugi et al., 2007).

   Individuals with WS have well-developed verbal skills (verbal IQ) and poorly developed visual-spatial skills (performance IQ). Rourke et al. (2002) found individuals with WS share many processing deficits with children who have nonverbal learning disabilities (NLD) evident in right hemisphere dysfunction.

"Hypersociability, including overfriendliness and heightened approachability towards others, combined with anxiety relating to new situations and objects and a difficulty forming and maintaining friendships with peers" can be evident (Bellugi et al., 2007, p. 99). Bellugi et al. (2007) found an intense preoccupation with faces even in toddlers with WS, who were more interested in gazing at and interacting with researchers than engaging with toys. Hypersensitivity to sound and enhanced musical ability have also been found in individuals with WS.

Fragile X syndrome   Mild to moderate levels of IDD are associated with **Fragile X syndrome** resulting from a defect in the Fragile X MR1 (FMR1) gene which produces a protein necessary for normal brain development. Children may demonstrate challenging behaviors (aggression in males, withdrawal in females), based on the degree of damage to the gene (Hall, De Bernardis, & Reiss, 2006).

Phenylketonuria (PKU)   **PKU** is caused by two recessive genes that carry **inborn errors of metabolism (IEM)**. Infants lack the enzyme required for amino acid conversion necessary to produce phenylalanine which is essential for body functioning. If not detected within the first year of life, irreversible damage can result. Routine screening for PKU at birth is conducted globally (e.g., in the United States, Canada, the United Kingdom). In the United Kingdom, annually 60–70 infants (of 793,000 births) test positive for PKU (Thomason et al., 1998). Early detection and placement on a low phenylalanine diet can reverse the effects and return intelligence to normal.

Subtypes and prevalence: etiology of environmental origins   Environmental toxins (**teratogens**) can cross the placenta and compromise the embryo, especially between three and eight weeks' gestation, when the nervous system and vital organs undergo significant development.

Substance use/abuse   Drugs (such as cocaine, crack) can increase risks for physical defects, brain dysfunction (hemorrhages and seizures), low birth weight, and damage to the central nervous system (Espy, Kaufmann, & Glisky, 1999; Richardson, Hamel, & Goldschmidt, 1996). **Fetal alcohol syndrome (FAS)** or **fetal alcohol effects** (**FAE**, a milder form of FAS) can be the end result of maternal alcohol consumption during pregnancy. Approximately 33% of infants born to mothers who consume excessive alcohol will develop FAS (Streissguth, Bookstein, & Barr 2004). Facial features include an underdeveloped upper lip, widely spaced eyes, and a small head, which will be less pronounced over time. However, cognitive deficits, hyperactivity, and impaired motor coordination often persist (Schonfeld, Mattson, & Lang, 2001).

Lead-based paint   Children can be exposed to lead-based paint by eating paint chips or living in residences where peeling paint releases toxins. Prenatal exposure can result in brain damage and other side effects (Davis, Change, Burns, Robinson, & Dossett, 2004). Higher lead levels are associated with increased need for special education resources and problems in attention, memory, learning, and behavior (Coppens, Hunter, & Bain, 1990; Davis et al., 2004).

Rubella   If a mother is exposed to **rubella** during the embryonic period (three to eight weeks' gestation), there is a 50% risk that the embryo will develop **congenital rubella syndrome** which can result in multiple handicaps, including: sensory deficits (hearing, vision), reduced mental capacity, aggressive tendencies, and/or self-injurious behaviors (Carvill & Marston, 2002; Eberhart-Phillips, Frederick, & Baron, 1993).

Birth trauma   Problems encountered during birth or delivery can result in **anoxia** (oxygen deprivation), which can cause deficits in intellectual functioning.

Health and injuries   Reduced mental capacity can result from contracting **encephalitis** or **meningitis**, poor prenatal care, severe malnutrition, or acquired brain injuries through accidents.

Assessment   Evaluation and identification of IDD will often involve a mental health team composed of a number of professionals. A full developmental, familial, and medical history can provide information about the etiology, severity, and specific nature of IDD and any comorbid features. Goals of the assessment will be to determine areas of weakness in order to establish intervention strategies, and to identify the child's strengths which can increase the success of the intervention program.

An individually administered intelligence test will determine the level of the child's cognitive functioning, pattern of strengths and weaknesses, and whether the child meets the criteria for diagnosis. Several intellectual assessment instruments are available depending on the child's age, and any cultural or second language considerations. Some of the most common assessments are presented in Table 7.1.

While some of the measures incorporate language-based components, a number of instruments are available for assessment of individuals who would be penalized if language were a requirement. These instruments are either language-free (Leiter International Performance Scale; Raven's Progressive Matrices) or contain a nonverbal ability scale (Differential Abilities Test). In addition to the assessment of cognitive functioning, assessments of adaptive functioning would also be administered. Some common adaptive instruments are also listed in Table 7.1.

Early intervention and prevention

Early intervention (EI)   In the formative years, the brain is highly plastic and has the potential for rapid development (Kolb, Brown, Witt-Lajeunesse, & Gibb, 2001). Early intervention programs (in the first five years) can act to halt further cognitive declines (Guralnick, 1998), and improve future school success (Stattin & Klackenberg-Larsson, 1993). Roberts, Mazzucchelli, Studman, and Sanders (2006) found parents who participated in a behavioral family intervention program (*Stepping Stones Triple P*) reported a reduction in stress and improvements in both maternal and paternal parenting style, while preschoolers demonstrated fewer behavior problems than controls.

School- and home-based programs   In the United States, numerous federally funded **Head Start Programs** were launched in the 1960s with various degrees of success. One of the most successful programs was the **High/Scope Perry Preschool Project**

Table 7.1 Common assessment instruments for neurodevelopmental disorders

Instrument	Age levels	Assesses
Individual intellectual assessments		
Bayley Scales of Infant and Toddler Development-III (Bayley, 2005)*	1–42 months	Five developmental domains: cognition, language, social-emotional, motor, and adaptive behavior
Wechsler Preschool & Primary Intelligence Test (WPPSI-III) (Wechsler, 2002a)*	2 years 6 months– 7 years 3 months	Full scale IQ, verbal IQ, performance IQ
Wechsler Intelligence Scale for Children (WISC-IV) (Wechsler, 2002b)*	6–16 years	Verbal comprehension, perceptual reasoning, processing speed, working memory index scores and full scale IQ
Stanford Binet, 5th Edition (Roid, 2003)	2–85 years	Full scale IQ, verbal IQ, performance IQ
Differential Ability Scales, 2nd Edition (DAS II) (Elliott, 2007)	2 years 6 months– 17 years 11 months	Verbal ability, non-verbal ability, spatial ability, general cognitive ability (GCA)
Leiter International Performance Scales-Revised (Roid, Gale, & Miller, 1997)	2–20 years	Reasoning, visualization, attention, and memory (language-free)
Raven's Standard Progressive Matrices (SPM/MHV) (Raven, Raven, & Court, 2004)*; **Raven's Colored Progressive Matrices (CPM/CVS)** (Raven, 2003)*	SPM: 7–18 years CPM: 4–11 years	Progressive matrices are either Standard (SPM) or Colored (CPM) and accompanied by Mill Hill Vocabulary (MHV) or Crichton Vocabulary Scale (CVS)
Adaptive behavior scales		
Vineland Adaptive Behavior Scales, Second Edition (Vineland-II) (Balla, Cicchetti, & Sparrow, 2005)	Birth–18 years 11 months	Development in four domains: communication, daily living, socialization, and motor skills
Adaptive Behavior Assessment System (ABAS II) (Harrison & Oakland, 2003)	Birth–21 years	Assesses 10 adaptive skills (DSM) plus three general areas (American Association of Mental Retardation)
Autism spectrum		
Autism Spectrum Rating Scales (ASRS) (Goldstein & Naglieri, 2010)	2–5 years; 6–18 years	Socialization, social/emotional reciprocity, atypical language, stereotypical/rigid behaviors
Autism Diagnostic Interview, Revised (ADI-R) (Rutter, LeCouteur, & Lord, 2003)	2 years +	Diagnosis/differential diagnosis and treatment planning; language, social reciprocity, atypical behaviors
Childhood Autism Rating Scale – 2nd Edition (CARS 2) (Schopler, Van Bourgondien, Wellman, & Love, 2010)	2 years +	Parent and teacher ratings of autistic behaviors for low- to high-functioning autism

Note: *UK norms available.

which followed 123 high-risk African American children living in poverty between 1962 and 1967 (58 were assigned to the program; 65 served as controls with no intervention). The average IQ for all children was between 70 and 85. Children attended the preschool for 2.5 hours per day, five days a week, over the course of two years. The preschool teachers made weekly home visits of 1.5 hours.

High/Scope Perry Preschool Project

Academically, 15% of children in the program required special education compared to 34% of controls, and 71% graduated from high school compared to 54% of controls. By 27 years of age, those in the control group had twice the number of arrests, while social assistance was required by 32% of the controls, compared to 15% of the program group (Schweinhart, Barnes, & Weikart, 1993). A cost-benefit analysis revealed that the public benefitted at a rate of $7.16 for each dollar invested in the program (Barnett, 1993).

During 2003–2004, the European Agency for Development in Special Needs Education (EADSNE, 2005) compiled a summary report on early childhood intervention (ECI) based on information provided by 19 countries. The report discussed the applicability of the **ecologic-systemic model** (Porter, 2002) to ECI programs in the United States and Europe. The model draws on several perspectives already discussed (attachment, social learning theory, and transactional/ecological) and focuses on child development as:

- **holistic** (competencies in all areas);
- **dynamic** (interactive and responsive to changing developmental needs);
- **transactional** (changes are reciprocal and on-going);
- **singular** (individual differences result in individual perspectives).

How many children need and receive special education services?

In the United States, six million children (aged three to 21 years) receive special education services (Wilmshurst & Brue, 2005). In the United Kingdom, an estimated 1.7 million pupils in schools have special educational needs, while 250,000 have Statements of special educational need, the majority of whom are disabled (Department of Health, 2002).

Prevention programs   There are several levels of prevention programs available to reduce potential risk factors, namely: primary, secondary, and tertiary prevention.

Primary prevention   Dissemination of information concerning appropriate nutrition in pregnancy to prevent low birth weight babies is an example of **primary prevention**. Programs are normally **universal** (i.e., targeting all women of child-bearing age).

Secondary prevention programs   **Secondary prevention programs** focus on high-risk populations and offer **selective prevention** targeting specific needs; for example, training parents to promote social engagement for inhibited children.

Tertiary prevention programs   **Tertiary prevention programs** provide **indicated prevention** specific to the area of need (e.g., parent behavioral management programs for problem behaviors) and target a population who already exhibit problems with the goal of reducing or preventing the problems from getting any worse.

Autism spectrum disorders (pervasive developmental disorders)

The category of **pervasive developmental disorders (PDD)** in the ICD and DSM has traditionally housed five disorders (autism, Asperger disorder (AD), childhood disintegrative disorder or other disintegrative disorder, Rett syndrome, and pervasive developmental disorder not otherwise specified (PDDNOS)). The disorders share features of qualitative impairments in communication, social reciprocity, and range of interests/activities (stereotypical patterns of behavior). The ICD and DSM criteria have met with criticism for failure to distinguish effectively between AD and autism (Woodbury-Smith, Klin, & Volkmar, 2005), and growing discontent with increased numbers of children diagnosed with PDDNOS based on limited criteria (Scheeringa, 2001). Currently, criteria for AD require ruling out communication delay or impairment; however, researchers have found children who meet criteria for AD but who have language problems (Eisenmajer et al., 1998), while others have found children with autism who do not demonstrate language delay (Miller & Ozonoff, 2000). Furthermore, some feel that communication problems in social pragmatics in those with AD are not adequately recognized by the current criteria (Klin, Volkmar, Sparrow, Cicchetti, & Rourke, 1995; Woodbury-Smith et al., 2005).

As a result, current revision plans for the ICD and DSM include potentially conceptualizing autism, AD, and PDDNOS and child disintegrative disorder as the **autism spectrum disorders** based on "significant and early-arising difficulties in basic aspects of social-communication and restricted, repetitive behaviors or interests" which are "the commonalities that strongly define this group" (Lord & Bishop, 2010, p. 4). With this in mind, the two defining criteria would include: social/communicative deficits and fixated/repetitive behaviors. Conceptually, social communicative behaviors would represent one cluster of symptoms instead of two.

ASD: nature and course   Deficits in social communication and social interaction are evident in the following three areas:

- deficits in reciprocal social-emotional responses; children with ASD often do not initiate or engage in social conversation, share interests, or participate in social referencing;

- deficits in nonverbal communication such as eye contact, social gestures, body language, facial expressions, and poor integration of verbal and nonverbal communication;
- lack of interest in or development of age-appropriate relationships with others (excluding the caregiver); lack of sharing, imaginative play, or imitation.

Restricted range of activities and engagement in repetitive patterns of behavior are evident in two of the following areas:

- repetition of behavior, such as repetitive speech, motor movements (hand flapping, rocking), or perseverance with objects (lining up objects or playing with parts of objects, such as spinning the wheel of a car);
- rigid adherence to routines, repetitive need for sameness (food, routines), and extreme resistance to change;
- restricted range of interests and intense preoccupation with themes (such as numbers, maps, and so on) or attachment to objects;
- hyper- or hypo-reactivity to environmental stimuli of a sensory nature (such as lights, sounds, textures, smells); possible adverse reactions to certain sensory input.

Developmental features   Children with ASD lack social interaction skills such as **social referencing**, or sharing interests with others (**joint attention behavior**). Communication may be minimal, or marked with oddities such as pronoun reversals, echolalia (repeating rather than responding), and robotic in nature. Social play is limited or non-existent. There is often a preoccupation with nonfunctional routines (lining things up), or other forms of **self-stimulation** that increase isolation from others. There can be an **insistence on sameness** (**IS**) (rigidity of routines, inflexibility to environmental changes, compulsions/rituals) that adds to child management issues, or **repetitive sensory and motor behaviors** (**RSMB**) (unusual sensory interests, self-stimulation, rocking, and repetitive acts) that tend to disengage children from the outside world. Szatmari et al. (2006) found that children who engaged in more RSMB behaviors were more delayed, while those with the IS factor demonstrated higher intellectual functioning.

Intellectual functioning   It was initially thought that 70% of individuals with autism have comorbid IDD, with 30% in the mild to moderate range, and 40% in the severe to profound range (Fombonne, 2003). However, more recent reports suggest that IDD may occur in only 50% of cases (CDC, 2000).

Autism and IQ: a biased report?

Concerns have been raised that reports of IQ deficits may be overestimated. IQ test scores may be inaccurate due to lack of motivation and deficits in language skills in individuals with autism (Edelson, 2006; Freeman & Van Dyke, 2006).

The term **high functioning autism** (**HFA**) has been used to refer to individuals with autism with an IQ score of above 70 (Klin, Volkmar, & Sparrow, 2000). Males are nine times more likely to have HFA compared to females (Volkmar, Szatmari, & Sparrow, 1993), and are four times more likely than females to be diagnosed with autism (CDC, 2000).

Asperger disorder (AD)   The category of AD has been controversial. While some suggest that AD represents a less severe form of autism on the spectrum, others support retaining the separateness between these two disorders, since children with AD present with "fewer symptoms and have a different presentation" (Volkmar et al., 1994, p. 1365). For example, while those with more severe autism perseverate on parts of objects (such as spinning a wheel), the child with AD perseverates on themes or topics of interest (such as dinosaurs or cars) and can become quite knowledgeable in these **"savant skills"** (Klin & Volkmar, 1997). Some children with AD may be preoccupied with numbers or letters and some can be **hyperlexic**, decoding words at a very early age. Although able to form attachments to family members, these skills do not transfer to peers. A pedantic monologue often replaces two-way conversations. Deficits in understanding social pragmatics can be painfully obvious when they attempt to join peer groups in adolescence (Klin & Volkmar, 1997). Their awkward gait and lack of coordination also may set them apart from their peers.

Rourke et al. (2002) found shared traits in those with AD and nonverbal learning disabilities (NLD): verbal strengths (left hemisphere) and deficits in right hemisphere processing (weaknesses in social interaction, complex reasoning, and nonverbal communication).

Woodbury-Smith et al. (2005) suggest conceptualizing autism and AD as two different types of social disability with their own unique patterns of behaviors and communication deficits. This would reinforce the need to recognize that communication abnormalities do exist in those with AD (in the form of pragmatic communication impairments) that "interfere with the ability to initiate and sustain a conversation," even though deficits are "fundamentally different from the type of language and communication impairments described in autism in which the language is delayed, echolalic, idiosyncratic and repetitive" (Woodbury-Smith et al., 2005, p. 238).

Theory of mind

Daria loves chocolate. When Daria leaves the room, Molly watches her teacher replace the chocolate in her lunch box with crackers. The teacher asks Molly: "When Daria returns to the room, what will she think is in the lunch box?

Theory of mind   Researchers have studied theory of mind problems, such as in the example in the box, and found varied success rates for those with autism, HFA, and AD. Successfully solving the dilemma requires awareness that others have a "mental set," or belief system based on their own perceptions. When faced with the dilemma, children with AD continually perform better than those with autism or HFA (Ozonoff, Rogers, & Pennington, 1991).

ASD: prevalence rates and etiology   Four to five times more males are diagnosed with autism and AD; however, females diagnosed with autism tend to be more severely affected (APA, 2000). Prevalence rates for autism are four times that of AD (Fombonne, 2003).

Autism: a growing concern

Prevalence rates for autism initially ranged from five to 25 cases per 10,000 (APA, 2000). However, rates have escalated, globally. In California, rates jumped from 44/100,000 in 1980 to 208/100,000 in 1994 (Dales, Hammer, & Smith, 2001). In the United Kingdom, cumulative incidence ratings rose from 7/10,000 in 1988, to 28/10,000 in 1993, and 33/10,000 in 1996 (Jick & Kaye, 2003).

The most recent reports from the Centers for Disease Control and Prevention (CDC, 2000) suggest that the prevalence rate for ASD in the United States is 1/70 for boys and 1/315 for girls, with an overall rate of 1/110 (CDC, 2009). These rates are very similar to those reported by Baird et al. (2006) concerning children in south-west London (United Kingdom), suggesting proportions of global concern. Recent reviews suggest that PDDNOS is now the most highly diagnosed category of ASD, with twice as many cases reported compared to autism (Fombonne, 2009).

Given the dramatic increase in rates for autism, some have questioned whether a childhood vaccine (particularly the **MMR vaccine** against measles, mumps, and rubella), or a preservative (**thiomersal**), in vaccines might be implicated. However, evidence is not supportive, and Jick and Kaye (2003) suggest increases are likely due to improved practices for identification of the disorder. Coincidentally, the MMR vaccine is typically administered around the time that symptoms of autism become more evident (12 to 15 months; and three to five years).

Etiology: genetics, brain structure, and function   There is an increased risk for autism linked to increased age of the parent (mothers and fathers) at the time of conception (Grether, Anderson, Croen, Smith, & Windham, 2009). If one sibling has autism, there is a 3–6% risk to the other siblings (Nicholson & Szatmari, 2003). About 25% of those with autism have elevated levels of serotonin (Klinger & Dawson, 1996). Increased head circumference has been reported, albeit the **corpus callosum** (lateralization of function) is reduced. In social cognitive situations, there is limited activity of the **amygdale** (processing emotion), while parts of the brain are activated that are most often associated with processing objects, rather than people (Pierce, Muller, Ambrose, Allen, & Courchesne, 2001). Recent investigations of adults with ASD have found atypical amygdale responses with poor connectivity to associated neural pathways (Gaigg & Bowler, 2007), and reduced receptors in the serotonergic (5-HT) system responsible for "modulating social behaviour, amygdale response to facial emotion and repetitive behaviours" (Murphy et al., 2006, p. 934).

In a recent study conducted in London, Ecker et al. (2010) analyzed brain scans (obtained through functional magnetic resonance imaging) of 20 adults with ASD using a pattern classification technique previously used in facial recognition studies. Compared to controls and adults with ADHD, Ecker et al. (2010) were able to predict, with 90% accuracy, the scans belonging to the group with ASD due to a consistent pattern of increased thickness of tissue in grey matter located in areas of the frontal and parietal lobes that are associated with specific behaviors and language. If the study is replicated with children, it may provide a "biomarker" for ASD which has been elusive to date.

ASD: assessment   The assessment and diagnosis of ASD is currently based on matching descriptions and observations to criteria as set out in the DSM or ICD. However, as Lord and Bishop (2010) point out, currently there are few "developmental referents" to guide professionals in defining symptoms for different ages and skill levels for this complex and diverse disorder. In addition, although a number of instruments and rating scales are available, some of which are presented in Table 7.1, there is no prescribed protocol for assessment. However, based on best practices, the National Autism Center (2009) suggests that assessment of autism should include:

- detailed developmental history;
- evaluation of the child's developmental cognitive, adaptive, and behavioral functioning;
- direct observation of the child's play, language, and social interaction;
- a physical examination.

Among the instruments that have been used to identify ASD, the Autism Diagnostic Observation Schedule (ADOS; Lord et al., 1989) is an instrument that has stood the test of time, with a recent replication of results confirming initial rates for prediction and validity (Gothman et al., 2008). The instrument has been available commercially since 2001 through Western Psychological Services (WPS). ADOS is accepted as the "gold standard of autism diagnosis ... based on a combination of results gleaned from a diagnostic interview and clinical judgment of an autism expert"; this developmental play-based assessment protocol "involves the systematic observation of key features associated with ASD" (Wilczynski et al., 2011, pp. 569–570). The instrument takes about 45 minutes to complete and requires fairly extensive training to administer. Another play-based assessment, also requiring trained practitioners, is the Screening Tool for Autism (STAT; Stone, Coonrod, & Ousley, 2000). The Modified Checklist for Autism in Toddlers (M-CHAT; Robins, Fien, Barton, & Green, 2001) is a screening device for ADS developed primarily for pediatricians to obtain parent ratings at their 24-month visit.

ASD: treatment and intervention   The need for early identification and intensive intervention has been well supported by research (Dawson et al., 2009; Lovaas, 1987). In addition to pharmacological treatment that may accompany interventions for ASD, the National Autism Center (2009) conducted a comprehensive review of empirically based intervention practices and comprehensive treatment models. The report suggests a number of intervention practices, including behavioral methods, such as conducting a functional behavioral analysis to link interventions to target behaviors, modeling, peer training, self-management strategies, and the use of story-based interventions. Given the diversity of ASD, it is important that behavioral packages be developed to address a student's individual needs and to incorporate family into the process (Lord & Bishop, 2010; National Autism Center, 2009; Wilczynski et al., 2011).

Lovaas: the UCLA ABA Program   Ivar Lovaas (1987) developed the UCLA treatment program for autism based on principles of **applied behavioral analysis (ABA)**. The program involved 40 hours of home and clinic intervention per week, over three years (from two-and-a-half to five-and-a-half years of age). By seven years of age, almost half (47%) of the children in this intense intervention increased their IQ by 37 points and were attending regular school programs.

The UCLA model was replicated in a community setting, using a quasi-experimental design, since assignment to group was not random, but based on parents' preference. Results revealed that the experimental group (21 children) achieved significantly higher IQ and adaptive scores relative to controls (21 children) receiving regular special education assistance (Cohen, Amerine-Dickens, & Smith, 2006).

The Schopler Program: TEACCH   TEACCH (treatment and education for autistic and related communication handicapped children) originated from Duke University, in North Carolina (Schopler, 1994). The program targets communication problems to reduce behavioral problems resulting from frustration, by developing skills in **intentional communication**. The theory is that children will become motivated to communicate based on internal drives and needs (e.g., the child will be motivated to learn the word water, if he or she is thirsty). Empirically, the TEACCH program has been successful in reducing self-injurious behaviors (Norgate, 1998), and more effective than non-specific educational alternatives (Panerai, Ferrante, & Zingale, 2002).

The Early Start Denver Model: ESDM   The ESDM model (Dawson et al., 2009) was a rigorously designed manualized program using ABA methods for children with ASD under 30 months of age who were randomly assigned to the ESDM or a community treatment control. The ESDM involved an intensive 15 hours of home-based intervention focusing on interpersonal skills and verbal and nonverbal communication. Parents were trained in behavioral strategies (positive reinforcement, use of positive affect) and were instructed to use these skills for at least five hours per week (although the average use was 16.3 hours per week). Program participants increased their IQ by 17 points compared to controls who demonstrated a seven-point increase in IQ.

Childhood disintegrative disorder (CDD)   There is limited information about CDD, a very rare condition afflicting approximately 2/100,000 males (Fombonne, 2009). The onset of the condition occurs between two and 10 years of age, following at least two years of normal functioning. CDD is often accompanied by severe IDD and possibly **metachromatic leukodystrophy** (**MLD**).

Metachromatic leukodystrophy (MLD)

The **myelin sheath**, a fatty covering that acts as an insulator around the nerve fibers, increases the efficiency of neurotransmitter message transmission. MLD is a lipid storage disease that impairs the development of myelin and is responsible for a toxic build-up of lipids in the nervous system, liver, and kidneys and is possibly responsible for loss of bladder function.

Children with CDD experience a progressive loss of function in several areas that can include: language, social/adaptive skills, bowel or bladder function, and play or motor skills. Atypical functioning in areas common to other ASD is also evident (social communication, and a restricted range of activities/repetitive and stereotypical patterns of behavior).

Etiology and treatment Little is known about the cause of CDD; however, a higher incidence of epilepsy is reported relative to those with autism (Kurita, Koyama, Setoya, Shimizu, & Osada, 2004). A phase of markedly fearful, anxious behavior can accompany the regressive period which includes loss of motor coordination, loss of physical skills (dressing, toileting, self-feeding, and the development of ataxia or drooling) and other neurological symptoms (Rogers, 2004). Treatments include medications to control seizures and behavioral programs similar to those used for children with ASD.

Children with speech, language, and communication problems

Speech and language impairments: nature of disorders Children who have a **language impairment** (**LI**) perform below age expectations in language, including: the acquisition of spoken language (expression, production, and comprehension) and written language, and language usage (vocabulary, grammar, and pragmatics). Language difficulties may shift based on the child's age and it may be difficult to determine whether a child is experiencing **late language emergence** (**LLE**), a **specific language impairment** (**SLI**), or **selective mutism**. Although it is suggested that LI can exist comorbid with other disorders (such as ASD, LD, and selective mutism), LLE and SLI are considered to be mutually exclusive. However, it is possible for a child to begin with a diagnosis of LI and be later diagnosed with SLI. Language impairment can cause a functional limitation in areas of communication, social engagement, academic achievement, and career.

Late language emergence (LLE) For children who demonstrate LLE, delay in language onset will be determined prior to four or five years of age by comparing rates of acquisition to expected language milestones (e.g., vocabulary, word combinations, ability to follow directions, use of gestures, and so on). Children with LLE are at risk for other developmental disorders, such as ASD, IDD, SLI, social communication disorder, or specific learning disabilities. Although the majority of children with LLE are not reclassified as having SLI, at least one study found that 20% of children identified as having LLE at 24 months continued to perform below the norm on language ability tests at seven years of age, compared to only 11% of controls (Rice, Taylor, & Zubrick, 2008). Risk factors for LLE include being male (males have three times the risk of females), having low birth weight (twice the risk), and having a family history of late onset speech (Zubrick, Taylor, Rice, & Slegers, 2007).

Specific language impairment (SLI)   In keeping with classical definitions of specific learning disabilities (which will be addressed in the next chapter), determining the existence of SLI entails a two-step process:

1. indication of below normal functioning on a standardized assessment of language functioning, usually 1 sd below average (Tomblin, Records, & Zhang, 1996);
2. a determination that the SLI is not due to other impairments, such as lack of opportunity to learn language, hearing deficits, or other pervasive disorders (such as IDD or ASD).

However, whether nonverbal scores should be at least in the average range or expanded to include nonverbal scores in the 70–85 range is an area of debate (Francis, Fletcher, Shaywitz, Shaywitz, & Bourke, 1996). The controversy regarding the requirements for nonverbal functioning have serious implications, conceptually and psychometrically, since studies have shown lower prevalence rates for cases where nonverbal intelligence is within the norm (Tomblin et al., 1997).

Specific language impairment (SLI) or auditory processing disorder (APD)?

APD refers to "deficits in the neural processing of non speech sounds that do not result from deficits in general attention, language or cognitive processes" (Ferguson, Hall, Riley, & Moore, 2011, p. 211). Differential diagnoses of APD and SLI have been problematic due to inconsistencies in definitions and lack of consistency in diagnostic assessments for APD. Furthermore, children diagnosed with SLI by speech and language pathologists and children diagnosed with APD by ENT or audiology professionals often present with similar and overlapping symptoms. In their recent comparative analysis of children diagnosed with SLI or APD, Ferguson et al. (2011) found no difference between these two groups on any of the audiological, language, or cognitive assessments conducted or any of the parent questionnaires. The authors suggest that differential diagnosis was based on "referral route" rather than any "actual differences."

It can be difficult to reliably identify language impairments in very young children (Dale, Price, Bishop, & Plomin, 2003). However, when SLIs are identified in the later preschool years, they tend to be more persistent (Law, Boyle, Harris, Harkness, & Nye, 2000; Tomblin, Zhang, Buckwalter, & O'Brien, 2003). In addition, children with SLI are at increased risk for longer-term negative outcomes academically (e.g., Catts, Fey, Tomblin, & Zhang, 2002; Young et al., 2002) and in psychosocial areas (e.g., Tomblin, Zhang, Buckwalter, & Catts, 2000; Beitchman et al., 2001).

Social communication disorder (SCD)   This category has been referred to by many different designations, including "semantic pragmatic disorder" which has been used primarily in the United Kingdom (Bishop & Rosenbloom, 1987), and refers to language problems resulting from difficulties with the semantics and pragmatics of social communication. There has been significant debate as to whether the disorder is part of ASD or a language disability in its own right. For example, Rapin and Allen (1998) suggest that although the disorder can often occur in children with ASD, it can also appear in children with other disorders such as hydrocephalus, Williams syndrome, and other brain conditions. More recently there has been increasing support for considering social communication as a language disorder that is separate from other language impairments involving syntactical qualities of speech, and that can also exist in populations without ASD (Bishop & Norbury, 2002; Tomblin, Zhang, Weiss, Catts, & Ellis Weismer, 2004). Because deficits in social communication are part of the criteria for ASD, the category of SCD would rule out those with ASD and would be reserved for children with otherwise intact language skills, who experience specific deficits in comprehension and communication in social situations based on poor ability to recognize and respond to subtle social nuances and understand non-literal interpretation of conversational speech (e.g., the use of idioms).

Issues of fluency and voice   In addition to impairments in language, some children also experience problems of speech fluency, e.g., production of speech sounds (phonological errors of articulation, substitutions or omissions), stuttering, cluttering (rate, clarity or organization of speech) or voice problems involving vocal pitch, loudness, tone and quality. In a community-based study, Beitchman, Nair, Clegg, and Patel (1986) estimated that 4.6% of five-year-olds with fluency issues had comorbid speech and language disorders.

Although the consequences of having speech sound disorders may not be as significant as for SLI, fluency problems can increase the risk for reading, and other academic and social problems (Raitano, Pennington, Tunick, Boada, & Shriberg, 2004). In clinical populations, high rates of comorbidity have been reported among stuttering, speech sound disorders, and SLI (Blood, Ridenour, Qualls, & Hammer, 2003). Onset of stuttering often occurs in the preschool years and may remit spontaneously, although it can persist. Due to the embarrassment often associated with stuttering, issues of self-confidence may result in restriction of social and vocational activities (Kroll & Beitchman, 2005).

Prevalence rates and etiology

Prevalence rates   Prevalence rates across studies vary widely. Epidemiological studies suggest that between 13 and 19% of children will demonstrate LLE by 24 months of age (Zubrick et al., 2007). Concerning SLI, Beitchman et al. (1986) found a prevalence rate of 12.6% for five-year-olds, using a definition that did not require normal nonverbal intelligence, while Tomblin et al. (1997) reported a prevalence rate of 7.4% for SLI when other disabilities were excluded and nonverbal intelligence was required to be in the normal range. Among six- and seven-year-old children, Law et al. (2000) found median prevalence estimates of 5.5% for the more exclusive and 3.1% for the less rigorous definitions of SLI.

In order to clarify the nature of speech, language, and communication needs (SLCN) of children living in the United Kingdom, the government commissioned a report, the Bercow Report (Bercow, 2008), to review data collected in the United Kingdom (Lindsay et al., 2008) with the goal of evaluating and improving services to meet the needs of children with SLCN. Based on data generated for this report, Lindsay et al. (2008) report that "a significant proportion of children in both primary and secondary school with special educational needs have SLCN as their primary need" (p. 14). Based on their data gathered in 2007, Lindsay et al. (2008) found that approximately 50% of children in some socio-economically disadvantaged populations have speech and language skills that are significantly lower than those of other children of the same age. In addition, approximately 7% of five-year-olds (40,000) in England had significant difficulties with speech and/or language, likely needing intervention at some point, while approximately 1% of five-year-olds (5500) had the most severe and complex speech, language, and communication needs (Desforges & Lindsay, 2010).

Prevalence rates for fluency disorders also vary by study. Studies of community samples in North America have reported a rate of 15.6% for speech sound disorders in three-year-olds (Campbell et al., 2003), and 3.8% for six-year-olds (Shriberg, Tomblin, & McSweeny, 1999).

In an Australian study of over 10,000 children (kindergarten through grade six) McKinnon, McLeod, and Reilly (2007) found a rate of 1.06% for speech sound disorders, and estimate 0.33% for stuttering, based on conservative procedures. Although rates differ based on definitions and procedures used, studies are consistent in revealing a reduction in prevalence rates with increased age (Shriberg, Kwiatkowski, & Gruber, 1994). Overall population rates for stuttering are less than 1%, ranging from a high of approximately 1.4% for children two to 10 years of age to a low of roughly 0.37% in adult populations (Bloodstein, 1995).

Etiology   Genetic factors have been prominent in studies of the etiology of SLI, and most SLIs can be linked to family history. Chromosome 6, 16, and 19 have been implicated in SLI, while chromosome 6 has also been linked to dyslexia (Falcaro et al., 2008; Rice, Smith, & Gayan, 2009). Children who have a first-degree biological relative with a stutter are three times more likely to stutter than the norm (APA, 2000). In their study of SLNC in children and adolescents in the United Kingdom, Lindsay et al. (2008) suggest three areas most likely to be associated with SLCN: the existence of a primary disorder in the area; cases where SLCN are secondary to another primary factor such as a significant hearing impairment which impedes speech, language, and communication; or lack of opportunity and exposure to adequate language models as a result of social disadvantage.

Assessment and treatment   Assessment and treatment of SLIs are primarily conducted by speech therapists and speech pathologists trained in the evaluation and treatment of deficits and delays in speech, language, and communication. Therapy can be provided in individual or small group sessions. Elaboration of the specific instruments and therapeutic interventions available to speech therapists is beyond the scope of this book;

however, Lindsay et al. (2008) suggest that, given the high prevalence rates for speech, language, and communication problems among school children, a multi-tiered system of intervention/universal prevention should be implemented, similar to response to intervention (RTI) procedures used in the United States (Reschly & Ysseldyke, 2002). The model would represent four tiers of service: language enrichment for all children, as part of early development; language enrichment and targeted support for half the population who experience language difficulties; targeting and specialist support for those with significant primary impairments in speech, language, and communication (7%); and complex and long-term support from specialists, in addition to targeted and universal applications for the most severe cases (Lindsay et al., 2008, pp. 14–15).

Other early onset childhood disorders

Eating and feeding disorders of infancy and early childhood

Feeding disorder   **Feeding disorder** is often characterized by "food refusal" or restricted food intake with the possible outcome of **failure to thrive** (**FTT**). Forty percent of young children evidence eating problems (Manikam & Perman, 2000), although "picky" eaters often compensate by eating larger quantities of preferred foods (Reau, Senturia, Lebailly, & Christoffell, 1996). However, children with FTT represent 3–4% of children six years of age and younger who fail to meet weight expectations; demonstrate symptoms of irritability, withdrawal, and possible developmental delays; and are responsible for between 1% and 5% of infant hospital admissions. Although abuse and/or neglect were initially thought to be a causal factor, recent research has shed doubt on this theory (Wright & Birks, 2000). Children with the disorder evidence feeding disturbance by repeated avoidance of food or by restricting intake. Sharp, Jaquess, Morton, and Herzinger (2010) found that behavioral interventions resulted in significant improvements in feeding behaviors, based on tracking antecedent and consequent conditions as part of the regime for successful intervention.

Pica   Children with **pica** repeatedly crave non-nutritive and non-food substances, with younger children most likely to consume paint, cloth, plaster, and string, while older children may eat sand, pebbles, leaves, and animal droppings. Adolescents may eat clay or soil. Pica is often associated with IDD (which may include adult populations), and can be a symptom of ASD but also may exist in young children who have normal intelligence. It is important to rule out cultural variations, since in some cultures eating non-nutritive substances (clay) is sanctioned (APA, 2000).

Rumination disorder   **Rumination** involves repeated regurgitation and re-chewing of food. Later onset is often associated with mental retardation. Although the DSM (APA, 2000) considers this a separate disorder, the ICD (WHO, 1996) considers rumination as a possible symptom of feeding disorder, rather than a separate disorder. If onset is between three and 12 months, rumination is most likely associated with stressful conditions, or neglect. Weight loss can be severe, and even fatal in 25% of cases.

Selective mutism (SM) Children with selective mutism (DSM) or elective mutism (ICD) are characterized by a failure to speak in specific social situations (school, groups), while being able to speak in other situations (family, siblings, or close peers). The mean age for SM is between 2.7 and 4.1 years (Bogels et al., 2010). There is a quandary as to where SM should be clustered in classification systems, due to a poor understanding of the etiology of the disorder, and as a result four different directions have been suggested:

1. SM is a type of anxiety disorder, such as a variant of social phobia (SP) or social anxiety disorder (SAD) (Bogels et al., 2010). This rationale is based on overlapping symptoms (anxiety and avoidance); the high rate of comorbidity between these two disorders (65% of children with SM also meet criteria for SAD; Black & Uhde, 1992; Kristensen, 2000); and the fact that fluoxetine which is successful in the treatment of SAD (Kristensen, 2000) also is successful in improving symptoms of SM (Bogels et al., 2010).
2. SM is an avoidant behavior pattern, similar to school refusal, which the child acquires over time and is reinforced through refusal to speak which reduces anxiety (Bogels et al., 2010).
3. SM is a strategy for emotion regulation by avoidance of speech, which serves to lower the level of emotional arousal (Scott & Beidel, 2011). Parent reports of the child's shy temperament and Kagan's (2001) research on inhibited children provide support for this premise.
4. SM is part of the externalizing or oppositional disorders (Black & Uhde, 1992).
5. SM is a type of language disorder or impairment because 30–38% of children with SM also exhibit speech and language disorders (Steinhausen & Juzi, 1996).

Assessment and treatment The majority of treatment investigations for SM have been in the form of case studies, which, although providing rich information, reduces the generalizability of results. However, success has been noted in studies using behavioral methods, such as shaping, systematic desensitization, and modeling (Pionek Stone, Kratochwill, Sladezcek, & Serlin, 2002).

References

Aman, M. G., Hammer, D., & Rohahn, J. (1993). Mental retardation. In T. H. Ollendick & M. Hersen (Eds.), *Handbook of child and adolescent assessment* (pp. 321–345). Needham Heights, MA: Allyn and Bacon.

American Psychatric Association (APA). (2000). *The diagnostic and statistical manual of mental disorders* (4th ed., text revision). Washington, DC: Author.

Baird, G., Simonoff, E., Pickles, A., Chandler, S., Loucas, T., & Meldrum, D. (2006). Prevalence of disorders of the autism spectrum in a population cohort of children in South Thames: The Special Needs and Autism Project (SNAP). *The Lancet, 368*(9531), 210–215.

Balla, D. A., Cicchetti, D. V., & Sparrow, S. S. (2005). *Vineland Adaptive Behavior Scales, 2nd edition: Vineland-II*. Circle Pines, MN: American Guidance Service.

Barnett, W. (1993). Benefit-cost analysis of preschool education: Findings from a 25-year follow-up. *American Journal of Orthopsychiatry, 63*, 25–50.

Bayley, N. (2005). *Bayley Scales of Infant and Toddler Development-III*. San Antonio, TX: Pearson.

Beitchman, J. H., Nair, R., Clegg, M., & Patel, P. G. (1986). Prevalence of speech and language disorders in 5-year-old kindergarten children in the Ottawa-Carleton region. *Journal of Speech and Hearing Disorders, 51*, 98–110.

Beitchman, J. H., Wilson, B., Johnson, C. J., Atkinson, L., Young, A., Adlaf, E.,... Douglas, L. (2001). Fourteen-year follow-up of speech/language impaired and control children: psychiatric outcome. *Journal of the American Academy of Child and Adolescent Psychiatry, 40*, 75–82.

Bellugi, U., Jarvinen-Pasley, A., Doyle, T., Reilly, J., Reiss, A., & Korenberg, J. (2007). Affect, social behavior and the brain in Williams syndrome. *Current Directions in Psychological Science, 10*, 99–104.

Bercow, J. (2008). *The Bercow Report: A review of services for children and young people (0–19). with speech, language and communication needs.* Nottingham: DCSF. Retrieved from https://www.education.gov.uk/publications/eOrderingDownload/Bercow-Report.pdf

Bishop, D. V. M., & Norbury, C. F. (2002). Exploring the borderlands of autistic disorder and specific language impairment: A study using standardised diagnostic instruments. *Journal of Child Psychology and Psychiatry, 43*(7), 917–929.

Bishop, D. V. M., & Rosenbloom, L. (1987). Classification of childhood language disorders. In W. Yule & M. Rutter (Eds.), *Language development and disorders. Clinics in developmental medicine* (pp. 16–41). London, Mac Keith Press.

Black, B., & Uhde, T. W. (1992). Elective mutism as a variant of social phobia. *Journal of the American Academy of Child and Adolescent Psychiatry, 31*, 1090–1094.

Blood, G. W., Ridenour, V. J., Qualls, C. D., & Hammer, C. S. (2003). Co-occurring disorders in children who stutter. *Journal of Communication Disorders, 36*, 427–448.

Bloodstein, O. (1995). *A handbook on stuttering* (5th ed.). San Diego, CA: Singular.

Bogels, S. M., Alden, L., Beidel, D. C., Clark, L. A., Pine, D. S., Stein, M. B., & Voncken, M. (2010). Social anxiety disorder: Questions and answers for the DSM-V. *Depression and Anxiety, 27*, 168–189.

Campbell, T. F., Dollaghan, C. A., Rockette, H. E., Paradise, J. L., Feldman, H. M., Shriberg, & L. D. (2003). Risk factors for speech delay of unknown origin in 3-year-old children. *Child Development, 74*, 346–357.

Carvill, S., & Marston, G. (2002). People with intellectual disability, sensory impairments and behavior disorder: A case series. *Journal of Intellectual Disability Research, 26*, 264–272.

Catts, H. W., Fey, M. E., Tomblin, J. B., & Zhang, X. Y. (2002). A longitudinal investigation of reading outcomes in children with language impairments. *Journal of Speech, Language, and Hearing Research, 45*, 1142–1157.

Centers for Disease Control and Prevention (CDC). (2000). *Prevalence of autism in Brick Township, New Jersey, 1998: Community report.* Atlanta: US Department of Health and Human Services.

Centers for Disease Control and Prevention (CDC). (2009). Prevalence of autism spectrum disorders—autism and developmental disabilities monitoring network, United States, 2006. *Morbidity and Mortality Weekly Report, 58*(SS10). 1–20.

Chapman, R. S., & Hesketh, L. J. (2000). Behavioral phenotype of individuals with Down syndrome. *Mental Retardation and Developmental Disabilities Research Review, 6*, 84–95.

Cohen, H., Amerine-Dickens, M. A., & Smith, T. (2006). Early intensive behavioural treatment: Replication of the UCLA Model in a community setting. *Journal of Developmental and Behavioural Pediatrics, 27*, S145–S155.

Coppens, N. M., Hunter, P. N., & Bain, J. A. (1990). The relationship between elevated lead levels and enrollment in special education. *Family and Community Health, 12*, 39–46.

Dale, P. S., Price, T. S., Bishop, D. V. M., & Plomin, R. (2003). Outcomes of early language delay: I. Predicting persistent and transient language difficulties at 3 and 4 years. *Journal of Speech, Language, and Hearing Research, 46,* 544–560.

Dales, L., Hammer, S. J., & Smith, N. J. (2001). Time trends in autism and MMR immunization coverage in California. *Journal of the American Medical Association, 285,* 1183–1185.

Davis, D. W., Change, F., Burns, B., Robinson, J., & Dossett, D. (2004). Lead exposure and attention regulation in children living in poverty. *Developmental Medicine and Child Neurology, 46,* 825–831.

Dawson, G., Rogers, S., Munson, J., Smith, M., Winter, J., Greenson, J., … Varley, J. (2009). Randomized, controlled trial of an intervention for toddlers with autism: The Early Start Denver Model. *Pediatrics, 125*(1), e17–e23.

Desforges, M., & Lindsay, G. (2010). *Procedures used to diagnose a disability and to assess special educational needs: An international review.* NCSE Research Report No. 5. Trim, Ireland: National Council for Special Education. Retrieved from http://ebook browse.com/gdoc.php?id=103355156&url=cb9ba546bf36dd545bd25ff3859814ac

Department of Health (2002). Valuing people: A new strategy for learning disability for the 21st century: A white paper. Retrieved from http://www.archive.official-documents. co.uk/document/cm50/5086/5086.pdf

Dykens, E. M., & Cassidy, S. B. (1995). Correlates of maladaptive behaviour in children and adults with Prader-Willi syndrome. *Neuropsychiatric Genetics, 60,* 546–549.

European Agency for Development in Special Needs Education (EADSNE). (2005). *Early-childhood intervention. Analysis of situations in Europe, key aspects and recommendations.* Middelfart: EADSNE.

Eberhart-Phillips, J. E., Frederick, P. D., & Baron, R. C. (1993). Measles in pregnancy: A descriptive study of 58 cases. *Obstetrics and Gynecology, 82,* 797–801.

Ecker, C., Rocha-Rego, V., Johnston, P., Mourao Miranda, J., Marquand, A., Daley, E. M., … MRC AIMS Consortium (2010). Investigating the predictive value of whole-brain structural MR scans in autism: A pattern classification approach. *Neuroimage, 49,* 44–56.

Edelson, M. G. (2006). Are the majority of children with autism mentally retarded? A systematic evaluation of the data. *Focus on Autism and other Developmental Disabilities, 21,* 66–83.

Eisenmajer, R., Prior, M., Leekam, S., Wing, L., Ong, B., Gould, J., & Welham, M. (1998). Delayed language onset as a predictor of clinical symptoms in pervasive developmental disorders. *Journal of Autism and Developmental Disorders, 28*(6), 527–533.

Elliott, C. D. (2007). *Differential Ability Scales, 2nd edition: DAS-II.* San Antonio, TX: Psychological Corporation.

Espy, K. A., Kaufmann, P. M., & Glisky, M. L. (1999). Neuropsychologic function in toddlers exposed to cocaine in utero: A preliminary study. *Developmental Neuropsychology, 15,* 447–460.

Falcaro, M., Pickels, A., Newbury, D. F., Addis, L., Banfield, E., Fisher, E. E., … SLI Consortium (2008). Genetics and phenotypic effects of phonological short-term memory and grammatical morphology in specific language impairment. *Genes, Brain and Behavior, 7,* 393–402.

Ferguson, M. A., Hall, R. L., Riley, A., & Moore, D. R. (2011). Communication, listening, cognitive and speech perception skills in children with auditory processing disorder (APD). or specific language impairment (SLI). *Journal of Speech, Language, and Hearing Research, 54,* 211–227.

Fombonne, E. (2003). Epidemiological surveys of autism and other pervasive developmental disorders: An update. *Journal of Autism and Developmental Disorders, 33,* 365–382.

Fombonne, E. (2009). Epidemiology of pervasive developmental disorders. *Pediatric Research, 65*(6), 591–598.

Francis, D. J., Fletcher, J. M., Shaywitz, B. A., Shaywitz, S. A., & Bourke, B. P. (1996). Defining learning and language disabilities: Conceptual and psychometric issues with the use of IQ tests. *Language, Speech, and Hearing Services in Schools, 27,* 132–143.

Freeman, B. J., & Van Dyke, M. (2006). Are the majority of children with autism mentally retarded? Invited commentary. *Focus on Autism and Other Developmental Disabilities, 21,* 86–88.

Gaigg, S., & Bowler, D. (2007). Differential fear conditioning in Asperger's syndrome: Implications for an amygdale theory of autism. *Neuropsychologia, 45,* 2125–2134.

Goldstein, S., & Naglieri, J. A. (2010). *Autism Spectrum Rating Scales: ASRS.* Tonawanda, NY: Multi-Health Systems Inc.

Gothman, K., Risi, S., Dawson, G., Tiger-Flusberg, H., Joseph, R., & Carter, A. (2008). A replication of the autism diagnostic observation schedule (ADOS). Revised algorithms. *Journal of the American Academy of Child and Adolescent Psychiatry, 47*(6), 642–651.

Grether, J., Anderson, M., Croen, L., Smith, D., & Windham, G. (2009). Risk of autism and increasing maternal and paternal age in a large North American population. *American Journal of Epidemiology, 1870*(9), 1118–1126.

Guralnick, M. J. (1998). Effectiveness of early intervention for vulnerable children: A developmental perspective. *American Journal of Mental Retardation, 102,* 319–345.

Hall, S., De Bernardis, M., & Reiss, A. (2006). Social escape behaviors in children with fragile X syndrome. *Journal of Autism and Developmental Disorders, 36,* 935–947.

Harrison, P., & Oakland, T. (2003). *Adaptive Behavior Assessment System: ABAS-II.* San Antonio, TX: Psychological Corporation.

Horsler, K., & Oliver, C. (2006). The behavioral phenotype of Angelman syndrome. *Journal of Intellectual Disability Research, 50,* 33–53.

Jick, H., & Kaye, J. (2003). Epidemiology and possible causes of autism. *Pharmacotherapy, 23,* 1524–1530.

Kagan, J. (2001). Temperamental contributions to affective and behavioral profiles in children. In S. G. Hofmann & P. M. DiBartolo (Eds.), *From social anxiety to social phobia: Multiple perspectives* (pp. 216–234). Needham Heights, MA: Allynand Bacon.

Klin, A., & Volkmar, F. R. (1997). Asperger's syndrome. In D. Cohen and F. R. Volkmar (Eds.), *Handbook of autism and pervasive developmental disorders* (2nd ed.) (pp. 94–122). New York: John Wiley & Sons, Ltd.

Klin, A., Volkmar, F. R., & Sparrow, S. (2000). *Asperger disorder.* New York: Guilford.

Klin, A., Volkmar, F. R., Sparrow, S. S., Cicchetti, D. V., & Rourke, B. P. (1995). Validity and neuropsychological characterization of Asperger syndrome: Convergence with nonverbal learning disabilities syndrome. *Journal of Child Psychology and Psychiatry, 36,* 1127–1140.

Klinger, L. G., & Dawson, G. (1996). Autistic disorder. In E. J. Mash & R. A. Barkley (Eds.), *Child psychopathology* (pp. 311–313). New York: Guilford.

Kolb, B., Brown, R., Witt-Lajeunesse, A., & Gibb, R. (2001). Neural compensations after lesions of the cerebral cortex. *Neural Plasticity, 8,* 1–16.

Kristensen, H. (2000). Selective mutism and comorbidity with developmental disorder/delay, anxiety disorder, and elimination disorder. *Journal of the American Academy of Child and Adolescent Psychiatry, 39,* 249–256.

Kroll, R., & Beitchman, J. H. (2005). Stuttering. In B. Sadock & V. Sadock (Eds.), *Kaplanand Sadock'scomprehensive textbook of psychiatry* (8th ed.) (pp. 3154–3159). Baltimore, MD: Lippincott Williams and Wilkins.

Kurita, H., Koyama, T., Setoya, Y., Shimizu, K., & Osada, H. (2004). Validity of childhood disintegrative disorder apart from autistic disorder with speech loss. *European Child and Adolescent Psychiatry, 13,* 221–226.

Law, J., Boyle, J., Harris, F., Harkness, A., & Nye, C. (2000). Prevalence and natural history of primary speech and language delay: Findings from a systematic review of the literature. *International Journal of Language and Communication Disorders, 35*(2), 165–188.

Lindsay, G., Desforges, M., Dockrell, J., Law, J., Peacey, N., & Beecham, J. (2008). Effective and efficient use of resources in services for children and young people with speech, language and communication needs. Retrieved from http://www.ican.org.uk/~/media/Ican2/Whats%20the%20Issue/Evidence/ICAN_TalkSeries9.ashx

Lord, C., & Bishop, S. L. (2010). Autism spectrum disorders: Diagnosis, prevalence and services for children and families. *Social Policy Report. Society for Research in Child Development, 24*(2).

Lord, C., Rutter, M., Goode, S., Heemsbergen, J., Jordan, H., Maawhood, L., & Schopler, E. (1989). Autism diagnostic observation schedule: A standardized observation of communicative and social behavior. *Journal of Autism and Developmental Disorders, 19*(2), 185–212.

Lovaas, O. I. (1987). Behavioral treatment and normal educational and intellectual functioning of young autistic children. *Journal of Consulting and Clinical Psychology, 55*, 3–9.

Manikam, R., & Perman, J. (2000). Pediatric feeding disorders. *Journal of Clinical Gastroenterology, 30*, 34–46.

McKinnon, D. H., McLeod, S., & Reilly, S. (2007). The prevalence of stuttering, voice, and speech-sound disorders in primary school students in Australia. *Language, Speech, and Hearing Services in Schools, 38*, 5–15.

Miller, J., & Ozonoff, S. (2000). The external validity of Asperger disorder. Lack of evidence from the domain of neuropsychology. *Journal of Abnormal Psychology, 109*(2), 227–238.

Milner, K. M., Craig, E. E., Thompson, R., Veltman, W. M., Thomas, N. S., Roberts, S., . . . Bolton, P. F. (2005). Prader-Willi syndrome: Intellectual abilities and behavioral features by genetic subtype. *Journal of Child Psychology and Psychiatry, 46*, 1089–1096.

Murphy, D., Daly, E., Schmitz, N., Toal, F., Murphy, K., & Curran, S. (2006). Cortical serotonin 5-HT$_{24}$ receptor binding and social communication in adults with Asperger's syndrome: An in vivo SPECT study. *American Journal of Psychiatry, 163*, 934–936.

National Autism Center (2009). National Standards Project – addressing the need for evidence-based practice guidelines for autism spectrum disorders. Retrieved from http://www.nationalautismcenter.org/about/national.php

Nicholson, R., & Szatmari, P. (2003). Genetic and neurodevelopmental influences in autistic disorder. *Canadian Journal of Psychiatry, 48*, 526–537.

Norgate, R. (1998). Reducing self injurious behavior in a child with severe learning difficulties: Enhancing predictability and structure. *Educational Psychology in Practice, 14*, 176–182.

Ozonoff, S., Rogers, S. J., & Pennington, B. F. (1991). Asperger's syndrome: Evidence of an empirical distinction from high-functioning autism. *Journal of Child Psychology and Psychiatry, 32*, 1107–1112.

Panerai, S., Ferrante, L., & Zingale, M. (2002). Benefits of the treatment and education of autistic and communication handicapped children (TEACCH) program as compared with a non-specific approach. *Journal of Intellectual Disability Research, 46*, 318–327.

Pennington, B. F., Moon, J., Edgin, J., Stedron, J., & Nadel, L. (2003). The neuropsychology of Down syndrome: Evidence of hippocampal dysfunction. *Child Development, 74*, 74–93.

Pierce, K., Muller, R. A., Ambrose, J., Allen, G., & Courchesne, E. (2001). Face processing occurs outside the fusiform "face area" in autism: Evidence from functional MRI. *Brain, 124*, 2059–2073.

Pionek Stone, B., Kratochwill, T. R., Sladezcek, I., & Serlin, R. C. (2002). Treatment of selective mutism: A best-evidence synthesis. *School Psychology Quarterly, 17*, 168–190.

Porter, L. (2002). *Educating young children with special needs.* London: Paul Chapman Publishing.

Raitano, N. A., Pennington, B. F., Tunick, R. A., Boada, R., & Shriberg, L. D. (2004). Pre-literacy skills of subgroups of children with speech sound disorders. *Journal of Child Psychology and Psychiatry, 45*, 821–835.

Rapin, I., & Allen, D. A. (1998). The semantic-pragmatic deficit disorder: Classification issues. *International Journal of Language and Communication Disorders, 33*(1), 82–87.

Raven, J. (2003). *Manual for the Raven's Colored Matrices.* San Antonio, TX: Harcourt Assessment.

Raven, J., Raven, J. C., & Court, J. H. (2004). *Manual for Raven's Progressive Matrices and Vocabulary Scales.* San Antonio, TX: Harcourt Assessment.

Reau, N. R., Senturia, Y. D., Lebailly, S. A., & Christoffell, K. K. (1996). Infant and toddler feeding patterns and problems: Normative data and a new direction. *Journal of Developmental and Behavioral Pediatrics, 17,* 149–153.

Reschly, D. J., & Ysseldyke, J. E. (2002). Paradigm shift: The past is not the future. In A. Thomas & J. Grimes (Eds.), *Best practices in school psychology IV* (pp. 3–20). Washington, DC: National Association of School Psychologists.

Rice, M. L., Smith, S. D., & Gayan, J. (2009). Convergent genetic linkage and associations to language, speech and reading measures in families of probands with specific language impairment. *Journal of Neurodevelopmental Disorders, 1,* 264–282.

Rice, M. L., Taylor, C. L., & Zubrick, S. R. (2008). Language outcomes of 7-year-old children with or without a history of late language emergence at 24-months. *Journal of Speech, Language, and Hearing Research, 51,* 394–407.

Richardson, G., Hamel, S. C., & Goldschmidt, L. (1996). The effects of prenatal cocaine use on neonatal neurobehavioral status. *Neurotoxicology and Teratology, 18,* 519–528.

Roberts, C., Mazzucchelli, T., Studman, L., & Sanders, M. (2006). Behavioural family interventions for children with developmental disabilities and behavioural problems. *Journal of Clinical Child and Adolescent Psychology, 35,* 180–193.

Robins, D. L., Fien, D., Barton, M. L., & Green, J. A. (2001). The modified checklist for autism in toddlers: An initial study investigating the early detection of autism and pervasive developmental disorders. *Journal of Autism and Pervasive Developmental Disabilities, 3*(2), 131–144.

Rogers, S. J. (2004). Developmental regression in autism spectrum disorders. *Mental Retardation and Developmental Disabilities Research Reviews, 10,* 139–143.

Roid, G. H. (2003). *Stanford Binet* (5th ed.). Itasca, IL: Riverside Publishing.

Roid, G. H., Gale, H., & Miller, L. J. (1997). *The Leiter International Performance Scales – Revised.* Wood Dale, IL: Stoelting.

Rourke, B. P., Ahmad, S., Collins, D., Jayman-Abello, B., Hayman-Abello, S., & Warriner, E. M. (2002). Child clinical/pediatric neuropsychology: Some recent advances. *Annual Review of Psychology, 53,* 309–339.

Royal College of Psychiatrists. (2012). The child with general learning disability: Factsheet for parents and teachers. Retrieved from http://www.rcpsych.ac.uk/mentalhealthinfo/mentalhealthandgrowingup/learningdisability.aspx

Rutter, M., LeCouteur, A., & Lord, C. (2003). *Autism Diagnostic Interview, Revised.* San Antonio, TX: Pearson.

Sattler, J. M. (2001). *Assessment of children: Cognitive applications* (2nd ed.). San Diego, CA: Jerome M. Sattler.

Sattler, J. M., & Hoge, R. D. (2006). *Assessment of children: Behavioral, social and clinical foundations* (5th ed.). San Diego, CA: Jerome M. Sattler.

Scheeringa, M. S. (2001). The differential diagnosis of impaired reciprocal social interaction in children: A review of disorders. *Child Psychiatry and Human Development, 32*(1), 71–89.

Schonfeld, A., Mattson, S. N., & Lang, A. (2001). Verbal and nonverbal fluency in children with heavy prenatal alcohol exposure. *Journal of Studies on Alcohol, 62,* 239–246.

Schopler, E., Van Bourgondien, M., Wellman, G., & Love, S. (2010). *Childhood Autism Rating Scale – 2nd edition (CARS 2).* Los Angeles, CA: Western Psychological Services.

Schopler, R. (1994). A statewide program for the treatment and education of autistic and related communication handicapped children (TEACCH). *Psychology and Pervasive Developmental Disorders, 3,* 91–103.

Schweinhart, L. J., Barnes, H. V., & Weikart, D. P. (1993). *Significant benefits: The High/Scope Perry Preschool Study through age 27. Monographs of the High/Scope Educational Research Foundation,* no. 10. Ypsilanti, MI: High/Scope Press.

Scott, S., & Beidel, D. C. (2011). Selective mutism: An update and suggestions for futureresearch. *Current Psychiatry Reports, 13,* 251–257.

Sharp, W. G., Jaquess, D. L., Morton, J. F., & Herzinger, C. V. (2010). Pediatric feeding disorders: A quantitative synthesis of treatment outcomes. *Clinical Child and Family Psychology Review, 13*, 348–365.

Shriberg, L. D., Kwiatkowski, J., & Gruber, F. A. (1994). Developmental phonological disorders II: Short-term speech sound normalization. *Journal of Speech and Hearing Research, 37*, 1127–1147.

Shriberg, L. D., Tomblin, B. J., & McSweeny, J. L. (1999). Prevalence of speech delay in 6-year-old children and comorbidity with language impairment. *Journal of Speech, Language, and Hearing Research, 42*(6), 1461–1481.

Stattin, H., & Klackenberg-Larsson, I. (1993). Early language and intelligence development and their relationship to future criminal behavior. *Journal of Abnormal Psychology, 102*, 369–378.

Steinhausen, H., & Juzi, C. (1996). Elective mutism: An analysis of 100 cases. *Journal of the American Academy of Child and Adolescent Psychiatry, 35*, 606–614.

Stone, W., Coonrod, E. E., & Ousley, O. Y. (2000). Brief report: Screening tools for autism in two year olds (STAT) developmental and preliminary data. *Journal of Autism and Pervasive Developmental Disabilities, 30*(6), 607–612.

Streissguth, A. P., Bookstein, F. L., & Barr, H. M. (2004). Risk factors for adverse life outcomes in fetal alcohol syndrome and fetal alcohol effects. *Journal of Developmental and Behavioral Pediatrics, 25*, 228–238.

Szatmari, P., Stelios, G., Bryson, S., Zwaigenbaum, L., Roberts, W., Mahoney, W., . . . Tuff, L. (2006). Investigating the structure of the restricted, repetitive behaviors and interests domain of autism. *Journal of Child Psychology and Psychiatry, 47*, 582–590.

Thomason, M. J., Lord, J., Bain, M. D., Chalmers, R. A. Littlejohns, P., Addison, G. M., . . . Seymour, C. A. (1998). A systematic review of evidence for the appropriateness of neonatal screening programmes for inborn errors of metabolism. *Journal of Public Mental Health, 20*, 331–343.

Tomblin, J. B., Records, N. L., Buckwalter, P., Zhang, X., Smith, E., & O'Brien, M. (1997). Prevalence of specific language impairment in kindergarten children. *Journal of Speech and Hearing Research, 40*(6), 1245–1260.

Tomblin, J. B., Records, N. L., & Zhang, X. (1996). A system for the diagnosis of specific language impairment in kindergarten children. *Journal of Speech and Hearing Research, 39*(6), 1284–1294.

Tomblin, J. B., Zhang, X. Y., Buckwalter, P., & Catts, H. (2000). The association of reading disability, behavioral disorders, and language impairment among second grade children. *Journal of Child Psychology and Psychiatry and Allied Disciplines, 41*, 473–482.

Tomblin, J. B., Zhang, X. Y., Buckwalter, P., & O'Brien, M. (2003). The stability of language disorder: Four years after kindergarten diagnosis. *Journal of Speech, Language, and Hearing Research, 46*, 1283–1296.

Tomblin, J. B., Zhang, X., Weiss, A., Catts, H., & Ellis Weismer, S. (2004). Dimensions of individual differences in communication skills among primary grade children. In M. L. Rice & S. F. Warren (Eds.), *Developmental language disorders: From phenotypes to etiologies* (pp. 53–76). Mahwah, NJ: Erlbaum.

Vicari, S. (2006). Motor development and neuropsychological patterns in persons with Down syndrome. *Behavior Genetics, 36*, 355–364.

Volkmar, F. R., Klin, A., Siegel, B., Szatmari, P., Lord. C., & Campbell, M. (1994). Field trial for autistic disorder in DSM–IV. *American Journal of Psychiatry, 151*(9), 1361–1367.

Volkmar, F. R., Szatmari, P., & Sparrow, S. (1993). Gender differences in pervasive developmental disorders. *Journal of Autism and Developmental Disorders, 23*, 579–591.

Wechsler, D. (2002a). *Wechsler Preschool and Primary Intelligence Test: WPPSI-III.* San Antonio, TX: Pearson.

Wechsler, D. (2002b). *Wechsler Intelligence Scale for Children: WISC-IV.* San Antonio, TX: Pearson.

Wigren, M., & Hansen, S. (2005). ADHD symptoms and insistence on sameness in Prader-Willi syndrome. *Journal of Intellectual Disability Research, 49*, 449–456.

Wilczynski, S. M., Fisher, L., Sutro, L., Bass, J., Mudgal, D., Zeiger, V., . . . Logue, J. (2011). Evidence-based practice and autism spectrum disorders. In M. A. Bray & T. J. Kehle (Eds.), *The Oxford handbook of school psychology* (pp. 567–592). New York: Oxford University Press.

Wilmshurst, L., & Brue, A. (2005). *A parent's guide to special education.* New York: AMACOM.

Woodbury-Smith, M., Klin, A., & Volkmar, F. (2005). Asperger's syndrome: A comparison of clinical diagnoses and those made according to the ICD-10 and DSM-IV. *Journal of Autism and Developmental Disorders, 35*, 235–240.

World Health Organization (WHO). (1996). *ICD-10 guide for mental retardation.* Geneva: Author.

Wright, C., & Birks, E. (2000). Risk factors for failure to thrive; A population-based survey. *Child Care, Health and Development, 26*, 5–16.

Young, A., Beitchman, J. H., Johnson, C. J., Atkinson, L., Escobar, M., Douglas, L., & Wilson, B. (2002). Young adult academic outcomes in a longitudinal sample of speech/language impaired and control children. *Journal of Child Psychology and Psychiatry and Allied Disciplines, 43*(5), 635–645.

Zubrick, R. R., Taylor, C. L., Rice, M. L., & Slegers, D. (2007). Late language emergence at 24 months: An epidemiological study of prevalence and covariates. *Journal of Speech, Language and Hearing Research, 50*, 1562–1592.

8

Problems of Learning and Attention

Clinical and Educational Child Psychology, First Edition. Linda Wilmshurst.
© 2013 John Wiley & Sons, Ltd. Published 2013 by John Wiley & Sons, Ltd.

Chapter preview and learning objectives

In *Chapter 7*, readers were introduced to intellectual disabilities and pervasive develop-mental disorders (autism spectrum disorders) that pose life-long challenges to children and adolescents. Readers were also acquainted with communication disorders and impairments that influence speech and language, often accompanying other disorders or representing a more specific area of impairment in their own right. In this chapter, we look more closely at disorders that can have far-reaching implications, socially, behaviorally, and emotionally, but whose main impact is evident in the specific chal-lenges associated with unique types of learning difficulties. Children and adolescents with specific learning disabilities (SLD) often have average intelligence and can have above-average skills in some areas, relative to significant weaknesses in others. As a result, children with learning disabilities are not a homogeneous group and can present a complex mix of characteristics. Even within categories of disabilities, unique patterns of strengths and weaknesses can be evident. Readers will gain an increased understanding of the nature of the different types of learning disabilities; how they influence learning at different developmental levels; as well as the causes, prevalence, and interventions that can help children with SLD at home and at school.

Children with SLD often experience other comorbid disorders, such as attention deficit hyperactivity disorder (ADHD), which will also be discussed at length in this chapter. Although most individuals are familiar with the hyperactive-impulsive form of the disorder, fewer realize that there are three variants of ADHD, and that some children only have the inattentive type of ADHD. After reading this chapter, readers will have an increased appreciation of the challenges facing individuals with ADHD.

Specific learning disabilities: an overview

The area of specific learning disabilities (SLD) has inspired debates concerning how the disability is best defined and how children with SLD are best identified. Children with a SLD have problems learning specific types of information, while their skills remain intact in areas unrelated to their disability. For our purposes, after a general discussion of the global nature and course of SLD, there will be a more detailed discussion of five specific types of SLD: disorders of reading, disorders of written expression, disorders of mathematics, nonverbal learning disabilities, and disabilities related to motor skills (dyspraxia, or developmental coordination disorder).

Definition of specific learning disabilities   The following definition of a SLD is dictated by federal special education law in the United States and has remained unchanged since its inception in the mid-1970s. As such, a SLD is defined as:

> a disorder in one or more of the basic psychological processes involved in understanding, or in using language, spoken or written, that may manifest itself in the imperfect ability to listen, think, speak, read, write, spell or do mathematical calculations, including conditions such as perceptual disabilities, brain injury, minimal brain dysfunction, dyslexia and developmental aphasia. Specific learning disability does not include learning problems that are primarily the result of visual, hearing or motor disabilities, of mental retardation, of emotional disturbance, or of environmental, cultural or economic disadvantage.
>
> (*Federal Register*, 2006, 300.8 (10), p. 46757)

SLD: nature and course

Hallahan and Mercer (2001) chronicle the history of specific learning disabilities (SLD), from Kussmaul's discovery of "word blindness" in an otherwise intact individual in 1897, to Hinshelwood's publication on congenital word blindness in 1917 that ushered in an era of investigation and discussions surrounding the nature and course of SLD. Because reading problems were found to exist, in spite of average ability, the importance of using intelligence as the benchmark for judging performance relative to ability became an integral part of the definition of SLD. As a result, the use of the discrepancy criterion became the main tool to identify the existence of SLD (the difference between a student's ability and expected achievement, relative to actual achievement). The discrepancy criterion has been recognized by the DSM (APA, 2000) and the ICD (WHO, 1993) as the definitive means of identifying children with SLD based on a significant discrepancy between achievement and IQ, with achievement "substantially below" IQ, which "is usually defined as a discrepancy of more than 2 standard deviations" (APA, 2000, p. 49). Exclusionary criteria require that the disorder not be due to a sensory deficit, or go beyond what would be expected given a sensory deficit. In the ICD-10 (WHO, 1993), specific developmental disorders of scholastic skills (SDDSS) recognizes learning problems in three academic areas (reading, spelling, and arithmetic skills). As for the on-going revisions of the DSM-5 and ICD-11, it is uncertain whether the DSM will shift criteria to align better with the Individuals with Disabilities Education Act (IDEA), and if so, how this might influence revisions of ICD-11. The current status of the debate will be revisited shortly, when the results of the Expert Panel White Paper (LDA, 2010) are addressed. But first, it is important to review some of the initial concerns surrounding exclusive use of the discrepancy criterion in the identification of students with SLD in the United States.

Issues in identification

The discrepancy criteria   Growing discontent regarding the exclusive use of the discrepancy criteria in the identification of SLD was based on a number of difficulties, including: lack of consistency in definitions and application (the lack of a universal protocol resulted in wide variations in the actual discrepancies used); an inherent bias towards the extremes (older children and those with higher IQs were more likely to meet the discrepancy criteria than younger children and those with lower IQs); use of a failure-based model; Matthew effects (poor readers acquire cumulative deficits lowering overall IQ; Stanovich, 1986); and lack of research support for the discrepancy criteria (Stanovich, 1991).

As a result, the latest revision of the law (IDEA, 2004) added an alternative method of identification for SLD, termed response to intervention (RTI), which allowed for the option of identification of SLD based on the child's failure to respond to a scientific, research-based intervention (*Federal Register*, 2006, 300.307(a), p. 46789).

Response to intervention (RTI) The proposed RTI system met with criticism, including concerns that RTI fractured the connection between the historical definition of SLD as a disorder in "the basic psychological processes" (IDEA, 2004) and the proposed identification procedures which in essence ignored assessment of cognitive processing deficits. According to Kavale (2005), "changes to the operational definition (RTI) without changes to the formal definition are indefensible" and result in a "disconnect between the formal definition and the operational definition" (p. 553). Semrud-Clikeman (2005) noted that RTI ignored intellectual ability which was crucial to developing an appropriate intervention, and that RTI was a failure-based system of identification based on a student's failure to respond to intervention.

Current conceptualizations The Learning Disabilities Association of America (LDA) responded to changes in legislation by preparing a working paper, the Expert Panel White Paper (LDA, 2010), based on responses from 56 professionals recognized by their peers for expertise in the area of SLD. The report addresses altered identification procedures for SLD which allow for bypassing consideration of the cognitive nature of the disorder in the decision-making process, and for determination of lack of achievement based on age or grade level criteria, rather than ability. The report suggests a number of recommendations, including: strengthening identification procedures to match the definition of SLD; recognition that students with SLD require individualized interventions, not more intensive general interventions (i.e., more of the same); and the use of cognitive and neuropsychological assessments to identify strengths and weaknesses for the purposes of developing interventions based on the learning profile.

Specific types of learning disabilities

Prevalence rates for SLD have been estimated to be somewhere between 2% and 10% of the population (APA, 2000). The following discussion will focus on five different types of disabilities, evident in disabilities in reading, writing, mathematics, nonverbal learning, and motor skills (coordination, including handwriting). A summary of these variations is available in Table 8.1.

Specific reading disability (dyslexia)

Traditionally, children with a reading disability (dyslexia) experience a significant discrepancy between general cognitive ability (IQ which is usually in the average range or above) and achievement in reading (which is significantly below IQ, by about 2 standard deviations). The disability is not the result of inadequate teaching, impaired sensory processes (vision or hearing problems), or second language factors. Reading problems can occur in **decoding** words (the recognition of sound/symbol association), and/or reading **comprehension** (understanding the meaning). Either or

Table 8.1　Types of specific learning disability

Disability	Nature of disability	Associated problems
Dyslexia	Reading disability	Problems with decoding, comprehension, fluency of reading. Associated problems may also be evident in spelling and speaking.
Dysgraphia	Disability in written expression	Problems in executing written responses, organizing information, sequencing ideas, grammatical structure, and handwriting.
Dyscalculia	Disability in mathematics	Problems with "number sense," estimation of quantity, money, spatial configurations, concept of time, recall for number facts, and problem solving using numbers.
Nonverbal learning disability	Disability in visuospatial areas	Problems associated with right hemisphere dysfunction, evident in poor mathematics ability, poor interpretation of symbols (numbers, graphs, charts), and poor sense of proprioception (sense of body in space), balance, and social pragmatics.
Dyspraxia	Developmental coordination disorder (DCD)	Problems with fine and gross motor skills, physical coordination, posture, eye–hand coordination, balance, and manual dexterity.

both of these processes can significantly influence reading *fluency* (the ability to read with appropriate speed and in an uninterrupted manner).

Definition of reading disability　Dyslexia (a specific reading disability) is defined as:

> a specific learning disability that is neurobiological in origin. It is characterized by difficulties with accurate and/or fluent word recognition and by poor spelling and decoding abilities. These difficulties typically result from a deficit in phonological component of language that is often unexpected in relation to other cognitive abilities and the provision of effective classroom instruction.
>
> (Lyon & Shaywitz, 2003, p. 2)

Although identification of low academic achievement (in, for example, reading, written expression, or mathematics) is the hallmark of a SLD (Johnson, Humphrey, Mellard, Woods, & Swanson, 2010), how intelligence and underlying cognitive processes influence the development and course of SLD remains an area of enquiry. In their longitudinal study of 232 children in grades 1 through 12, Ferrer et al. (2010) found that while *typical readers* evidence a bidirectional influence between IQ and reading, *compensated readers* (who eventually master reading, but are not fluent readers) and *persistently poor readers* demonstrate a "disruption in the interconnection between IQ and reading over time" (p. 99). Ferrer et al. (2010) suggest that in typical readers there is a naturally occurring feedback loop (coupling) between IQ and reading, as reading opens the door for the acquisition of increased vocabulary and general knowledge which in turn enhances IQ. However, for those who are *compensated readers* or *persistently poor readers*, the "Matthew effect" (Stanovich, 1986) takes over, producing an ever widening gap between good and poor readers. Furthermore, poor reading may also negatively impact the development of language and intellectual functioning.

Characteristics of dyslexia are most evident in problems of **accuracy** in decoding skills in the primary grades; however, by adolescence and adulthood, even if accuracy improves, **fluency** issues (slow and labored reading) become the signature characteristic of dyslexia (Ferrer et al., 2010). Shaywitz and Shaywitz (2008, p. 1343) suggest that fluency issues justify the need for extra time on "high stakes standardized tests such as the SATs, GMAT, GRE" since students with dyslexia are at "a disadvantage compared to nondyslexic peers."

Nature and course

Developmental characteristics   Younger children may experience problems with pre-reading skills, such as learning the alphabet; recognizing letters, numbers, or shapes; word retrieval; and rhyming tasks. Reading instruction in the primary grades may be halted due to the child's inability to attach the correct sound to a letter, tendency to blend sounds together or confuse similar-looking words (mirror reading or writing; for example, saw for was), or difficulty in sequencing letters correctly. Because there are wide variations in skills and abilities due to different levels of exposure to reading materials, some children may demonstrate lags and then "catch up," while others continue to fall further and further behind. By third grade, reading problems become more noticeable, and in subsequent grades children with dyslexia will often begin to use avoidance to escape the embarrassment of reading out loud. As reading demands increase, children may become overwhelmed with the pace of reading demonstrated by their peers. If they are able to master decoding and word recognition, they may not be able to read for comprehension due to problems processing information in a way that retains the sequence of information in a meaningful way. Other difficulties that can be exhibited by children with dyslexia include problems following directions and responding to questions in an organized and timely manner.

Children and adolescents with dyslexia also often exhibit executive functioning deficits (working memory, self-monitoring, self-regulation (inhibition), and metacognitive skills), the identification of which can be instrumental in developing successful interventions (Semrud-Clikeman, 2005).

Prevalence and etiology

Prevalence   The prevalence rates for dyslexia range from 5% to 17%, depending on the definitions used and the populations sampled (Ferrer et al., 2010). Although the majority of sources report dyslexia accounts for 80% of all SLD (APA, 2000; Lerner, 1989), Mayes and Calhoun (2007) have challenged this assumption based on results from a clinical population (containing 485 children) that revealed written expression (92%) as the most common form of SLD.

Genetic influences   Dyslexia is a highly heritable disorder with at least half (50%) of the variance in the disorder explained by genetics (Olson & Byrne, 2005), with recent investigations focusing on the influence of DCDC2 contained on chromosome 6 (Schumacher, Anthoni, Dahdou, Konig, & Hillmer, 2006). Between 23% and 65% of children with dyslexia have parents with dyslexia, while 40% of children with dyslexia have a sibling with the disorder (Pennington & Gilger, 1996). Although more boys are referred and identified, there are a significant number of girls who also are dyslexic (Flynn & Rahbar, 1994).

Neurological systems and dyslexia   Several studies have pinpointed deficits in phonological processing in children with dyslexia, and interventions targeting weaknesses in the area have met with success (Torgesen, 2000). Other cognitive processing deficits associated with dyslexia include: expressive and receptive language, processing speed (Flanagan, Ortiz, Alfonso, & Dynda, 2006; Pennington, 2009), and verbal working memory (Swanson, 2009). In their meta-analysis of 32 studies investigating cognitive processes associated with SLD, Johnson et al. (2010) suggest that based on the magnitude of effect sizes, future studies should focus on: working memory, processing speed, executive function, and receptive and expressive language.

Using functional magnetic resonance imaging (fMRI) technology, researchers have found that normal readers access three areas of the left hemisphere of the brain to accomplish specific tasks: phoneme recognition (**anterior system: left frontal gyrus**); mapping sound to letter form (**posterior system: parietotemporal region**); and storage of sight vocabulary for rapid identification in the future (**posterior system: occipitotemporal region**). The occipitotemporal region, also termed the **visual word-form area (VWFA**; Cohen et al., 2000), is an integral component of reading fluency. Developmentally, neural pathways for reading mature from the posterior regions (visual perceptual processes, letter and word naming) to the frontal regions (activated in reading comprehension), and from the right hemisphere to the left. However, individuals with dyslexia show low activation of the left posterior systems and compensate by using both the left and right anterior systems, and the right posterior VWFA (Shaywitz & Shaywitz, 2008). See Figure 8.1 for an illustration.

Attention and dyslexia   Based on the discrepancy criteria used, prevalence rates for comorbid ADHD and dyslexia are reported to be as high as 38–45% (Dykman & Ackerman, 1991). Reynolds and Besner (2006) have focused on the attentional aspects of reading, and suggest that attention is crucial to the reading process and essential to translating print into speech for fluent reading. The neurological system that maintains attention, particularly the prefrontal cortex, is regulated by the release of catecholamines (dopamine, norepinephrine). Compared to controls, children with ADHD show less activity in the prefrontal and frontal cortex, caudate nucleus, cerebellum, and parietal cortex (Casey, Nigg, & Durston, 2007; Epstein et al., 2007). The posterior parietal cortex plays a significant role in both the regulation of attention and dyslexia through its connection to the prefrontal cortex. In this way, activation of the prefrontal areas may serve to active the posterior reading systems. Shaywitz and Shaywitz (2008, p. 1343) suggest that contemporary research has demonstrated that "attentional mechanisms play a critical role in reading and that disruption of these attentional mechanisms plays a causal role in reading difficulties."

Assessment and treatment/intervention

Assessment   An initial assessment for dyslexia includes an evaluation of reading achievement in decoding, fluency, and reading comprehension. Whether an

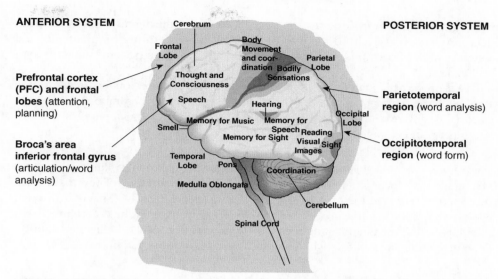

Figure 8.1 Neural systems involved in reading. Normal readers access the left hemisphere: an anterior system (inferior frontal gyrus) and posterior systems (parietotemporal region and occipitotemporal region). Individuals with dyslexia compensate for poor processing in the left hemisphere by increased activation of the inferior frontal gyrus and occipitotemporal regions in the right hemisphere.

assessment should include measures of cognitive ability has been a matter of debate among educators, researchers, professionals, and policy makers. As emphasized by Johnson et al. (2010), the importance of identifying the underlying deficits in cognitive processes is at the basis of the definition of and eventual intervention for SLD. In their paper, Johnson et al. (2010) recommend cognitive assessments for reading disability (RD) are needed to detect:

- normal psychometric intelligence;
- below-normal achievement in reading;
- below-normal performance in specific cognitive processes;
- deficits in isolated cognitive processes that persist despite exposure to evidence-based instruction;
- that cognitive processing deficits are not directly caused by environmental factors or contingencies (e.g., low socio-economic status).

Intervention   Although RTI has been suggested as the first line of intervention, there is evidence from meta-analytic sources (Tran, Sanchez, Arellano, & Swanson, 2011) that children with higher IQ scores than reading scores are less responsive to treatment than children whose IQ and achievement scores share the same lower range. Furthermore, research shows that reading difficulties persist and do not subside with time. According to Shaywitz, Morris, & Shaywitz (2008), this important finding "should put an end to the unsupported, but unfortunately, too widely held notion that reading problems are outgrown or somehow represent a developmental lag" (p. 470).

Shaywitz and Shaywitz (2008) questioned whether neural systems involved in reading could be malleable and change given the appropriate reading intervention. In an experiment involving dyslexic readers in the second and third grades, the researchers demonstrated that given 50 minutes of daily individual tutoring on phonemes and sound symbol associations, subjects increased brain activation patterns similar to typical readers.

Based on a meta-analysis of empirically supported interventions for reading, the Report of the National Reading Panel (2000) highlights five components that are essential to any reading instruction program: phonemic awareness, phonics, fluency, vocabulary, and reading comprehension.

Early intervention/prevention   Programs that target children in kindergarten and first grade and focus on phonemic awareness and the meaning of text have been successful in reducing the rates of at-risk students to less than 5% (Shaywitz, Morris, & Shaywitz, 2008). These programs have offered instruction in the classroom (Fuchs & Fuchs, 2005), or pullout programs (Vellutino, Scanlon, Small, & Fanuele, 2006), or some combination of the two (Vaughn, Linar-Thompson, & Hickman, 2003).

Later interventions   Results with older children and adolescents are not as promising as those for early intervention, and although accuracy may be improved considerably, fluency often remains a serious issue. Programs which have been successful in improving accuracy include those focusing on direct instruction (phonological analysis) and metacognitive strategies (Lovett, Barron, & Benson, 2003).

The majority of programs that address fluency issues use a repeated readings approach (Meyer & Felton, 1999) which involves reading a passage repeatedly, timing the speed of reading and accuracy by recording the reading on tape. Repeated readings with scaffolding (support by peers or teachers) have been successful in improving fluency for children with dyslexia (Kuhn & Stahl, 2003). Comprehension-focused instruction often emphasizes strategies and critical thinking skills related to reading for meaning.

Disorders of written expression (dysgraphia)

Compared to research on reading disorders, investigation concerning written expression has lagged far behind (Hooper, Swartz, Wakely, de Kruif, & Montgomery, 2002), especially regarding the nature of neurocognitive processes involved in executing written tasks.

Definition of disorders of written expression   Part of the difficulty in amassing information about problems in written expression is the difficulty in defining and assessing the problem area. According to the DSM (APA, 2000), a disorder of written expression includes the "composition of written texts (e.g., writing grammatically correct sentences and organized paragraphs," which may include multiple spelling errors and poor handwriting but excludes "a disorder in spelling or handwriting alone, in the absence of other difficulties of written expression" (p. 56). Measurement of the discrepancy between ability and achievement in written expression is similar to the criteria used for measurement of achievement in reading and includes "an individually administered standardized test, *or functional assessment.*" The reason for inclusion of the "functional assessment" is that evaluation may include a review of samples of a child's written schoolwork. Furthermore, the DSM states that "if poor handwriting is due to impairment in motor coordination, then a diagnosis of developmental coordination disorder should be considered" (APA, 2000, p. 56).

Nature and course   Disabilities in written expression may manifest in a number of different errors, including: sentences with punctuation and grammatical errors; poor organizational presentation; and delays in initiating written responses. Early warning signs may be evident in poor ability to copy words correctly, or in letter reversals or transpositions; however, identification can be delayed since demands for written work are often minimal in the first grade program, and delays may remit in some children. Often children with problems in written expression experience reading disorders, mathematics disorders, or both (Mayes & Calhoun, 2007). The process of writing is complex and involves a number of stages and composite skills, including: planning, generating content, organizing the composition, translating content into written language, and revising and improving the writing (Reid & Ortiz Lienemann, 2006).

In their study of the writing process, Berninger and Rutberg (1992) found that young children's early fine motor planning and control were related to success or lack of it in later written expression. Other neurological factors and executive functions that have been implicated in the writing process include: memory, attention, graphomotor output, sequential processing, and higher order verbal and visual-spatial functions (Hooper et al., 2002). In particular, executive functions associated with the prefrontal cortex have been of increased interest to researchers investigating written expression. Given this direction, it is not surprising to see a number of studies that have investigated written expression in children with ADHD which is primarily a disorder of executive function. Children with ADHD have been found to have significantly more problems in transcription skills (handwriting, copying) and spelling than their non-disabled peers (Imhof, 2004; MTA Cooperative Group, 1999).

Prevalence and etiology   According to Mayes and Calhoun (2007), prevalence rates for problems of written expression have been underestimated, especially in clinical populations, where written problems were the most prevalent form of learning disability. Developmentally, prevalence rates for writing problems escalate from 1.3–2.7% in primary-grade children (Berninger & Hart, 1992), to 6–22% of middle school children (Hooper et al., 2002). Although research into the root causes of dyslexia has been prolific, few studies have explored the etiology of disabilities in written expression, and, as a result, little is known about potential causes of the disorder.

Assessment and intervention

Assessment   Identification of written expression problems can depend on the assessment instrument used. Mayes, Calhoun, and Lane (2005) compared results from the Woodcock-Johnson (1989) *Written Language Subtests* (which measures achievement for the production of single words and single sentences) with results from the Wechsler Individual Achievement Test (WIAT; Psychological Corporation, 1992) *Written Expression Subtest* (which assesses compositional writing skills). While the Woodcock-Johnson identified 35% of children as having significant writing problems, the WIAT identified 78% of the sample as having significant problems in written expression. The authors suggest that compositional writing is a more complex task and should be assessed in determining whether an individual has significant problems in written expression.

Intervention   Direct instruction in writing strategy (planning) using prompts and mnemonics with guided feedback and self-regulatory procedures can improve the quality of writing for students with writing disabilities (Vaughn, Gersten, & Chard, 2000; Graham, Harris, & Larsen, 2001). In students with ADHD and comorbid writing disabilities, Reid and Ortiz Lienemann (2006) found that the use of a Self-Regulated Strategy Development (SRSD) model, stressing goal setting and self-monitoring, was instrumental in increasing the amount and quality of written work produced by children with ADHD who had comorbid writing problems.

Accommodations that circumvent the writing process can also be beneficial for children with severe writing problems and who would otherwise not be able to disseminate their ideas. For these students, dictated passages have been found to be superior to written essays (Graham, Harris, & Larsen, 2001) and students may also benefit from using speech recognition software (Reid & Ortiz Lienemann, 2006), or keyboards and word processors (Graham et al., 2001; MacArthur, 2000). Accommodations such as providing access to class notes, use of a scribe, study guides, outlines, and modified test taking through increased time or reduced written content (filling in blanks, multiple choice, oral exams) can also increase students' opportunities for academic success (Reid & Ortiz Lienemann, 2006).

Specific mathematics disability/mathematics learning disability (MLD/dyscalculia)

Definition   Children with dyscalculia have limitations in mathematical areas involving "number sense," problem solving, and fluency in retrieving mathematical facts (Geary, Brown, & Samaranayake, 1991). Research into cognitive processing deficits that impact performance in mathematics are not as readily available as those in reading; however, deficits have been suggested in a number of areas associated with executive functions, including: visual and verbal working memory, processing speed, and attention (Fuchs et al., 2005; Geary, 2004; Swanson & Jerman, 2006).

Nature and course   Geary, Hamson, and Hoard (2000) suggest that problems in charting the course and in the identification of MLD are compounded by variability in performance and the types of assessment instruments used. For example, some students may show low achievement levels in one grade but average levels in another. The variability may be related to the specific concept taught (e.g., some may struggle with division, others with fractions), or other factors (such as emotional difficulties). Furthermore, instruments that use composite scores for evaluating mathematical performance may not be sensitive to severe gaps and weaknesses in specific areas. Compared to those with intermittent performance, children who have MLD experience mathematics problems as a result of cognitive or memory deficits, which are persistent, and often treatment-resistant. These problems are evident in deficits in **calculation fluency** (Gersten, Jordan, & Flojo, 2005) and early acquisition of **number sense** (the ability to estimate, judge quantity, and sequence).

Prevalence and etiology   Estimates suggest that 5–10% of children enrolled in the educational system will meet criteria for MLD (Barbaresi, Katusic, Collagin, Weaver, & Jacobsen, 2005; Shalev, Manor, & Gross-Tsur, 2005). The two main approaches to understanding MLD involve a domain-general approach and a domain-specific approach (Mazzocco, Feigenson, & Halberda, 2011). The former approach seeks to answer questions about how and why some children develop MLD and focuses on cognitive systems and executive functions such as phonological skills, working memory, long-term memory, visuospatial processing (Geary, 1993), and genetic pre-dispositions to MLD (Plomin & Kovas, 2005). Other researchers focus on specific processing deficits, such as number processing skills or "number sense," and how these skill deficits relate to MLD (Dehaene, Piazza, Pinel, & Cohen, 2003; Mazzocco, Feigenson, & Halberda, 2011).

Findings from domain-general research   Heritability rates for general mathematics disability (43%) and reading disability (47%) suggest far more genetic than environmental influence (Kovas et al., 2007; Plomin & Kovas, 2005). Plomin and Kovas (2005) suggest a "Generalist Genes Hypothesis" of learning abilities and disabilities based on twin studies that have demonstrated high genetic correlations (averaging 0.68) between reading and mathematics ability, suggesting extensive genetic overlap. However, since the correlation is not perfect, Kovas, Harlaar, Petrill, and Plomin (2005) estimate that approximately a third of the genetic variance in mathematics is independent of reading and general intelligence (g).

Inherent in MLD are processing problems, such as problems of executive functions (attention, short-term memory) and deficits in visual-spatial functioning, that may contribute to poor alignment of numbers or faulty understanding of place value systems, or charts and maps (Geary, 2003). Children who repeatedly use their fingers for counting may be using this strategy to make up for deficits in working memory (Geary, 2000).

Findings from domain-specific research   Mazzocco, Feigenson, and Halberda (2011) investigated deficits in the Approximate Number System (ANS) in 71 ninth graders. The ANS is an implicit system that is universally evident at an early age in normally developing children and involves the use of "number sense" in making judgments about the relative size or quantity of one array compared to another. In their paper describing the process, Mazzocco et al., (2011) use the example of "selecting a checkout line" in a store based on the number of people lined up. Results from their study suggest that children with MLD demonstrated significantly poorer ANS acuity compared to peers without MLD, even when controlling for more general cognitive abilities.

Assessment and intervention/prevention   There has been a consolidated effort to develop and research valid early screening measures for mathematics proficiency (Gersten, Jordan, & Flojo, 2005). The *Number Knowledge Test* (Okamoto & Case, 1996) is a screening device that provides good predictive validity for early skills in basic mathematical concepts, operations, number sense, and counting.

Because mathematics is a cumulative area of knowledge, emphasis has focused on early identification and prevention. Morgan, Farkas, and Wu (2011) recently investigated the learning trajectories for a large sample of children (7400) from kindergarten to grade 5, in children with LD (specific learning disabilities, in reading and/or mathematics), SLI (speech and language impairment), and controls. Results revealed Matthew effects (i.e., the poor get poorer) for children with MLD but not for those with reading disabilities, suggesting the importance of early intervention/prevention in this population.

Results from early intervention programs and prevention initiatives have found that significant time and practice must be devoted to strengthening mathematical concepts. For example, in one study, small-group first grade intervention, four days per week for 15 minutes per session over the course of 18 weeks, yielded no significant effect on mathematics ability for students in the program (Bryant, Bryant, Gersten, Scammacca, & Chavez, 2008). However, in a follow-up study, extending the time to 20-minute sessions four days per week over the course of 23 weeks did reveal a significant positive effect (Bryant, Bryant, Gersten, Scammacca, Funk et al., 2008). Other studies have had mixed results. For example, Fuchs et al. (2006) found that their computer fact retrieval system increased student facility for addition facts, but not subtraction. In their review of intervention programs, Gersten et al. (2005) stress the importance of assessment and intervention in areas of discrimination of quantity (such as using number lines) and identification of numbers.

Nonverbal learning disabilities (NLD)

Definition   Rourke and colleagues (Rourke, 1982, 2000; Rourke, Hayman-Abello, & Collins, 2003) have distinguished a type of learning disability which is distinct from other learning disabilities due to an emphasis on the nonverbal aspects of information processing, compared to problems resulting from a **basic phonological processing disorder** (**BPPD**) associated with reading and writing disabilities. As a result, children with a **nonverbal learning disability** (**NLD**) will evidence right hemisphere dysfunction (Mattson, Sheer, & Fletcher, 1992) and problems in visual-spatial processing, unlike those with BPPD who demonstrate deficits in the left hemisphere. The syndrome is characterized by "significant primary deficits in some dimensions of tactile perception, visual perception, complex psychomotor skills and in dealing with novel circumstances" (Rourke et al., 2002, p. 311). The disability has also been referred to in the literature as **developmental right-hemisphere syndrome** (Gross-Tsur, Shalev, Manor, & Amir, 1995) and **visuospatial learning disability** (Cornoldi, Venneri, Marconato, Molin, & Montinari, 2003).

Nature and course   Characteristics of children with NLD may include clumsiness, poor coordination, and a poor sense of spatial awareness, especially of their body in space and social/personal space. In their study of children with NLD, Gross-Tsur et al. (1995) found the vast majority experienced problems with slow processing speed both cognitively and motorically (80%), graphomotor impairment (90%), and dyscalculia (67%). Visual memory, including immediate memory for faces, was also impaired for children with NLD (Liddell & Rasmussen, 2005). In their study of measures of social perception, Semrud-Clikeman, Walkowiak, Wilkinson, and Minne (2010) found that children with NLD and Asperger disorder evidenced impairment in reading social and emotional cues and were more likely to exhibit sadness and social withdrawal compared to controls. Studies have demonstrated that children with NLD experience many deficits in social functioning, including poor ability to understand social rules, pragmatic language, eye contact, and facial expressions (Gross-Tsur et al., 1995).

Reluctance to engage in novel situations or tasks, and social withdrawal, can have negative long-term outcomes for individuals with NLD, resulting in increased risk for depression and suicide (Rourke, 1995). Comorbid ADHD is not uncommon in those with NLD.

Prevalence and etiology The prevalence of NLD is rare (0.1%); however, cases may remain undiagnosed or misdiagnosed (e.g., as Asperger disorder) due to the lack of understanding or familiarity with of this type of learning disability. Unlike other learning disabilities, the male to female ratio is equal for NLD. While other forms of learning disabilities have a strong genetic component, NLD is related more to brain structure and function.

The white matter model

According to Rourke (1982, 1995), the etiology of NLD is best explained by deficits (destruction or dysfunction) in the white matter that impairs the ability to access the right hemisphere to integrate information cross-modally.

Assessment and treatment/intervention Given the neurological basis for NLD, a neuropsychological examination is recommended which evaluates functioning in a wide range of areas tapping motor and psychomotor functions, including: grip strength, eye tracking, visual-spatial organization, and other neuropsychological functions. Assessment of cognitive ability, problem solving, and set shifting (category test), as well as academic and behavioral evaluations, are also recommended. Cornoldi et al. (2003) have developed a visuospatial questionnaire to assist in the identification of students with visuospatial disabilities which may also be of value in identifying NLD.

It is important for intervention programs to target weak academic areas (especially mathematics skills) as well as social challenges facing children with NLD. Direct instruction in social pragmatics (social skills, social communication, emotion recognition) can assist children to improve social competence. The majority of children with NLD (72%) will experience significant math difficulties both in calculation and problem solving (Rourke, 1995, 2000), and many will need practice to improve handwriting skills.

Dyspraxia (developmental coordination disorder)

Definition Dyspraxia and developmental coordination disorder (DCD) are terms that have been used interchangeably to refer to problems children experience with posture, movement, and coordination. While dyspraxia is more commonly used in the United Kingdom, in the United States DCD is the term most frequently used.

Historically, several terms have been used to describe children who exhibit *movement difficulties,* such as "congenital clumsiness," "child or **developmental dyspraxia**" (Vaivre-Douret et al., 2011), or **developmental coordination disorder** (**DCD**). The term DCD was introduced in the DSM-III-R (APA, 1987) and is the only version that is supported by diagnostic criteria. Overall, it is the most widely used term (Sugden,

Kirby, & Dunford, 2008). Children with DCD satisfy two inclusionary (A, B) and two exclusionary criteria (C, D):

A. The ability to perform tasks requiring motor coordination is significantly below the norm.
B. The disturbance significantly impedes activities of daily living or academic achievement.
C. The disturbance is not due to a medical condition (e.g., cerebral palsy).
D. If IDD is also present, the disturbance is beyond what would be expected given the IDD. (APA, 2000, p. 58)

Disturbances of motor coordination may include: delay in motor milestones (crawling, walking), tendency to drop items, general "clumsiness," and poor performance in athletics or academics due to poor handwriting. There are high rates of comorbidity among children with DCD and developmental dyslexia, ADHD, SLI, and ASD (Sugden et al., 2008). After conducting a substantive review of the research concerning dyspraxia and DCD, Gibbs, Appleton, and Appleton (2006) state that: "the terminology of coordination disorders has been confused but in practice dyspraxia and DCD should be regarded as synonymous" (p. 537).

Dyspraxia versus apraxia

While the term **dyspraxia** refers to the failure to develop the ability to perform age-appropriate fine or gross motor skills, the term **apraxia** is used in adult populations to refer to the loss of function previously acquired (e.g., loss of movement through stroke).

Currently, the DSM does not consider DCD as a learning disorder, per se, but as a motor skills disorder, and states that when considering disorders of written expression, "if poor handwriting is due to impairment in motor coordination, a diagnosis of DCD should be considered" (APA, 2000, p. 56). However, given the impact of the disorder on learning and achievement, for purposes of this book, DCD will be discussed along with the other learning disorders.

Nature and course   Children with DCD have difficulties planning, controlling, and coordinating motor activities in the absence of any neurological or physical condition (Bowens & Smith, 1999). Recent investigations have found that in children with ADHD, comorbidity rates with DCD can be as high as 50% (Kadesjo & Gillberg, 1998), leading some to suggest the existence of a combined disorder, atypical brain disorder (Gilger & Kaplan, 2001), or deficits in attention, motor control, and perception (DAMP; Gillberg, 1992). However, recent investigation of cognitive profiles of children with ADHD and comorbid ADHD and DCD reveal that while those with ADHD alone do not demonstrate deficits in visuospatial ability, those with DCD performed significantly weaker on the Perceptual Reasoning Index of the WISC-IV compared to individuals with ADHD alone, leading researchers to suggest that the two disorders have different etiology (Loh, Piek, & Barrett, 2011).

Developmentally, children with DCD often demonstrate a history of delayed motor milestones, poor ability to dress themselves (buttons and shoe laces), poor ability to catch or throw a ball, and immaturities in art work (cutting, coloring). In primary school, motor skills will continue to be delayed with slow and labored attempts at handwriting and copying from the board.

Perceptual reasoning and intelligence

The Wechsler Intelligence Scale for Children (WISC-IV; Wechsler, 2002) has four major scales that are used to derive an overall IQ score, namely: Verbal Comprehension, Perceptual Reasoning, Working Memory, and Processing Speed. Perceptual reasoning involves the ability to derive solutions to problems based on visual conceptual reasoning and the analysis and synthesis of visual information (such as reproducing block designs), and working with complex visual designs (matrix reasoning).

Prevalence and etiology It has been estimated that as many as 6% of children (five to 11 years of age) may meet criteria for DCD (APA, 2000). The exact cause of DCD is not known but several suggestions have been made to account for central nervous system dysfunction, including: premature birth, impairment in the dominant cerebral hemisphere, sensory integration disorder, or birth complications, such as anoxia or hyponoxia (Vaivre-Douret et al., 2011). Pinpointing the origins is further complicated due to bidirectional influences from biological, cognitive, and behavioral facets of the disorder (Barnett, 2008). Although DCD has been associated with the development of internalizing behaviors in older children and adolescents (Cantell & Kooistra, 2002), more recent reports suggest that signs of internalizing problems in this population may be evident as early as three and four years of age (Piek, Bradbury, Elsley, & Tate, 2008). Sequences of genetic codes for dopamine receptors DRD1–DRD5 and dopamine transporter DAT1 that have been identified in children with ADHD have also been uncovered in those who have comorbid ADHD and DCD. Piek et al. (2008) found that individuals with comorbid ADHD and DCD had significantly higher depression scores than those with either disorder in isolation. Furthermore, studies of students in college and university with motor difficulties have found that 50% reported continued handwriting difficulties as a major source of difficulty for them, while 52% also reported problems in areas of executive functioning, such as organizational skills, time management, and decision making (Kirby, Sugden, Beveridge, & Edwards, 2008).

Assessment and treatment Although it is beyond the goals of this book to provide a review of potential assessment and treatment techniques that can be applied to DCD, interested readers are urged to read Barnett's (2008) article which provides an excellent summary of screening and assessment tools for DCD.

According to Sugden et al. (2008), challenges for the future will be to investigate the needs of adolescents and adults who are attending higher education, and how to assess DCD appropriately in these populations who may require disability services in order to be academically successful. Since a diagnosis of DCD requires the assessment of motor skill deficits, the overall goals of occupational therapists are often centered on targeting areas of sensorimotor impairment for intervention. However, Sugden et al. (2008) emphasize the importance of targeting "participation" as an overall goal for children with DCD, within a more ecological framework, engaging students in areas of schoolwork, recreational activities, and self-care tasks.

Problems of impulsivity, hyperactivity, and inattention

Attention deficit hyperactivity disorder (ADHD)

Definition   There is global consensus that extreme forms of impulsivity, overactivity, and inattention constitute features of a disorder which can cause significant impairment in functioning (International Consensus Statement on ADHD, 2002). However, while the ICD-10 (WHO, 1993) defines the syndrome of **hyperkinetic disorder (HKD)** using a narrow set of parameters, the DSM (APA, 2000) classifies **attention deficit hyperactivity disorder (ADHD)** as a more broadly defined disorder with three variations: **inattentive, hyperactive-impulsive, or combined subtypes.** Both systems require symptoms to be pervasive (evident in two different situations; for example, home and school), although for the ICD-10, full criteria must be met in both situations. The disorder is persistent with onset usually prior to five (ICD-10) or seven years of age (DSM).

The ICD-10 defines HKD as one disorder comprised of symptoms of inattention **and** overactivity, while the DSM defines three versions of the disorder depending on whether conditions are met for **inattentive type** (six of nine inattentive symptoms), **hyperactive-impulsive type** (six of nine hyperactive-impulsive symptoms), **or a combined type** (meeting criteria for both the inattentive and hyperactive-impulsive type).

Conceptual differences between the ICD-10 and DSM

The major conceptual difference between these two classification systems is that the ICD-10 does not recognize the inattentive subtype or the hyperactive-impulsive subtype. The combined subtype is closest to the diagnostic criteria for HKD; however, while the DSM requires that symptoms are pervasive across more than one situation (e.g., home and school), the ICD is more stringent in requiring that the full criteria must be met across two different situations.

Although symptoms are similar for both classification systems, differences in criteria have resulted in variations in prevalence rates. Furthermore, the ICD-10 discourages comorbidity of HKD, other than within the confines of **hyperkinetic conduct disorder**, while the DSM emphasizes that high rates of comorbidity exist for ADHD with other disorders (ODD, CD, anxiety and mood disorders, and DCD).

Nature and course

Birth to toddler period   Parent reports of infant patterns of excessive activity, poor sleep habits, irritability, and being difficult to soothe (Barkley, 1998) have been associated with increased risk for ADHD. Diagnosis is difficult in the toddler period due to normally high levels of activity and lower levels of self-control.

Preschool age (three to six years)   By three years of age, children who do not regulate behaviors and emotions as expected are seen as more demanding and stressful than peers. As a result, they evidence increased problems in unsupervised situations (Altepeter & Breen, 1992), and in relationships with peers, preschool teachers, and parents (Campbell & Ewing, 1990).

School age (six to 10 years)   Difficulties are more evident as children face increased academic and social demands. Problems of inattention, distractibility, organization, and task completion place children at greater risk for academic problems. Socially, overactive and impulsive behaviors, intrusive behaviors, excessive talking, and noisy play can be disruptive in social circles. Risk of accidental injury at this stage is evident in bicycle accidents, pedestrian injuries, and head injuries (Barkley, 1998).

Adolescence   Adolescents with ADHD are more likely to evidence the lingering effects of inattention, evident in ease of distractibility and poor ability to sustain their focus at a time when the educational setting is becoming more complex (multiple teachers), is more demanding (increased workload), and requires more self-discipline and organization.

Although individuals with ADHD are at a disadvantage for graduating from high school (Barkley, Fischer, Edelbrock, & Smallish, 1990), increased recognition of the potential impact of ADHD on academic performance over the past 30 years has resulted in improvements in support services and modifications to programming for children and youth with disabilities. As a result, there has been an increase in the number of students with "hidden disabilities," such as ADHD and learning disabilities, who are now seeking admission to colleges across the United States (Wolf, 2001), and the enrollment of college students with ADHD is steadily increasing (Shaw-Zirt, Popali-Lehane, Chaplin, & Bergman, 2005). It has been estimated that 2–4% of the college student population would meet criteria for a diagnosis of ADHD (DuPaul et al., 2001; Weyandt, Linterman, & Rice, 1995). College students with ADHD represent 20% of students in college who have disabilities and one-quarter of those receiving support services (Guthrie, 2002; Henderson, 1999).

Adolescents and adults with ADHD are at risk for lower educational achievement, increased unemployment or underemployment, problematic interpersonal relationships, and less stability of residence, and a higher incidence of psychiatric disorders, substance use disorders, and antisocial behavior (Grenwald-Mayes, 2002). In adolescence, lack of academic success and concomitant social problems can lead to a host of comorbid externalizing and internalizing problems (Biederman, Faraone, & Lapey, 1992). One of the major tasks of adolescents is identity formation and the development of a positive self-concept based on peer acceptance, gained through increasingly refined social skills. However, adolescents with ADHD often experience low self-concept and poor levels of acceptance from peers, and are vulnerable to bouts of depression. Mannuzza and Klein (2000) found that children who demonstrate deficits in social skills and self-esteem continue to experience difficulties in these areas throughout adolescence and adulthood.

Stimulant medication and future risk

Although parents often express concern that stimulant medication can be a "gateway drug" leading to the abuse of other substances, research finds the opposite to be true. Adults with ADHD who did not have the benefit of stimulant medication are at greater risk for later substance abuse than those whose ADHD was successfully managed, medically (Biederman, Wilens, Mick, Spencer, & Faraone, 1999).

Prevalence and etiology

Prevalence   Due to the narrower criteria, the ICD-10 identifies fewer individuals with HKD, while the broader criteria of the DSM leads to the identification of more individuals with ADHD (Foreman, Foreman, Prendergast, & Minty, 2001). Lee et al. (2008) compared the predictive validity of the two systems and found only 11% out of the 419 cases that met criteria for ADHD also met criteria for HKD due to the more rigid criteria of pervasiveness in the ICD-10 (requiring the full criteria to be met in more than one situation). The authors support previous results (Lahey et al., 2006) suggesting that the ICD-10 criteria under-identify those with significant impairment. However, a study conducted by the UK Office of National Statistics reported that ADHD was the most common referral to specialist child and adolescent mental health services (CAMHS) across the United Kingdom (Meltzer, Gatward, Goodman, & Ford, 2000), while in the United States, it is reported that approximately 30–50% of referrals involve children with ADHD (Barkley, 1998).

Although the majority of children who are diagnosed with ADHD (90%) have the more obvious forms of the disorder (*hyperactive-impulsive* or *combined hyperactive-impulsive–inattentive type*), children with the *inattentive type* are likely to be identified much later, or remain undiagnosed. While lack of self-control (disinhibition) associated with hyperactive-impulsive and combined types is likely to improve with age, inattention remains relatively stable over time (Hart, Lahey, Loeber, Applegate, & Frick, 1995).

The disorder is more frequent in males than females with ratios ranging from 2:1 to 9:1 (APA, 2000, p. 90); however, research suggests that females with ADHD are significantly more impaired than males with ADHD and controls in areas of psychosocial functioning, including: depression, anxiety, self-esteem, and overall stress levels (Rucklidge & Tannock, 2001). Since 90% of those diagnosed with ADHD have either the impulsive/hyperactive or combined type, it is possible that gender differences among children may represent differences in type. Whether there are male/female differences in the subtypes of ADHD symptoms continues to be an area of debate. At least one study found females were twice as likely to have the inattentive type (Biederman, Mick, & Faraone, 2002), although research with college students has demonstrated significantly less gender disparity (Weyandt, Linterman, & Rice, 1995).

It is estimated that between one-third and two-thirds of children with ADHD will continue to demonstrate ADHD symptoms throughout their lifetime (Wender, Wolf,

& Wasserstein, 2001), while approximately 2–6% of the adult population will meet criteria for diagnosis (Wender, 1995).

Etiology Complex interactions between biological factors and environmental factors are at the core of ADHD. There is high heritability, with 50% of parents with ADHD having a child with the disorder (Biederman et al., 1995). One study demonstrated that if children and parents shared high ADHD symptoms, the children demonstrated no improvement in the program, suggesting that it may be necessary to treat the parent prior to intervention, in cases such as these (Sonuga-Barke, Daley, Thompson, Laver-Bredbury, & Weeks, 2001).

Brain structures and brain function

Modern technology, positron emission tomography (PET), magnetic resonance imaging (MRI), functional magnetic resonance imaging (fMRI), and single-photon emission computed tomography (SPECT) brain scans have focused on three sites relevant to ADHD: **prefrontal cortex** (*executive functions, planning ability*), **cingulated gyrus** (*focusing of attention and response selection*), and **basal ganglia** (*time perception*).

Neurotransmitters The **catecholamines** (dopamine, norepinephrine, epinephrine) are neurotransmitters that have been associated with attention and motor activity. Medications that have been successful in treating the disorder, such as **Dexedrine** (dextroamphetamine), **Ritalin** (methlyphenidate), and **Cylert** (pemoline), work to increase the number of catecholamines in the brain (Barkley, 1998).

According to Barkley (1997), **behavioral inhibition** (the ability to inhibit a response, interrupt a current response, or block a distractor) is an essential step that allows sufficient time for higher functioning (executive functions) to take place. This delay allows the necessary time to process information in four major areas: **working memory** (*planning skills*), **internalization of speech** (*analysis*), **self-regulation of affect** (*goal direction and sustained attention*), and **reconstitution** (synthesis). Individuals with ADHD, especially the hyperactive-impulsive variant, evidence poor behavioral inhibition.

Video games versus homework

Why is it that children with ADHD can play video or computer games for hours, yet cannot do homework? Barkley (1997) addresses the issue by distinguishing between **sustained attention** (effortful attention in a low interest task, such as homework) versus **contingency based attention** (focusing on a task that in inherently rewarding, such as a video game). Children with ADHD have problems sustaining goal-directed behavior for low interest tasks that are not rewarding.

Assessment and treatment/intervention   Assessment for ADHD can involve a number of different procedures depending on the professional involved. A family physician can diagnose the disorder based on an evaluation of symptoms and medical/developmental history. A psychologist may observe the child in the classroom, have parents and teachers complete a number of behavioral questionnaires, and administer a battery of individual tests (of cognitive ability, executive functions, and academic achievement), most of which have been previously discussed.

Treatment will vary based on the nature and severity of the problem, and the child's developmental level. Determining the correct type of medication and dosage may be difficult and frustrating. In addition to stimulant medications that target the catecholamines, **Strattera**, a selective norepinephrine reuptake inhibitor (NRI), has recently been found effective in the treatment of ADHD.

Although medication is often the treatment of choice, there are times when medication either is ineffective or produces unwanted side effects. Alternative treatment methods, such as behavior management programs, can be devised through observations at school and at home and by conducting a functional behavioral assessment to target behaviors for intervention (e.g., to increase on-task behavior). Examples of functional behavioral assessments are available in *Chapter 5*. Other classroom interventions that have been successful include peer tutoring and computer-assisted instruction (DuPaul & Eckert, 1998; Hoffman & DuPaul, 2000). Parent training programs can also improve parent management, help reduce parent stress, and increase positive behaviors (Barkley, 1997; Forehand & McMahon, 1981).

References

Altepeter, T. A., & Breen, M. J. (1992). Situational variation in problem behavior at home and school in attention deficit disorder with hyperactivity: A factor analytic study. *Journal of Child Psychology and Psychiatry, 33*, 741–748.

American Psychiatric Association (APA). (1987). *Diagnostic and statistical manual of mental disorders* (3rd rev. ed.). Washington, DC: Author.

American Psychiatric Association (APA). (2000). *Diagnostic and statistical manual of mental disorders* (4th ed., text revision). Washington, DC: Author.

Barbaresi, W. J., Katusic, S. K., Collagin, R. C., Weaver, A. L., & Jacobsen, S. J. (2005). Math learning disorder: Incidence in a population-based birth cohort, 1976–82, Rochester, Minn. *Ambulatory Pediatrics, 5*, 281–289.

Barkley, R. A. (1997). Behavior inhibition, sustained attention and executive function. *Psychological Bulletin, 121*, 65–94.

Barkley, R. A. (1998). *Attention deficit hyperactivity disorder: A handbook for diagnosis and treatment* (2nd ed.). New York: Guilford.

Barkley, R. A., Fischer, M., Edelbrock, C. S., & Smallish, L. (1990). The adolescent outcome of hyperactive children diagnosed by research criteria. An 8-year perspective follow-up study. *Journal of the American Academy of Child and Adolescent Psychiatry, 32*, 233–256.

Barnett, A. L. (2008). Motor assessment in DCD: From identification to intervention. *International Journal of Disability, Development and Education, 55*(2), 113–129.

Berninger, V. W., & Hart, T. M. (1992). A developmental neuropsychological perspective for reading and writing acquisition. *Educational Psychologist, 27*(4), 415–434.

Berninger, V., & Rutberg, J. (1992). Relationship of finger function to beginning writing: Application to diagnosis of writing disabilities. *Developmental Medicine and Child Neurology, 34*, 198–215.

Biederman, J., Faraone, S., & Lapey, K. (1992). Comorbidity of diagnosis in attention-deficit hyperactivity disorder. In G. Weiss (Ed.), *Child and adolescent psychiatry clinics in North America: Attention deficit disorder* (pp. 335–360). Philadelphia: W.B. Saunders.

Biederman, J., Mick, E., & Faraone, S. V. (2002). Influence of gender on attention deficit hyperactivity disorder in children referred to a psychiatric clinic. *American Journal of Psychiatry, 159,* 36–42.

Biederman, J., Wilens, T., Mick, E., Spencer, T., & Faraone, S. V. (1999). Pharmacotherapy of attention-deficit/hyperactivity disorder reduces risk for substance use disorder. *Pediatrics, 104,* e20.

Biederman, J., Wozniak, J., Kiely, K., Ablon, S., Faraone, S., & Mick, E. (1995). CBCL clinical scales discriminate prepubertal children with structured-interview-derived diagnosis of mania from those with ADHD. *Journal of the American Academy of Child and Adolescent Psychiatry, 34,* 464–471.

Bowens, A., & Smith, I. (1999). *Childhood dyspraxia: Some issues for the NHS. Nuffield Portfolio Programme Report No. 2.* Leeds: Nuffield Institute for Health.

Bryant, D. P., Bryant, B. R., Gersten, R., Scammacca, N., & Chavez, M. (2008). Mathematics intervention for first- and second-grade students with mathematics difficulties. The effects of Tier 2 intervention delivered as booster lessons. *Remedial and Special Education, 29,* 20–32.

Bryant, D. P., Bryant, B. R., Gersten, R., Scammacca, N., Funk, C., Winter, A., . . . Pool, C. (2008). The effects of Tier 2 intervention on first-grade mathematics performance of first-grade students who are at risk for mathematics difficulties. *Learning Disability Quarterly, 31,* 47–63.

Campbell, S. B., & Ewing, L. J. (1990). Follow-up of hard to manage preschoolers: Adjustment at age 9 and predictors of continuing symptoms. *Journal of Child Psychology and Psychiatry, 31,* 871–889.

Cantell, M., & Kooistra, L. (2002). Long term outcomes of developmental coordination disorder. In S. Cermak & D. Larkin (Eds.), *Developmental coordination disorder* (pp. 23–38). Albany, NY: Thomas Learning.

Casey, B., Nigg, J., & Durston, S. (2007). New potential leads in the biology and treatment of attention deficit-hyperactivity disorder. *Current Opinion in Neurology, 20,* 119–124.

Cohen, L., Dehaene, S., Naccache, L., Lehericy, S., Dehaene-Lambertz, G., & Henaff, M. A. (2000). The visual word form area: Spatial and temporal characterization of an initial stage of reading in normal subjects with posterior split-brain patients. *Brain, 123*(2), 291–307.

Cornoldi, C., Venneri, A., Marconato, R., Molin, A., & Montinari, C. (2003). A rapid screening measure for the identification of visuospatial learning disability in schools. *Journal of Learning Disabilities, 36,* 299–306.

Dehaene, S., Piazza, M., Pinel, P., & Cohen, L. (2003). Three parietal circuits for number processing. *Cognitive Neuropsychology, 20,* 487–506.

DuPaul, G., & Eckert, T. L. (1998). Academic interventions for students with attention-deficit/hyperactivity disorder: A review of the literature. *Reading and Writing Quarterly: Overcoming Learning Difficulties, 14,* 59–82.

DuPaul, G., Schaughency, E., Weyandt, L., Tripp, G., Kiesner, J., Ota, K., & Stanish, H. (2001). Self-report of ADHD symptoms in university students: Cross-gender and cross-national prevalence. *Journal of Learning Disabilities, 34,* 370–379.

Dykman, R. A., & Ackerman, P. T. (1991). Attention deficit disorder and specific reading disability: Separate but often overlapping disorders. *Journal of Learning Disabilities, 24,* 96–103.

Epstein, J. N., Cases, B. J., Toney, S. T., Davidson, M. C., Reilss, A. L., & Garrett, A. (2007). ADHD and medication-related brain activation effects in concordantly affected parent–child dyads with ADHD. *Journal of Child Psychology and Psychiatry, 48,* 899–913.

Federal Register. (2006). Retrieved from http://idea.ed.gov/download/finalregulations.pdf

Ferrer, E., Bennett, A., Shaywitz, J. M., Holahan, J. M., Marchione, K., & Shaywitz, S. E. (2010). Uncoupling of reading and IQ over time: Empirical evidence for a definition of dyslexia. *Psychological Science, 21*(93), 93–101.

Flanagan, D., Ortiz, S., Alfonso, V., & Dynda, A. (2006). Integration of response to intervention and norm-referenced tests in learning disability identification: Learning from the Tower of Babel. *Psychology in the Schools, 43*(7), 807–825.

Flynn, J., & Rahbar, M. (1994). Prevalence of reading failure in boys compared with girls. *Psychology in the Schools, 31*, 66–71.

Forehand, R., & McMahon, R. J. (1981). Predictors of cross setting behavior change in the treatment of child problems. *Journal of Behavior Therapy and Experimental Psychiatry, 12*, 311–313.

Foreman, D. M., Foreman, D., Prendergast, M., & Minty, B. (2001). Is clinic prevalence of 1CD-10 hyperkinesis underestimated? Impact of increasing awareness by a questionnaire screen in a UK clinic. *European Child and Adolescent Psychiatry, 10*(2), 130–134.

Fuchs, D., & Fuchs, L. (2005). Peer-assisted learning strategies: Promoting word recognition, fluency and reading comprehension in young children. *Journal of Special Education, 39*, 34–44.

Fuchs, L. S., Compton, D. L., Fuchs, D., Paulsen, K., Bryant, J. D., & Hamlett, C. L. (2005). Responsiveness to intervention: Preventing and identifying mathematics disability. *Teaching Exceptional Children, 37*, 60–66.

Fuchs, L. S., Fuchs, D., Hamlet, C. L., Powell, S. R., Capizzi, A. M., & Seethaler, P. M. (2006). The effects of computer-assisted instruction on number combination skill in at-risk first graders. *Journal of Learning Disabilities, 39*, 467–475.

Geary, D. C. (1993). Mathematical disabilities: Cognitive, neuropsychological, and genetic components. *Psychological Bulletin, 114*, 345–362.

Geary, D. C. (2000). Mathematical disorders: An overview for educators. *Perspectives, 26*, 6–9.

Geary, D. C. (2003). Learning disabilities in arithmetic. In H. L. Swanson, K. R. Harris, & S. Graham (Eds.), *Handbook of learning disabilities* (pp. 199–212). New York: Guilford.

Geary, D. (2004). Mathematics and learning disabilities. *Journal of Learning Disabilities, 37*(1), 4–15.

Geary, D., Brown, S., & Samaranayake, V. (1991). Cognitive addition: A short longitudinal study of strategy choice and speed of processing differences in normal and mathematically disabled children. *Developmental Psychology, 27*(S), 787–797.

Geary, D. C., Hamson, C. O., & Hoard, M. K. (2000). Numerical and arithmetical cognition: A longitudinal study of process and concept deficits in children with learning disability. *Journal of Experimental Child Psychology, 77*, 236–263.

Gersten, R., Jordan, N. C., & Flojo, J. R. (2005). Early identification and interventions for students with mathematics difficulties. *Journal of Learning Disabilities, 38*, 293–304.

Gibbs, J., Appleton, J., & Appleton, R. (2006). Dyspraxia or developmental coordination disorder? Unravelling the enigma. *Archives of Disease in Childhood, 92*, 534–539.

Gilger, J. W., & Kaplan, B. J. (2001). Atypical brain development: A conceptual framework for understanding developmental learning disabilities. *Developmental Neuropsychology, 20*, 465–481.

Gillberg, C. (1992). Deficits in attention, motor control and perception and other syndromes attributed to Minimal Brain Dysfunction. In J. Aircardi (Ed.), *Diseases of the nervous system in childhood. Clinics in developmental medicine* (pp. 115–118). London, Mac Keith Press.

Graham, S., Harris, K. R., & Larsen, L. (2001). Prevention and intervention of writing difficulties for students with learning disabilities. *Learning Disabilities Research and Practice, 16*, 74–84.

Grenwald-Mayes, G. (2002). Relationship between current quality of life and family of origin dynamics for college students with attention-deficit/hyperactivity disorder. *Journal of Attention Disorders, 5*, 211–222.

Gross-Tsur, V., Shalev, R. S., Manor, O., & Amir, N. (1995). Developmental right-hemisphere syndrome: Clinical spectrum of the nonverbal learning disability. *Journal of Learning Disabilities, 28*(2), 80–86.

Guthrie, B. (2002). The college experience. In K. Nadeau & P. Quinn (Eds.), *Understanding women with AD/HD* (pp. 288–312). Silver Spring, MD: Advantage.

Hallahan, D. P., & Mercer, C. D. (2001, August). Learning disabilities: Historical perspectives. Paper presented at the Learning Disabilities Summit: Building a Foundation for the Future, Washington, DC.

Hart, E., Lahey, B. B., Loeber, R., Applegate, B., & Frick, P. J. (1995). Developmental changes in attention deficit hyperactivity disorder in boys: a four-year longitudinal study. *Journal of Abnormal Child Psychology, 2*, 729–750.

Henderson, C. (1999). *College freshmen with disabilities: A statistical profile.* Washington, DC: HEATH Resource Center.

Hoffman, J., & DuPaul, G. J. (2000). Psychoeducational interventions for children and adolescents with attention-deficit/hyperactivity disorder. *Child and Adolescent Psychiatric Clinics of North America, 9*, 647–661.

Hooper, S. R., Swartz, C. W., Wakely, M. B., de Kruif, R. E., & Montgomery, J. W. (2002). Executive functions in elementary school children with and without problems in written expression. *Journal of Learning Disabilities, 35*(1), 57–68.

Imhof, M. (2004). Effects of color stimulation on handwriting performance of children with ADHD without and with additional learning disabilities. *European Child and Adolescent Psychiatry, 13*, 191–198.

Individuals with Disabilities Education Act (IDEA). (2004). Retrieved from http://idea.ed.gov/download/finalregulations.pdf

International Consensus Statement on ADHD. (2002). *Clinical Child and Family Psychology Review, 5*, 89–111.

Johnson, E. E., Humphrey, M., Mellard, D. F., Woods, K., & Swanson, H. L. (2010). Cognitive processing deficits and students with specific learning disabilities: A selective meta-analysis of the literature. *Learning Disability Quarterly, 33*, 3–18.

Kadesjo, B., & Gillberg, C. (1998). Developmental coordination disorder in Swedish 7-year-old children. *Journal of the American Academy of Child and Adolescent Psychiatry, 38*, 820–828.

Kavale, K. A. (2005). Identifying specific learning disability: Is response to intervention the answer. *Journal of Learning Disabilities, 38*, 553–562.

Kirby, A., Sugden, D. A., Beveridge, S., & Edwards, L. (2008). Support and identification of students with developmental co-ordination disorder (DCD) in further and higher education. *Journal of Research in Special Educational Needs, 3*(8), 120–131.

Kovas, Y., Harlaar, N., Petrill, S. A., & Plomin, R. (2005). Generalist genes and mathematics in 7-year-old twins. *Intelligence, 33*(5), 473–489.

Kovas, Y., Haworth, C. M., Harlaar, N., Petrill, S. A., Dale, P. S., & Plomin, R. (2007). Overlap and specificity of genetic and environmental influences on mathematics and reading disability in 10-year-old twins. *Journal of Child Psychology and Psychiatry, 48*(9), 914–922.

Kuhn, M., & Stahl, S. (2003). Fluency: A review of developmental and remedial practices. *Journal of Educational Psychology, 95*, 3–21.

Lahey, B. L., Pelham, W. E., Chronis, A., Massetti, G., Kipp, H., Ehrhardt, A., & Lee, S. S. (2006). Predictive validity of ICD-10 hyperkinetic disorder relative to DSM-IV attention-deficit/hyperactivity disorder among younger children. *Journal of Child Psychology and Psychiatry, 47*, 472–479.

Lee, S. I., Schachar, R. J., Chen, S. X., Ornstein, T. J., Charach, A., Barr, C., & Ickowicz, A. (2008). Predictive validity of DSM-IV and ICD-10 criteria for ADHD and hyperkinetic disorder. *Journal of Child Psychology and Psychiatry, 49*, 70–78.

Lerner, J. W. (1989). Educational interventions in learning disabilities. *Journal of the American Academy of Child and Adolescent Psychiatry, 28,* 326–331.

Learning Disabilities Association of America. (2010). The Learning Disabilities Association of America's white paper on evaluation, identification and eligibility criteria for students with specific learning disabilities. Retrieved from http://www.ldanatl.org/pdf/LDA%20White%20Paper%20on%20IDEA%20Evaluation%20Criteria%20for%20SLD.pdf

Liddell, G. A., & Rasmussen, C. (2005). Memory profile of children with nonverbal learning disability. *Learning Disabilities Research & Practice, 20*(3), 137–141.

Loh, P. R., Piek, J. P., & Barrett, C. (2011). Comorbid ADHD and DCD: Examining cognitive functions using the WISC-IV. *Research in Developmental Disabilities, 32,* 1260–1269.

Lovett, M., Barron, R. W., & Benson, N. (2003). *Effective remediation of word identification and decoding difficulties in school-age children with reading disabilities.* New York: Guilford.

Lyon, G. R., & Shaywitz, S. E. (2003). Part 1: Defining dyslexia, comorbidity, teachers' knowledge of language and reading. *Annals of Dyslexia, 53,* 1–14.

MacArthur, C. A. (2000). New tools for writing: Assistive technology for students with writing difficulties. *Topics in Language Disorders, 20,* 85–100.

Mannuzza, S., & Klein, R. G. (2000). Long-term prognosis in attention-deficit/hyperactivity disorder. *Child and Adolescent Psychiatric Clinics of North America, 9,* 711–726.

Mattson, A. J., Sheer, D. E., & Fletcher, J. M. (1992). Electrophysiological evidence of lateralized disturbances in children with learning disabilities. *Journal of Clinical and Experimental Neuropsychology, 14,* 707–716.

Mayes, S. D., & Calhoun, S. L. (2007). Challenging the assumptions about the frequency and coexistence of learning disability types. *School Psychology International, 28*(4), 437–448.

Mayes, S. D., Calhoun, S. L., & Lane, S. E. (2005). Diagnosing children's writing disabilities: Different tests give different results. *Perceptual and Motor Skills, 101,* 72–78.

Mazzocco, M. M., Feigenson, L., & Halberda, J. (2011). Impaired acuity of the approximate number system underlies mathematical learning disability (dyscalculia). *Child Development, 82*(4), 1224–1237.

Meltzer, H., Gatward, R., Goodman, R., & Ford, T. (2000). *Mental health of children and adolescents in Great Britain.* London: Stationery Office.

Meyer, M., & Felton, R. (1999). Repeated reading to enhance fluency: Old approaches and new directions. *Annals of Dyslexia, 49,* 283–306.

Morgan, P. J., Farkas, G., & Wu, Q. (2011). Kindergarten children's growth trajectories in reading and mathematics: Who falls increasingly behind? *Journal of Learning Disabilities, 44,* 472–488.

MTA Cooperative Group. (1999). A 14-month randomized clinical trial of treatment strategies for attention-deficit/hyperactivity disorder. *Archives of General Psychiatry, 56,* 1073–1086.

Okamoto, Y., & Case, R. (1996). Exploring the microstructure of children's central conceptual structures in the domain of number. *Monographs of the Society for Research in Child Development, 61,* 27–59.

Olson, R., & Byrne, B. (2005). Genetic and environmental influences on reading and language ability and disability. In H. Catts & A. Kamhi (Eds.), *The connections between language and reading disability* (pp. 173–200). Hillsdale, NJ: Erlbaum.

Pennington, B. (2009). *Diagnosing learning disorders: A neuropsychological framework* (2nd ed.). New York: Guilford.

Pennington, G., & Gilger, J. (1996). *How is dyslexia transmitted?* Baltimore, MD: York.

Piek, J. P., Bradbury, G. S., Elsley, S. C., & Tate, L. (2008). Motor coordination and social-emotional behaviour in preschool aged children. *International Journal of Disability, Development and Education, 55*(2), 143–151.

Plomin, R., & Kovas, Y. (2005). Generalist genes and learning disabilities. *Psychological Bulletin, 131*(4), 502–617.

Psychological Corporation. (1992). *Wechsler Individual Achievement Test (WIAT). Manual.* New York: Psychological Corp.

Reid, R., & Ortiz Lienemann, T. (2006). Self-regulated strategy development for written expression with students with attention deficit/hyperactivity disorder. *Exceptional Child, 73*(1), 53–68.

Report of the National Reading Panel. (2000). *Teaching children to read: An evidence-based assessment of the scientific research literature on reading and its implications for reading instruction.* Washington, DC: US Department of Health and Human Services, National Institute of Health, National Institute of Child Health and Human Development.

Reynolds, M., & Besner, D. (2006). Reading aloud is not automatic: Processing capacity is required to generate a phonological code from print. *Journal of Experimental Psychology: Human Perception and Performance, 32,* 1303–1323.

Rourke, B. P. (1982). Central processing deficiencies in children: Toward a developmental neuropsychological model. *Journal of Clinical Neuropsychology, 4,* 1–18.

Rourke, B. P. (1995). *Syndrome of nonverbal learning disabilities.* New York: Guilford.

Rourke, B. P. (2000). Neuropsychological and psycho-social subtyping: A review of investigations within the University of Windsor laboratory. *Canadian Psychology, 41,* 34–51.

Rourke, B. P., Ahmad, S., Collins, D., Jayman-Abello, B., Hayman-Abello, S., & Warriner, E. M. (2002). Child clinical/pediatric neuropsychology: Some recent advances. *Annual Review of Psychology, 53,* 309–339.

Rourke, B. P., Hayman-Abello, B. A., & Collins, D. W. (2003). Learning disabilities: A neuropsychological perspective. In B. S. Fogel, R. B. Schiffer, & S. M. Rao (Eds.), *Neuropsychiatry* (2nd ed.) (pp. 630–659). New York: Lippincott, Williams, and Wilkins.

Rucklidge, J. J., & Tannock, R. (2001). Psychiatric, psychosocial and cognitive functioning of female adolescents with ADHD. *Journal of the American Academy of Child and Adolescent Psychiatry, 40,* 530–540.

Schumacher, J., Anthoni, H., Dahdou, F., Konig, I., & Hillmer, A. (2006). Strong genetic evidence of DCDC2 as a susceptibility gene for dyslexia. *American Journal of Human Genetics, 78,* 52–62.

Semrud-Clikeman, M. (2005). Neuropsychological aspects for evaluating learning disabilities. *Journal of Learning Disabilities, 38,* 563–568.

Semrud-Clikeman, M., Walkowiak, J., Wilkinson, A., & Minne, E. P. (2010). Direct and indirect measures of social perception, behavior, and emotional functioning in children with Asperger's disorder, nonverbal learning disability or ADHD. *Journal of Abnormal Child Psychology, 38,* 509–519.

Shalev, R. S., Manor, O., & Gross-Tsur, V. (2005). Developmental dyscalculia: A prospective six-year follow-up. *Developmental Medicine and Child Neurology, 47,* 121–125.

Shaywitz, S. E., Morris, R., & Shaywitz, B. A. (2008). The education of dyslexic children from childhood to young adulthood. *Annual Review of Psychology, 59,* 451–475.

Shaywitz, S. E., & Shaywitz, B. A. (2008). Paying attention to reading: The neurobiology of reading and dyslexia. *Development and Psychopathology, 20,* 1329–1349.

Shaw-Zirt, B., Popali-Lehane, L., Chaplin, W., & Bergman, A. (2005). Adjustment, social skills, and self-esteem in college students with symptoms of ADHD. *Journal of Attention Disorders, 8*(3), 109–120.

Sonuga-Barke, E. J., Daley, D., Thompson, M., Laver-Bredbury, C., & Weeks, A. (2001). Parent-based therapies for preschool attention-deficit/hyperactivity disorder: A randomized, controlled trial with a community sample. *Journal of the American Academy of Child and Adolescent Psychiatry, 40,* 402–408.

Stanovich, K. E. (1986). Matthew effects in reading: Some consequences of individual differences in the acquisition of literacy. *Reading Research Quarterly, 21,* 360–407.

Stanovich, K. E. (1991). Discrepancy definitions of reading disability: Has intelligence led us astray? *Reading Research Quarterly, 26,* 7–29.

Sugden, D., Kirby, A., & Dunford, C. (2008). Issues surrounding children with developmental coordination disorder. *International Journal of Disability*, 2(55), 173–187.

Swanson, H. L. (2009). Neuroscience and RTI: A complementary role. In E. Fletcher-Janzen & C. R. Reynolds (Eds.), *Neuropsychological perspectives on learning disabilities in the era of RTI: Recommendations for diagnosis and intervention* (pp. 28–53). Hoboken, NJ: John Wiley & Sons, Ltd.

Swanson, H. L., & Jerman, O. (2006). Math disabilities: A selective meta-analysis of the literature. *Review of Educational Research*, 76, 249–274.

Torgesen, J. K. (2000). Individual differences in response to early interventions in reading: The lingering problem of treatment resisters. *Learning Disabilities Research and Practice*, 1, 55–64.

Tran, L., Sanchez, T., Arellano, B., & Swanson, H. L. (2011). A meta-analysis of the RTI literature for children at risk for reading disabilities. *Journal of Learning Disabilities*, 44(3), 283–295.

Vaivre-Douret, L., Lalanne, C., Ingster-Moati, I., Boddaert, N., Cabrot, D., Dufier, J., ... Falissard, B. (2011). Subtypes of developmental coordination disorder: Research on their nature and etiology. *Developmental Neurospychology*, 36(5), 614–643.

Vaughn, S., Gersten, R., & Chard, D. J. (2000). The underlying message in LD intervention research: Findings from research syntheses. *Exceptional Children*, 6, 99–114.

Vaughn, S., Linar-Thompson, S., & Hickman, P. (2003). Response to treatment as a way of identifying students with learning disabilities. *Exceptional Children*, 69, 391–409.

Vellutino, F. R., Scanlon, D. M., Small, S., & Fanuele, D. P. (2006). Response to intervention as a vehicle for distinguishing between children with and without reading disabilities: Evidence for the role of kindergarten and first-grade interventions. *Journal of Learning Disabilities*, 39, 157–169.

Wechsler, D. (2002). *Manual for the Wechsler Intelligence Scale for Children – WISC-IV*. San Antonio, TX: Psychological Corporation.

Wender, P. H. (1995). *Attention-deficit hyperactivity disorder in adults*. New York: Oxford University Press.

Wender, P. H., Wolf, L. E., & Wasserstein, J. (2001). Adults with ADHD: An overview. In J. Wasserstein, L. Wolf, & F. F. LeFever (Eds.), *Adult attention deficit disorder: Brain mechanisms and life outcomes* (pp. 1–16). New York: New York Academy of Sciences.

Weyandt, L. L., Linterman, I., & Rice, J. A. (1995). Reported prevalence of attention deficits in a sample of college students. *Journal of Psychopathology and Behavior Assessment*, 17, 293–304.

Wolf, L. (2001). College students with ADHD and other hidden disorders: Outcomes and interventions. *Annals of the New York Academy of Arts and Sciences*, 931, 385–395.

Woodcock, R. W., & Johnson, M. B. (1989). *Woodcock-Johnson Psycho-Educational Battery-Revised*. Allen, TX: DLM Teaching Resources.

World Health Organization (WHO). (1993). *The ICD-10 classification of mental and behavioral disorders. Clinical descriptions and diagnostic guidelines*. Geneva: Author.

9

Externalizing Problems and Disruptive Behavior Disorders

Chapter preview and learning objectives

While internalizing problems are often subtle and covert, externalizing problems are often disruptive and overt. In this chapter, the focus is on the continuum of aggressive behaviors, beginning with normal aggressive responses (instrumental aggression) and extending into those behaviors that have the capacity to inflict harm on others, in a number of different forms, whether they involve bullying, relational aggression, or reactive or callous acts of aggression. This chapter will provide readers with an increased understanding of:

- the various forms of aggression and the severity of each type;
- the etiology and prevalence of behavioral disorders;
- the bio-psycho-social conditions that can precipitate and maintain aggressive behaviors;

Clinical and Educational Child Psychology, First Edition. Linda Wilmshurst.
© 2013 John Wiley & Sons, Ltd. Published 2013 by John Wiley & Sons, Ltd.

- the qualitative and quantitative differences in the two major disruptive disorders: oppositional defiant disorder and conduct disorder;
- treatment and intervention programs that can assist in the management of behavioral disorders.

Externalizing problems: an overview

Early onset externalizing problems, such as aggressive, oppositional, and destructive behaviors, can increase a child's risk for developing serious problems (such as delinquency and conduct problems) later on (Campbell, 2002). In a study from the Netherlands, externalizing behaviors were identified as early as 12 months of age (van Zeijl et al., 2006). Harsh and inconsistent discipline practices, low parental monitoring, exposure to adult aggression, lack of family cohesion, and low parental warmth have all been linked to increased risk for externalizing behaviors, while a sense of connectedness to family and school has been identified as a protective factor (Patterson, Capaldi, & Bank, 1991; Resnick et al., 1997). The Conduct Problems Prevention Research Group (CPPRG, 2011) has constructed a dynamic cascade model of the development of antisocial behavior. In their model, which will be discussed shortly, they outline several risk factors that are targeted in their longitudinal Fast Track Prevention Program for high-risk youth. The intervention program identifies and targets eight risk factors for antisocial behavior:

- poor parent behavior management;
- weaknesses in social cognitive information processing;
- deficits in emotional coping skills;
- poor peer relationships;
- weak academic skills;
- classroom environments that are disruptive and rejecting;
- poor parental monitoring and supervision;
- poor home–school relations. (CPPRG, 2011, p. 332)

Results have demonstrated that early starters (those who evidence conduct problems early in life) are at the highest risk for life-long antisocial behaviors (Moffitt, 1993) and that having a number of the risk factors above can have a **multiplier effect**. In an early study, Rutter (1979) found that children who were exposed to two risk factors were at four times the risk for developing a disorder, while having four risk factors increased the risk tenfold. More recently, Herrenkohl, Maguin, and Hill (2000) found that if a 10-year-old were exposed to six or more risk factors, they would be 10 times more likely to engage in violent crime by 18 years of age, compared to peers who had been exposed to only one risk factor.

Given the wide range of disruptive behaviors that might be subsumed under the category of externalizing behaviors, it is not surprising to see that estimates for externalizing behaviors demonstrate considerable variability. As a result estimates of prevalence rates in community samples have ranged from 2% to 20% of the population (Brandenburg, Friedman, & Silver, 1990; Offord et al., 1987). In a longitudinal study of preschool children at two, four, and five years of age, Hill, Degnan, Calkins, and Keane (2006) found that 11% of girls and 9% of boys demonstrated clinical levels of externalizing behaviors. In this study, the authors found that inattention at two years of age was predictive of later externalizing problems.

Physical abuse has been found to be a significant risk factor for externalizing behaviors, such as aggression (Lansford, Criss, Pettit, Dodge, & Bates, 2003), conduct disorder (Lynch & Cicchetti, 1998), and juvenile delinquency (Attar, Guerra, & Tolan, 1994). Family poverty and living in violent neighborhoods have also been found to increase the risk of externalizing problems (Attar et al., 1994; Widom, 1989). Child characteristics, such as social competence, having positive peer relationships, and good social problem solving skills, have been found to be protective factors that reduce the risk of developing externalizing problems (Ladd, Kochenderfer, & Coleman, 1996; Lochman & Wells, 2002).

Aggressive behaviors

The importance of developing self-regulation and emotional control is an important developmental milestone. While children who are **fearful** often over-control behaviors to avoid situations that can heighten their arousal level (Kagan, Reznick, & Gibbons, 1989), children who are **fearless** often approach high-risk or emotionally charged situations without hesitation (Kagan, 1997).

The high cost of high emotionality and low emotion regulation

Rydell, Berlin, and Bohlin (2003) found that young children (five to eight years of age) who demonstrated high levels of emotional arousal and low emotion regulation often demonstrated poor social adaptation, regardless of whether the emotion-inducing situation was positive or negative. In negative situations, they were easily provoked to aggression, while in positive situations, their behaviors escalated out of control.

Definition and types of aggressive behaviors Definitions of "aggressive" behaviors can differ based on the degree to which intentionality is considered in the definition. While some theorists may consider any act of force to constitute an act of aggression (Cote, Vaillancourt, LeBlanc, Nagin, & Tremblay, 2006), others consider a behavior to be aggressive only if there is an intent to harm another individual (Dodge, Coie, & Lyman, 2006). Researchers who take a middle ground distinguish between two forms of aggression, **instrumental aggression** and **hostile aggression**. Additionally, hostile aggression can be further partitioned into two subtypes: acts of **overt aggression** (obvious forms of aggression, such as verbal threats, hitting, punching, pushing) or acts of **covert aggression** (hidden and less obvious forms of antisocial behaviors, such as lying, stealing, bullying). Overt forms of aggression can be exhibited as **proactive aggression**, motivated by the anticipation of a reward (Dodge & Coie, 1987; Little, Jones, Henrich, & Hawley, 2003); or **reactive aggression,** a response to perceived threats or provocation. Proactive forms of aggression can include characteristics

Table 9.1 Subtypes of aggression

Aggression: "an act of force"			
Hostile: *with intent to harm*			**Instrumental:** *with intent to obtain a goal*
Overt		Covert	
Hitting, punching, verbal threats		*Secretive, hidden*	
Proactive *(planned)* Sub-type: *Callous-unemotional*	Reactive *(defensive)* Sub-type: *Impulsive*	Covert destructive: *Violations of property* Covert non-destructive: *Status violations*	Relational: *Purposeful manipulations targeting peer groups*

of **callous-unemotional aggression** (Frick, Cornell, Barry, Bodin, & Dane, 2003), while reactive forms characteristically are represented by more impulsive and emotionally aggressive responses. Forms of covert aggression may include destructive acts of **property violation** (vandalism, breaking and entering), non-destructive acts of **status violation** (truancy, running away), or acts of **relational aggression**. See Table 9.1 for a list of aggressive subtypes.

Aggressive response patterns have also been subtyped according to neurophysiological profiles, comorbidity, overt versus covert patterns of behaviors, and age of onset.

There has been considerable research linking aggression to problems in social adjustment, such as peer rejection and social skills deficits, as well as associated problems in areas of academic difficulties, externalizing problems, and depressive symptoms (Barriga et al., 2002; Campbell, Spieker, Burchinal, & Poe, 2006). However, research has only recently begun to examine whether outcomes differ for the various subtypes of aggression, especially relational aggression. Compared to boys, females have been found to engage in more relationally aggressive behaviors than males, who are equally likely to use overt or relational aggression (Putallaz et al., 2007). Preddy and Fite (2012) investigated the impact of relational versus overt aggression on four psychosocial outcomes (academic performance, social problems, depression, and delinquency) in a community sample of 89 children (with a mean age of 10.4 years). Results revealed negative associations between relational aggression and academic performance and positive associations between overt aggression and delinquency. Furthermore, gender differences were significant, with social problems being related to overt aggression in males and relational aggression in females.

Instrumental aggression and hostile aggression The distinction between instrumental and hostile aggression is the nature of intent; instrumental aggression is goal-directed behavior that does not include an intent to harm another individual, while the intent of hostile aggression is to inflict harm on another (Hartup, 1974). Instrumental aggression is thought to increase in the second and third years due to the child's increasing cognitive and social awareness of intentionality and engagement in goal-directed behaviors (e.g., Campos et al., 2000); however, nonverbal or physical aggression decreases with age after this time, likely due to increased awareness of social rules and ability to solve conflicts verbally. Studies have shown that for toddlers, the use of physical aggression declines as their vocabulary increases (Dionne, Tremblay, Boivin, Laplante, & Perusse, 2003).

In preschool populations, a common area of peer conflict which can result in acts of instrumental aggression involves disputes regarding the possession of objects, such as toys, and attempts to defend or retrieve these possessions. According to Friedman and Neary (2008), this type of conflict is common because toddlers believe that ownership rests with the child who first possesses the toy. Hay, Hurst, Waters, and Chadwick (2011) observed the defensive responses of 200 infants and toddlers in a London sample ranging in age from nine months to 30 months. Behaviors were coded as: *resistance* (movement towards the object, gently trying to retrieve it); *verbal or vocal protests* (crying, verbal persuasion), or *physical force* (tugging at the object, using bodily force). Results revealed that developmentally, infants initially resisted when a possession was taken, but engaged in more active and vocal defense with increased age, and by two years of age were more likely than younger children to engage in instrumental aggression. Hay et al. (2011) suggest that these results support findings by Tremblay et al. (2004) of a peak in aggressive behaviors in toddlers at two years of age, but add that the spike in aggressive behavior may be due to an increase in instrumental aggression during this time. However, the authors also note that, similar to previous studies, the use of physical force was not the most common strategy used by toddlers, and that when used, the authors found no evidence of an intent to harm.

In studies that have looked at more hostile oriented aggressive patterns in early childhood, several family characteristics evident in the first three years of life were associated with increased risk for developing disruptive behavior disorders, including: caregiver depression, avoidant attachment pattern, stress, lack of quality care giving, and low socio-economic status (Aguilar, Sroufe, Egeland, & Carlson, 2000; Tremblay et al., 1999). Lacourse et al. (2006) found that kindergarten children from low income neighborhoods were at highest risk for deviant behavior in adolescence if they also were hyperactive, fearless, and low in prosocial behaviors.

Reactive aggression versus proactive aggression   Distinctions between reactive and proactive aggression have been made regarding the intent and function of the aggressive behavior. While reactive aggression refers to an individual's defensive response to a perceived threat or aggravation, proactive aggression refers to behavior that is planned or premeditated with a specific goal in mind, with the intention of personal gain or influence (e.g., a bully who wants to obtain another child's lunch money). Research has found different environmental contexts can be associated with these different aggressive patterns. While being subjected to harsh parenting practices may place a child at risk for reactive aggression (Dodge, Lochman, Harnish, Bates, & Pettit, 1997), Xu, Farver, and Zhang (2009) found that Chinese children who had an indulgent parent were at increased risk for proactive aggression. However, Vitaro, Barker, Boivin, Brendgen, and Tremblay, (2006) found that harsh and inconsistent parenting practices can be associated with both types of aggressive behaviors, which may suggest that hypervigilant children may respond to an increased bias towards threat, while proactive children may model the same behaviors. While studies have found that children with reactive aggression are more socially isolated compared to their proactive peers (Dodge et al., 1997), those with proactive aggression are more likely to engage in delinquent behaviors in mid-adolescence (Vitaro, Gendreau, Tremblay, & Oligny, 1998).

Reactive and proactive aggression

From a theoretical perspective, reactive aggression is best supported by the frustration aggression model (Berkowitz, 1978) and principles of negative reinforcement, since the aggressive act is intended to remove the perceived threat (Vitaro et al., 2006). Proactive aggression is best explained by using Bandura's (1973) social learning model, where aggressive acts can be modeled and positively reinforced through rewards such as increased status, power, and control.

Studies have also found that the two forms of aggression can be evident in the same individual, with approximately half of children demonstrating both forms of aggression, and just 15% demonstrating only one form (Barker, Tremblay, Nagin, Lacourse, & Vitaro, 2006; Crick & Dodge, 1996; Dodge et al., 1997).

Callous-unemotional (CU) aggressive traits   In adults, it has long been recognized that antisocial personality disorder includes a cluster of traits that characterize a lack of empathy or guilt, a lack of remorse, and a tendency to use others for personal gain. There is a continuum of severity within the disorder, with some individuals prone to more violent and chronic patterns of psychopathy (Comer, 2010). Similarly, youth who exhibit disruptive behavior disorders also represent a heterogeneous group, with some children exhibiting traits which have been associated with more severe, negative, and chronic outcomes.

Research has shown that children with behavior disorders who also exhibit CU traits do not process emotionally-based information or recognize positive or negative emotions in others, and exhibit less response at a physiological level to emotional cues, than peers without CU traits. Furthermore, these children are non-responsive to harsh parenting, engage in more high-risk behaviors, and demonstrate reduced activity in the amygdale which is responsible for emotional control, the fear response, and interpretation of nonverbal emotional expressions (Jones, Laurens, Herba, Barker, & Viding, 2009; Levenston, Patrick, Bradley, & Lang, 2000; Marsh, Gerber, & Peterson, 2008). Furthermore, the genetic impact for children with behavior disorders and CU traits is significantly higher (0.81) compared to youth with behavior disorders without CU traits (0.30), who are influenced more by environment than heredity (Viding, Blair, Moffitt, & Plomin, 2005; Viding, Jones, Frick, Moffitt, & Plomin, 2008).

Children who exhibit CU traits also demonstrate lower levels of behavioral inhibition and higher levels of behavioral dysregulation than other children with disruptive behavior disorders (Frick et al., 2003). These children are more likely to exhibit proactive aggressive patterns and decreased emotional reactivity, and to have a family history of antisocial personality disorder (Hubbard, Smithmyer, & Ramsden, 2002). Children with CU are most likely to exhibit early onset conduct disorder (CD) and further discussion of this subtype will be revisited later in this chapter.

Aggression and neurophysiological profiles   In addition to reduced activity in the amygdale of individuals with aggression and CU traits, researchers have also found immature P300 wave amplitudes in boys with a history of behavior problems involving

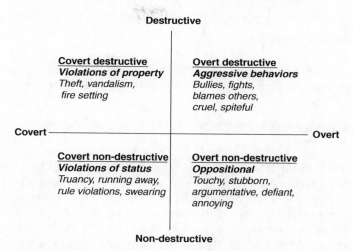

Figure 9.1   Overt/covert and destructive/non-destructive behaviors based on a meta-analysis (Frick et al., 1993).

rule violations (Bauer & Hesselbrock, 2003). In a study of delinquent adolescents, Teichner et al. (2000) found four clusters of deficits suggesting four different subtypes of aggressive behaviors: verbal–left hemisphere deficits, subcortical-frontal deficits, mild verbal deficits, and normals. The subcortical frontal cluster was associated with significantly higher scores on the thought problems and delinquent behavior scales of the Child Behavior Checklist (Achenbach & Rescorla, 2000). The biological basis of antisocial behaviors will be revisited in the discussion of CD later in this chapter.

Overt versus covert acts of aggression   In a meta-analytic study of 60 cases, Frick et al. (1993) identified four clusters of symptoms along two factor analytic dimensions: overt and covert forms of aggression, and destructive or non-destructive acts. Overt forms of aggression can be represented by destructive behaviors such as aggressive behaviors, bullying, fighting, blaming others, and being cruel and spiteful; or non-destructive behaviors, such as being oppositional, touchy, stubborn, argumentative, defiant, and annoying. The overt behaviors are more symptomatic of behaviors one associates with oppositional defiant disorder (ODD). On the other hand, covert behaviors in this model include destructive acts such as property violations, theft, vandalism, and fire setting, and non-destructive behaviors such as status violations, truancy, running away, and rule violations. The latter characteristics are more closely associated with symptoms of conduct disorder (CD). The four quadrants are displayed graphically in Figure 9.1.

When considering the prevalence of overt acts of aggression, males are typically seen as more aggressive than girls, and when considering severity of physical aggression, males are also seen as more severe at all ages from four to 18 years (Crick, Casas, & Mosher, 1997; Stranger, Achenbach, & Verhulst, 1997).

However, since Crick and Grotpeter (1995) introduced the concept of **relational aggression**, researchers have investigated the possibility that females may be more aggressive than initially thought, but that the form of this aggression may be different from the overt acts of physical aggression that we normally associate with aggressive behaviors.

Relational aggression

According to Crick and Grotpeter (1995, p. 711) relational aggression involves "harming others through purposeful manipulation and damage of their peer relationship."

Research since this time has suggested that the developmental trend for aggression moves from overt acts of physical aggression, to overt vocal displays (due to increased verbal skills), with relational aggression being more prevalent among older children and girls, due to their increased understanding of social skills (Björkqvist, 1994). While most studies support the fact that girls demonstrate more relational aggression than boys from middle childhood (Björkqvist, Österman, & Kaukiainen, 1992; Crick, 1995, 1996), there are opposing views as well (Dodge et al., 2006). One study of elementary school children found that relational aggression was related to depression and peer rejection for girls, but not for boys, although there was a negative correlation between prosocial behavior and relational aggression for all children in the study (Crick, Casas, & Mosher, 1997).

Aggression and age of age of onset   As previously noted, overt forms of aggression peak between two and four years of age and decline after that period (Tremblay et al., 1999). However, for some children, *early starters*, aggression remains a stable characteristic (Aguilar et al., 2000). Early signs that can predict the stability of aggressive behaviors include: tendencies to be fearless (Kagan, 1997), or having a difficult temperament (Vitaro et al., 2006). Children who demonstrate high levels of emotionality may have a lowered threshold for stimulation, and may react with a more intense level of response. The combination of high emotionality and low emotion regulation within the context of externalizing behaviors can result in intensified emotional arousal, reactivity, and escalation of disruptive behaviors (Rydell et al., 2003).

Later onset aggression is usually associated with more positive outcomes than early onset, and is more often triggered by environmental conditions, such as inadequate parental monitoring or affiliation with a deviant peer group (Patterson, Capaldi, & Bank, 1991). According to Dodge et al. (1997), *late starters* are more likely to engage in proactive forms of aggression or "socialized" aggression.

Bullying

Definition   Bullying is an act of aggression that asserts power over an individual who is repeatedly victimized (Olweus, 1995). Bullying can take several forms, including overt acts of **physical aggression**, **verbal aggression** (threats, name calling), **relational aggression** (rumors meant to isolate an individual from their social group), and, more recently, **cyber bullying** (text messaging, photos, or e-mails meant to harass, embarrass, or ostracize the recipient). Due to an unprecedented rise in the cases and awareness of bullying, there has been an associated rise in the number of articles appearing in peer-reviewed journals about the topic. Although fewer than

200 peer-reviewed articles on bullying could be found between 1980 and 2000, over 600 articles were published on the topic between 2000 and 2007 (Cook, Williams, Guerra, Kim, & Sadek, 2010). Researchers have investigated the nature of bullying (types of bullying), participants in the process (bullies and victims), and the efficacy of school-based prevention programs (such as the Olweus Bullying Prevention Program; Olweus, 1993). However, results concerning prevention programs have been disappointing, finding some mixed positive effects, but no overall effect (Bauer, Lozano, & Rivara, 2007), or initial gains dissipating at 12-month follow-up (Jenson, Dieterich, Brisson, Bender, & Powell, 2010).

Bullies, victims, and bully-victims   Research has investigated the nature of bullying and the outcomes to victims. Cook, Williams, Guerra, & Kim (2009) found three groups of youth involved in the act of bullying: **bullies**, **victims**, and **bully-victims**. Studies have confirmed that bullying increases as youth reach adolescence and that it is a worldwide problem. Negative outcomes for the victims can be evident in psychosocial concerns (loneliness, depression, low self-esteem, school avoidance) and can even result in suicide attempts (Hawker & Boulton, 2000; Rigby & Slee, 1999).

Based on their meta-analysis of 153 studies of bullying, Cook et al. (2010) suggest that the majority of studies conducted in the past 30 years focus on individual characteristics, without giving due recognition to the characteristics of the contextual settings in which bullying occurs.

Context as a moderating variable in bullying

In their study of self-esteem and bullying, Gendron, Williams, and Guerra (2011) found that school climate had a moderating effect on self-esteem. When high self-esteem was evident within the context of a negative school climate, it predicted bullying perpetration; however, when high self-esteem occurred within a school climate that was positive, it predicted lower levels of bullying perpetration.

In their meta-analysis, Cook and colleagues (2010, pp. 75–76) found a number of characteristics related to bullying for each of the three groups:

Bully   Youth in this category evidence comorbid externalizing and internalizing symptoms, experience problems socially and academically, and have a negative view of themselves, others, their community, and school. They have poor conflict resolution skills, and are negatively influenced by peers. Family characteristics of bullies were positive for family conflict, and poor parental monitoring.

Victims   Youth who are victims share a number of characteristics with bullies, including a mix of externalizing and internalizing symptoms, poor social skills, and negative self-view, although they are more likely to come from negative environments (family, school, community) and are openly rejected and isolated by peers.

Bully-victims This group of youth has all the same characteristics noted above for bullies and victims, sharing bullies' characteristics of low academic performance and being negatively influenced by peers, but, similar to victims, they are also noticeably rejected by peers. Although the group of bully-victims was not always included in the studies, the researchers suggest that bully-victims seem to be the group most in need of prevention and intervention programs.

In their investigation of bullying outcomes for adolescents in secondary schools in East London, Rothon, Head, Klineberg, and Stansfeld (2011) found that although a high level of parent support was associated with good mental health in general, high levels of support from friends served as the protective factor against adverse academic consequences in the wake of bullying. However, support from friends or family did not protect victims from the mental health consequences, such as depressive symptoms in males.

Due to the increase in bullying, there has been concentrated effort in the past 10 years not only to investigate the nature of this form of aggression, but also to develop school-based prevention programs.

Multifinality and equifinality

Cook et al. (2010) suggest that shared characteristics of bullies, victims, and bully-victims can be accounted for by the principle of **multifinality**. Recall that *multifinality* refers to similar beginnings but different outcomes, while **equifinality** refers to different beginnings but similar outcomes.

Cyber bullying Although having a large collection of "cyber friends" may provide a sense of social comfort and reduce feelings of social anxiety and loneliness (Ando & Sakamoto, 2008), there is also the potential for misuse and abuse of the internet as an instrument of social aggression. In their recent paper on cyber aggression, Schoffstall and Cohen (2011, p. 588) define cyber aggression as "intentional behavior aimed at harming another person or persons through computers, cell phones, and other electronic devices, and perceived as aversive by the victim." The authors elaborate the different forms that cyber aggression may take, including: "flaming (a brief heated exchange), harassment, denigration, impersonation, outing, trickery, exclusion/ostracism, stalking, and happy slapping (violence photographed via a camera phone)" (Schoffstall & Cohen, 2011, p. 588). The authors make the distinction between cyber aggression and cyber bullying, stating that while the intent of cyber aggression is to inflict harm, this process may not include one perpetrator and victim, nor does it imply that the behavior is necessarily repetitive. As a result, it is suggested that approximately only one-quarter (21–25%) of cyber harassment and aggression meets the criteria for bullying (Wolak, Mitchell, & Finkelhorn, 2007). Reports of bullying and cyber bullying continue to reach unprecedented levels. A survey of 177 grade seven students in an urban city in Canada revealed that 54% reported being bullied in the "traditional" sense, while over 25% reported being a victim of cyber bullying; furthermore, the majority of youth did not report these incidents to an adult (Li, 2007).

Cyber bullying can be perceived as more dangerous and threatening than "traditional" bullying because the perpetrator can remain anonymous. Cyber bullying has been used to threaten, embarrass, harass, and socially target and isolate victims (Hinduja & Patchin, 2009; Williams & Guerra, 2007). More recently, studies have focused on sexual harassment via cyber bullying, in the transmission of unsolicited messages or photos of a sexual nature, or propositions to engage in sexual acts (Hinduja & Patchin, 2009). Researchers have used qualitative methods such as focus groups (Mishna, Saini, & Solomon, 2009) and mixed methods research (Guerra, Williams, & Sadek, 2011) in an attempt to better understand the underlying dynamics from the students' points of view. Results have revealed the increasing tendency to use sexualized messages targeting victims in middle and secondary school (Guerra et al., 2011; Mishna, Saini, & Solomon, 2009).

Oppositional defiant disorder

There are two major disorders of childhood associated with excess aggression; however, the way in which these disorders are classified depends on the system used. The DSM-IV-TR specifies **oppositional defiant disorder** (ODD) and **conduct disorder** (CD) as separate disorders with individual symptom lists, requiring three out of a possible 15 symptoms for CD and four out of a possible eight symptoms for ODD. Of the two disorders, ODD is the less severe disorder. On the other hand, the ICD-10 conceptualizes ODD as a subtype of CD with a 23-item symptom list consisting of 15 more severe items (similar to the CD list of the DSM) and eight less severe items (resembling the DSM symptoms for ODD).

ODD and CD: two disorders or one?

There is on-going controversy whether ODD and CD represent a continuum, with ODD being a milder form of CD, or if they represent two distinct disorders. There are several arguments for retaining two distinct disorders, including age of onset (which is much earlier for ODD than CD). Also, the vast majority of those with ODD (75%) never develop CD and the disorders manifest qualitatively different forms of aggression. The ICD-10 states that "many authorities consider that ODD patterns of behavior represent a less severe type of CD rather than a qualitatively distinct type," although it does go on to say that "research evidence is lacking on whether the distinction is qualitative or quantitative" (WHO, 1992, p. 212).

Definition The age of onset for ODD is typically between four and eight years of age, and ODD represents a persistent pattern of defiant, disobedient, provocative, and negative behaviors. The behaviors are primarily directed towards authority figures, and include:

- loss of temper;
- spitefulness and vindictiveness;

- arguments and confrontations with adults;
- defiance and noncompliance;
- refusal to accept blame; blaming others;
- becoming irritated easily; touchiness;
- deliberate annoyingness;
- anger and resentfulness.

Symptoms are not better accounted for by CD, have onset within the developmental period (prior to 18 years of age), and are in excess of what would be anticipated given the age of the child. Clinicians are cautioned to exclude **transient oppositional behaviors** which can commonly occur at different stages of development, such as the increase in autonomous and demanding behaviors that accompany certain developmental transitions (e.g., the "terrible twos"; adolescence). Behaviors that include violations of societal norms, rules, or the rights of others will likely fall under CD. Developmentally, the behavior pattern must be beyond what would be anticipated, given the child's age. The DSM-IV-TR (APA, 2000) notes that transient oppositional behavior such as oppositional behaviors associated with increased autonomy is common in toddlers and teens and would not be considered atypical during those developmental periods, unless excessive.

Temper outbursts and temper dysregulation

There has been considerable controversy among professionals concerning how to categorize children with serious behavior problems and moods that vacillate between irritableness, grumpiness, and explosive angry outbursts. While many have been labeled as bipolar in recent years, the DSM-V is suggesting a new category of temper dysregulation disorder with dysphoria to classify children with this constellation of symptoms. The debate surrounding this proposed category will be discussed further in Chapter 11 in the section on bipolar disorder.

Nature and course   It was initially thought that ODD was a disorder that was specific to childhood and that children would either outgrow the disorder or the disorder would intensify culminating in conduct disorder. However, a more recent study by Biederman et al. (2008) revealed that over 16% (16.6%) of those with ODD continued to evidence symptoms at 25 years of age, while Harpold et al. (2007) found that 30% of those with ODD and comorbid ADHD the symptoms persisted into adulthood. This is a significant finding, because comorbidity rates for ODD and ADHD have been reported to be as high as 65% (Biederman et al., 1996; Petty et al., 2009). Given the high prevalence rate for this comorbid combination, it has been suggested that comorbid ODD and ADHD might represent a specific presentation of symptoms that is evident in some families (Petty et al., 2009). Children with earlier onset of ODD are at greater risk (30%) for developing CD (Connor, Glatt, Lopez, Jackson, & Melloni, 2002) which is three times greater than for those who have later onset.

Our understanding of ODD has been limited in the past by research that has tended to include both ODD and CD in the same samples of disruptive disorders, which has masked individual differences in the outcomes. Current research focus is on separating the two disorders in order to obtain more information specific to these individual disorders (Greene et al., 2002; Petty et al., 2009). Longitudinal studies have found that youth diagnosed with ODD are at greater risk for developing major depressive disorder than peers without the disorder (Biederman et al., 2008).

Prevalence and etiology   It is estimated that between 2% and 16% of the population would meet criteria for a diagnosis of ODD. Although gender differences are evident in childhood, with males having higher prevalence rates for ODD, by adolescence the rates equalize (APA, 2000). Although 75% of those with ODD never develop CD, 90% of those with CD have an initial diagnosis of ODD (Rey, 1993). Unfortunately, there is minimal information available regarding the etiology of ODD since there are no investigations of the origin of ODD separate from those systematic investigations of "behavior disorders" which clump ODD and CD together. The most that is known pertains to CD, which has been studied more exclusively because of the severity of the disorder, and will be discussed in the section on conduct disorder. Presently there is a widespread belief that ODD results from an interaction between complex risk and protective factors, although much more is known of the risks (AACAP, 2007).

Assessment and treatment/intervention

Assessment   There are a number of different methods and instruments available for assessing externalizing behaviors, such as ODD, which were previously discussed at length in *Chapter 5*. Instruments can include a variety of behavioral rating scales completed by parents, teachers, and the child, while methods can include such activities as direct observations of the child in the classroom or at playtime and diagnostic interviews.

Prevention/intervention   For preschoolers, some Head Start Programs have demonstrated positive outcomes in reducing future incarceration and delinquent behaviors (Connor et al., 2002; Greenspan, 1992). Other parenting programs, such as home visitation for families at high risk (Eckenrode et al., 2000), and group programs with discussions focusing on videotaped modeling, have also had positive outcomes (Webster-Stratton, 1994). Parent training programs seem to be the most successful for younger children with ODD, while cognitive behavioral methods seem more appropriate for school-age children and adolescents with ODD and CD (Brestan & Eyberg, 1998). Greene, Ablon, Goring, Fazio, and Morse (2004) have developed a program that focuses on emotion regulation, frustration tolerance, problem solving, and flexibility. The program, *Collaborative Problem Solving* (CPS), focuses on parent education (underlying parent/child dynamics) and interventions aimed at deficits in child information processing (cognitive distortions). Results have been very favorable. Other programs that have demonstrated success in assisting children to enhance problem-solving skills and manage anger include Problem Solving Skills Training (PSST: Kazdin, 1996) and Coping Power (Larson & Lochman, 2002). Coping Power is a 33-session program based on weekly small group sessions involving cognitive behavioral techniques (in vivo practice) designed to improve anger management.

Disorders of conduct

Definition   While children with ODD exhibit a persistent form of disobedience and defiance that typically has an onset prior to 10 years of age, youth with **conduct disorder** experience a more severe, repetitive, and persistent form of disordered behavior that involves a **violation of the rights of others**, or a **serious violation of social norms**.

There are four categories of symptoms that accompany this disorder, which have been evident within the past 12 months, with at least one symptom evident in the past six months. According to the DSM, at least three symptoms are required for a diagnosis, from a list of 15 potential symptoms:

Aggression to people and animals:
- bullies, threatens, or intimidates others;
- initiates fights;
- uses a weapon that can cause serious harm;
- physically cruel to others;
- cruel to animals;
- has stolen while confronting a victim (mugging, purse snatching);
- has forced someone into sexual activity.

Destruction of property:
- deliberate fire setting to cause serious damage;
- deliberately destroying others' property.

Deceitfulness or theft:
- has broken into someone's house, building, or car;
- lies to obtain goods or favors or to avoid obligations ("cons others");
- has stolen items of non-trivial value (shop lifting, forgery).

Serious rule violations:
- often stays out all night, beginning before 13 years of age;
- has run away from home, staying out overnight (twice, or once if lengthy);
- often truant from school, beginning before 13 years of age.

Given the wide range of symptoms, individuals with CD can present with a heterogeneous mix of characteristics, and severity. The DSM uses the specifiers mild, moderate, and severe to distinguish between youth who possess few symptoms and exhibit minor tendencies to harm from those who exhibit many symptoms of the disorder and can inflict significant harm on others.

Sub-types of CD   The DSM recognizes two subtypes of CD: **childhood-onset type** which refers to children who present with at least one symptom of CD prior to 10 years of age; and **adolescent-onset type** for youth who exhibit no symptoms prior to 10 years of age.

The ICD lists several subtypes of CD, including:

- **unsocialized conduct disorder:** behaviors occur in isolation, usually with rejection from peer groups, and evident in such acts as bullying, fighting, and assault;

- **socialized conduct disorder:** behaviors occur in the context of deviant peer group activity;
- **mixed disorders of conduct and emotions:** this classification is used for comorbid presentations. Youth with depressive conduct disorder would meet criteria for both CD and depressed mood (symptom criteria for depression include loss of interest and pleasure, misery, self-blame, hopelessness, and sleep and appetite disturbances). Other emotional combinations are also possible (e.g., anxiety, phobias, obsessions and compulsions, hypochondriasis, depersonalization, and so on).

Sub-types, systems, and comorbidity

Recall that a major difference between the DSM and ICD systems is that the ICD seeks to determine a predominant diagnosis, while the DSM allows for comorbidity for as many diagnoses that meet criteria (Kolvin & Trowell, 2002). Due to the high rates of comorbidity of CD with emotional disorders, the ICD has created sub-types of CD to address this issue.

Callous and unemotional traits   Some youth with CD exhibit traits that have been labeled as **callous and unemotional** (**CU**) to reflect the underlying lack of empathy and affect that accompany this type of CD (Frick & Viding, 2009). There has been significant research to support the identification of this cluster of traits as a unique subtype of CD (Lynam, Caspi, Moffitt, Loeber, & Stouthamer-Loeber, 2007). As a result, it has been suggested that the callous and unemotional specifier be used to label a unique sub-type of CD. This subtype would require at least two of the following criteria, with two having been demonstrated across at least two settings over the past 12 months:

- *lack of remorse or guilt:* does not feel bad or guilty when he/she does something wrong (except if expressing remorse when caught and/or facing punishment);
- *callous-lack of empathy:* disregards and is unconcerned about the feelings of others;
- *unconcerned about performance:* does not show concern about poor/problematic performance at school, at work, or in other important activities;
- *shallow or deficient affect:* does not express feelings or show emotions to others, except in ways that seem shallow or superficial (e.g., his/her emotions are not consistent with his/her actions); can turn emotions "on" or "off" quickly, or use emotions for gain (e.g., to manipulate or intimidate others (Scheepers, Buitelaar, & Matthys, 2011, p. 90).

Nature and course   As previously mentioned, Frick et al. (1993) found that behaviors most closely related to CD symptoms were more likely to be classified as covert rather than overt, and contained both destructive (property violations) and nondestructive acts (status violations). Youth with CD can exhibit a host of aggressive behaviors towards others in open acts of aggression (physical fights) but can also commit more covert acts of intimidation, issuing threats or gaining power through manipulation, lying, deceit, and failure to follow through on promises or obligations (APA, 2000).

Research has demonstrated that children exposed to poverty or stressful life events, or who have a history of parental psychopathology (especially antisocial personality disorder), are at increased risk for developing conduct problems. Poor monitoring and supervision, low levels of parent warmth and engagement, and harsh/inconsistent parenting have all been associated with increased aggression and behavior problems (Patterson, Reid, & Dishion, 1992), as has association with deviant peer groups (Fite, Colder, Lochman, & Wells, 2007). Neighborhoods that are violent and involve antisocial activity also provide an environment that increases the risk of youth developing CD (McCabe, Lucchini, Hough, Yeh, & Hazen, 2005).

Using an ecological and transactional model, the Conduct Problems Prevention Research Group (CPPRG, 2011) charts the potential course of behavioral difficulties in a child from the onset of minor conduct problems to the culmination in serious and violent behaviors, based on the child's interaction with forces in the immediate or proximal environment (family, peers, neighborhood, school, teachers) as depicted in Bronfenbrenner's (1979) microsystem. The developmental pathway is constructed based on our knowledge of the risk factors noted earlier. The trajectory begins with a difficult temperament evident in problems of impulse control and behavior regulation, within the context of a home where the parent is ill-equipped to manage the behavior, especially if living within the stressful conditions of a disadvantaged neighborhood with few resources, supports, or extra time. In these conditions, the research would predict that, by the time school age arrives, the child will likely be poorly prepared and lacking in the necessary skills to be successful academically or socially, and be at risk for peer rejection (Dodge, Coie, & Lyman, 2006) and conflict with teachers (Stormshak et al., 2000).

Within this type of scenario, children continue to follow the path towards CD based on their lack of social skills and problem-solving ability, eventually disengaging from a system that is a constant reminder of failure. Ultimately, the youth find support in a deviant peer group who share a sense of isolation and regain their power through aggression and violence (Dodge et al., 2006).

Lynam et al. (2007) investigated the interaction of impulsivity and neighborhood disadvantage and found that impulsive adolescents were at increased risk for engaging in delinquent activity, relative to peers with low impulsivity, if they lived in neighborhoods high in economic disadvantage. However, although both Lynam et al. (2007) and the CPPRG (2011) address the biological characteristic of impulsivity, neither of these papers addresses other biological factors that may have an impact on the outcome. The biological side of the interaction will be addressed next.

Prevalence and etiology Both biological and environmental factors have been implicated in the development of CD. Elevated levels of the hormone **testosterone** have been linked to the genetic transmission of aggressive impulses (Dabbs & Morris, 1990), while lower levels of Dopamine beta-hydroxylase (DBH), an enzyme that converts dopamine to norepinephrine, may produce increased risk taking and sensation seeking in youth (Quay, 1986). Behavioral theorists have studied parent–child interactions and have proposed a coercive model whereby patterns of noncompliance and coercive responses can result in an on-going and negatively reinforced pattern of behaviors (Patterson, Shaw, Snyder, & Yoerger, 2005). This is especially true when the temperament of the child (high emotion reactivity) and parent (inconsistent, impulsive) are a poor fit (Barkley, 1997).

Some of the highest levels of comorbidity with CD are seen in ADHD, substance abuse, and depression. Approximately half of youth diagnosed with CD will have comorbid bipolar disorder (Kovacs & Pollock, 1995) and half will also have a substance abuse problem (Reebye, Moretti, & Gulliver, 1995).

Assessment and treatment/intervention   Youth with serious behavioral disorders have been treated in a wide variety of settings and, depending on the degree of severity, interventions may take place in the school setting, in alternative schools, or in residential treatment centers. Community-based programs that have been empirically supported include: successful placements in specialized foster care (Chamberlain & Reid, 1998): successful treatment of juvenile offenders using Multisystemic Therapy (Schoenwald, Borduin, & Henggeler, 1998); and a five-day-a-week, in-home family preservation program using cognitive behavioral methods (Wilmshurst, 2002).

Fast Track Prevention Intervention   The CPPRG (2011) recently released the results of their 10-year intervention program involving 891 early-starting children (69% male; 51% African American) who were randomly assigned to intervention or control conditions (445 intervention; 446 control) involving four geographical locations across the United States, and 55 schools, selected on the basis of crime and poverty statistics. The study used a multi-gating screening procedure, involving screenings of ratings for disruptive behavior obtained from parents and teachers for all kindergarten children attending the 55 schools across three cohorts (1991–1993). Children who scored within the top 40% on teacher ratings were selected for home-based ratings. Intervention procedures were instituted in two phases: the elementary school phase (grades 1–5), consisting of opportunities for parent training, home visitations, academic tutoring, and child social skills training; and the middle and early high school phase (grades 6–10), offering a middle school transition program, groups for parents and youth concerning adolescent topics (such as positive involvement and monitoring), and youth forums (addressing topics such as peer pressure). Results from the multiple-gating screening procedure predicted an 82% likelihood of exhibiting an externalizing disorder by 18 years of age, for those children who were rated in the top 3 percentiles, on combined parent–teacher ratings. Involvement in the long-term prevention program reduced the risk to half of that predicted for this group. Furthermore, not only did participation in the prevention program prevent these children from being diagnosed with CD, the positive effects continued to remain when they were re-assessed two years after termination of the program. The authors suggest that the program had the biggest impact on those with the most severe forms of CD, which justifies the use of this prevention program for those at highest risk; however, effects were limited for groups in the study demonstrating more "moderate risk."

References

Achenbach, T. M., & Rescorla, L. A. (2001). *Manual for the ASEBA school-age forms and profiles.* Burlington, VT: University of Vermont, Research Center for Children, Youth and Families.

Aguilar, B., Sroufe, L. A., Egeland, B., & Carlson, E. (2000). Distinguishing the early-onset/persistent and adolescent-onset antisocial behavior types. From birth to 16 years. *Development and Psychopathology, 12*, 109–132.

American Academy of Child and Adolescent Psychiatry (AACAP). (2007). Practice parameter for the assessment and treatment of children and adolescents with oppositional defiant disorder. *Journal of the American Academy of Child and Adolescent Psychiatry, 46*(1), 126–141.

American Psychiatric Association (APA). (2000). *Diagnostic and statistical manual of mental disorders* (4th ed., text revision). Washington, DC: Author.

Ando, K., & Sakamoto, A. (2008). The effect of cyber-friends on loneliness and social anxiety: Differences between high and low self-evaluated physical attractiveness groups. *Human Behavior, 24,* 993–1009.

Attar, B. K., Guerra, N. G., & Tolan, P. H. (1994). Neighborhood disadvantage, stressful life events, and adjustment in urban elementary-school children. *Journal of Clinical Child Psychology, 23*(4), *Special issue: Impact of poverty on children, youth, and families,* pp. 391–400.

Bandura, A. (1973). *Aggression: A social learning theory analysis.* New York: Prentice Hall.

Barker, E. D., Tremblay, R. E., Nagin, D. S., Lacourse, E., & Vitaro, F. (2006). Development of male proactive and reactive aggression during adolescence. *Journal of Child Psychology and Psychiatry, 47,* 783–790.

Barkley, R. A. (1997). Behavior inhibition, sustained attention and executive function. *Psychological Bulletin, 121,* 65–94.

Barriga, A. Q., Doran, J. W., Newell, S. B., Morrison, E. M., Barbetti, V., & Robbins, B. D. (2002). Relationships between problem behaviors and academic achievement in adolescents: The unique role of attention problems. *Journal of Emotional and Behavioral Disorders, 10*(4), 233–240.

Bauer, L. O., & Hesselbrock, V. M. (2003). Brain maturation and subtypes of conduct disorder: Interactive effects on P300 amplitude and topography in male adolescents. *Journal of the American Academy of Child and Adolescent Psychiatry, 42,* 106–115.

Bauer, N. W., Lozano, P., & Rivara, F. P. (2007). The effectiveness of the Olweus bullying prevention program in public middle schools: A controlled trial. *Journal of Adolescent Health, 40,* 266–274.

Berkowitz, L. (1978). Whatever happened to the frustration-aggression hypothesis? *American Behavioral Scientist, 32,* 691–708.

Biederman, J., Faraone, S. V., Milberger, S., Carcia Jetton, J., Chen, J., & Mick, E. (1996). Is childhood oppositional defiant disorder a precursor to adolescent conduct disorder? Findings from a four-year follow-up study of children with ADHD. *Journal of the American Academy of Child and Adolescent Psychiatry, 35,* 1193–1204.

Biederman, J., Perry, C. R., Dolan, C., Hughes, S., Mick, E., & Montuteauz, M. C. (2008). The long-term longitudinal course of oppositional defiant disorder and conduct disorder in ADHD boys: Findings from a controlled 10-year prospective longitudinal follow-up study. *Psychological Medicine, 38,* 1027–1036.

Björkqvist, K. (1994). Sex differences in physical, verbal, and indirect aggression: A review of recent research. *Sex Roles, 30,* 177–188.

Björkqvist, K., Österman, K., & Kaukiainen, A. (1992). The development of direct and indirect aggressive strategies in males and females. In K. Björkqvist & P. Niemela (Eds.), *Of mice and women: Aspects of female aggression* (pp. 51–64). San Diego, CA: Academic Press.

Brandenburg, N. A., Friedman, R. M., & Silver, S. (1990). The epidemiology of childhood psychiatric disorders: Prevalence findings from recent studies. *Journal of the American Academy of Child and Adolescent Psychiatry, 29,* 76–83.

Brestan, E. V., & Eyberg, S. M. (1998). Effective psychosocial treatments of conduct disordered children and adolescents: 29 years, 82 studies and 5,272 kids. *Journal of Clinical Child Psychology, 27,* 180–189.

Bronfenbrenner, U. (1979). *The ecology of human development.* Cambridge, MA: Harvard University Press.

Campbell, S. B. (2002). *Behaviour problems in preschool children: Clinical and developmental issues.* New York: Guilford.

Campbell, S. B., Spieker, S., Burchinal, M., & Poe, M. D. (2006). Trajectories of aggression from toddlerhood to age 9 predict academic and social functioning through age 12. *Journal of Child Psychology and Psychiatry, 47*(8), 791–800.

Campos, J., Anderson, D., Barbu-Roth, M., Hubbard, E., Herrenstein, M., & Witherington, D. (2000). Travel broadens the mind. *Infancy, 1*, 149–219.

Chamberlain, P., & Reid, J. (1998). Comparison of two community alternatives to incarceration for chronic juvenile offenders. *Journal of Consulting and Clinical Psychology, 66*, 624–633.

Comer, R. J. (2010). *Abnormal psychology* (7th ed.). New York: Worth.

Connor, D. F., Glatt, S. J., Lopez, I. D., Jackson, D., & Melloni, R. H. (2002). Psychopharmacology and aggression: I. A meta-analysis of stimulant effects onovert/covert aggression-related behaviors in ADHD. *Journal of the American Academy of Child and Adolescent Psychiatry, 41*, 253–261.

Cook, C. R., Williams, K. R., Guerra, N., & Kim, T. (2009). Variability in the prevalence of bullying and victimization: A cross-national and methodological analysis. In S. R. Jimerson, S. M. Swearer, & D. L. Espelage (Eds.), *The international handbook of school bullying* (pp. 347–362). Mahwah, NJ: Erlbaum.

Cook, C. R., Williams, K. R., Guerra, N., Kim, T., & Sadek, S. (2010). Predictors of bully and victimization in childhood and adolescence: A meta-analytic investigation. *School Psychology Quarterly, 25*, 65–83.

Cote, S., Vaillancourt, T., LeBlanc, J. C., Nagin, D. S., & Tremblay, R. E. (2006). The development of physical aggression from toddlerhood to pre-adolescence: A nationwide longitudinal study of Canadian children. *Journal of Abnormal Child Psychology, 34*, 71–85.

Conduct Problems Prevention Research Group (CPPRG). (2011). The effects of the Fast Track Prevention Intervention on the development of conduct disorder across childhood. *Child Development, 82*, 331–345.

Crick, N. R. (1995). Relational aggression: The role of intent attributions, feelings of distress, and provocation type. *Development and Psychopathology, 7*, 313–322.

Crick, N. R. (1996). The role of overt aggression, relational aggression, and prosocial behavior in the prediction of children's future social adjustment. *Child Development, 67*, 2317–2327.

Crick, N. R., Casas, J. F., & Mosher, M. (1997). Relational and overt aggression in preschool. *Developmental Psychology, 33*, 579–588.

Crick, N. R., & Dodge, K. A. (1996). Social information-processing mechanisms in reactive and proactive aggression. *Child Development, 67*, 993–1002.

Crick, N. R., & Grotpeter, J. K. (1995). Relation alaggression, gender, and social-psychological adjustment. *Child Development, 66*, 710–722.

Dabbs, J., & Morris, R. (1990). Testosterone, social class and antisocial behavior in a sample of 4, 462 men. *Psychological Science, 1*, 209–211.

Dionne, G., Tremblay, R. E., Boivin, M., Laplante, D., & Perusse, D. (2003). Physical aggression and expressive vocabulary in 19-month-old twins. *Developmental Psychology, 39*, 261–273.

Dodge, K. A., & Coie, J. D. (1987). Social-information-processing factors in reactive and proactive aggression in children's peer groups. *Journal of Personality and Social Psychology, 53*, 1146–1158.

Dodge, K. A., Coie, J., & Lyman, D. (2006). Aggression and antisocial behavior in youth. In N. Eisenberg (Ed.), *Handbook of child psychology*, vol. 3 (series Eds. W. Damon and R. Lerner) (pp. 719–788). Chichester: John Wiley & Sons, Ltd.

Dodge, K. A., Lochman, J. E., Harnish, J. D., Bates, J. E., & Pettit, G. S. (1997). Reactive and proactive aggression in school children and psychiatrically impaired chronically assaultive youth. *Journal of Abnormal Psychology, 106*, 37–51.

Eckenrode, J., Ganzel,B., Henderson, C. R., Smith, E., Olds, D. L., Powers, J., . . . Cole, R. (2000). Preventing child abuse and neglect with a program of nurse home visitation: The limiting effects of domestic violence. *Journal of the American Medical Association, 284,* 1385–1391.

Fite, P. J., Colder, C. R., Lochman, J. E., & Wells, K. C. (2007). The relation between childhood proactive and reactive aggression and substance use initiation. *Journal of Abnormal Child Psychology, 36,* 261–271.

Frick, P. J., Cornell, A. H., Barry, C. T., Bodin, S. D., & Dane, H. E. (2003). Callousunemotional traits and conduct problems in the prediction of conduct problem severity, aggression, and self-report of delinquency. *Journal of Abnormal Child Psychology, 31,* 457–470.

Frick, P. J., Lahey, B. B., Loeber, R., Tannenbaum, L., Van Horn, Y, Christ, M. A., ... Hanson, K. (1993). Oppositional defiant disorder and conduct disorder: A meta-analytic review of factor analysis and cross validation in a clinical sample. *Clinical Psychology Review, 13,* 319–340.

Frick, P. J., & Viding, E. (2009). Antisocial behavior from a developmental psychopathology perspective. *Development and Psychopathology, 21,* 1111–1131.

Friedman, O., & Neary, K. R. (2008). Determining who owns what: Do children infer ownership from first possession? *Cognition, 107,* 829–849.

Gendron, B. P., Williams, K. R., & Guerra, N. G. (2011). An analysis of bullying among students within schools: Estimating the effects of individual normative beliefs, self-esteem and school climate. *Journal of School Violence, 10*(2), 150–164.

Greene, R. W., Ablon, J. S., Goring, J. C., Fazio, V., & Morse, L. R. (2004). Treatment of oppositional defiant disorder in children and adolescents. In P. M. Barrett & T. H. Ollendick (Eds.), *Handbook of interventions that work with children and adolescents* (pp. 369–393). Chichester: John Wiley & Sons, Ltd.

Greene, R. W., Biederman, J., Zerwas, S., Montuteaux, M. C., Goring, J. C., & Faraone, S. V. (2002). Psychiatric comorbidity, family dysfunction and social impairment in referred youth with oppositional defiant disorder. *American Journal of Psychiatry, 159,* 1214–1224.

Greenspan, S. I. (1992). *Infancy and early childhood: The practice of clinical assessment and intervention with emotional and developmental challenges.* Madison, CT: International Universities Press.

Guerra, N. G., Williams, K. R., & Sadek, S. (2011). Understanding bullying and victimization during childhood and adolescence: A mixed methods study. *Child Development, 82*(1), 295–310.

Harpold, T., BiedermanJ., Gignac, M., Hamamerness, P., Surman, C., & Potter, A. (2007). Is oppositional defiant disorder a meaningful diagnosis in adults? Results from a large sample of adults with ADHD. *Journal of Nervous and Mental Disease, 195,* 601–605.

Hartup, W. W. (1974). Aggression in childhood: Developmental perspectives. *American Psychologist, 29,* 336–341.

Hawker, D. S., & Boulton, M. J. (2000). Twenty years' research on peer victimization and psychosocial maladjustment: A meta-analytic review of cross-sectional studies. *Journal of Child Psychology and Psychiatry, 41,* 441–455.

Hay, D. F., Hurst, S., Waters, C. S., & Chadwick, A. (2011). Infants' use of force to defend toys: The origins of instrumental aggression. *Infancy, 16*(5), 471–489.

Herrenkohl, T. I., Maguin, E., & Hill, K. G. (2000). Developmental risk factors for youth violence. *Journal of Adolescent Health, 26*(7), 176–186.

Hill, A. L., Degnan, K. A., Calkins, S. D., & Keane, S. P. (2006). Profiles of externalizing behavior problems for boys and girls across preschool: The roles of emotion regulation and inattention. *Developmental Psychology, 42*(5), 913–928.

Hinduja, S., & Patchin, J. W. (2009). *Bullying beyond the schoolyard: Preventing and responding to cyberbullying.* Thousand Oaks, CA: Sage.

Hubbard, J. A., Smithmyer, C. M., & Ramsden, S. R. (2002). Observational, physiological and self-report measures of children's anger: Relations to reactive versus proactive aggression. *Child Development, 73,* 1101–1118.

Jenson, J. M., Dieterich, W. A., Brisson, D., Bender, K., & Powell, A. (2010). Preventing childhood bullying: Findings and lessons from the Denver Public Schools Trial. *Research on Social Work Practice, 20,* 509–517.

Jones, A. P., Laurens, K. R., Herba, C. M., Barker, G., & Viding, E. (2009). Amygdala hypoactivity to fearful faces in boys with conduct problems and callous-unemotional traits. *American Journal of Psychiatry, 166*(1), 95–102.

Kagan, J. (1997). Temperament and the reactions to unfamiliarity. *Child Development, 68,* 139–143.

Kagan, J., Reznick, J. S., & Gibbons, J. (1989). Inhibited and uninhibited types of children. *Child Development, 60,* 838–845.

Kazdin, A. E. (1996). Problem solving and parent management in treating aggressive and antisocial behavior. In E. S. Hibbs & P. S. Jensen (Eds.), *Psychosocial treatments for child and adolescent disorders: Empirically based strategies for clinical practice* (pp. 377–408). Washington, DC: APA.

Kolvin, I., & Trowell, J. (2002). Diagnosis and classification in child and adolescent psychiatry: The case of unipolar disorder. *Psychopathology, 35,* 117–121.

Kovacs, M., & Pollock, M. (1995). Bipolar disorder and comorbid conduct disorder in childhood and adolescence. *Journal of the American Academy of Child and Adolescent Psychiatry, 34,* 715–723.

Lacourse, E., Nagin, D. S., Vitario, F., Cote, S., Arseneault, L., & Tremblay, R. E. (2006). Prediction of early-onset deviant peer group affiliation: A 12-year longitudinal study. *Archives of General Psychiatry, 63*(5), 562–568.

Ladd, G., Kochenderfer, B., & Coleman, C. C. (1996). Friendship quality as a predictor of young children's early school adjustment. *Child Development, 67,* 1103–1118.

Lansford, J. E., Criss, M. M., Pettit, G. S., Dodge, K. A., & Bates, J. E. (2003). Friendship quality, peer group affiliation and peer antisocial behavior as moderations of the link between negative parenting and adolescent externalizing behaviour. *Journal of Research on Adolescence, 13*(2), 161–184.

Larson, J., & Lochman, J. E. (2002). *Helping school children cope with anger: A cognitive-behavioral intervention.* New York: Guilford.

Levenston, G. K., Patrick, C. J., Bradley, M. M., & Lang, P. J. (2000). The psychopath as observer: Emotion and attention in picture processing. *Journal of Abnormal Psychology, 109,* 373–385.

Li, Q. (2007). New bottle but old wine: A research of cyber bullying in schools. *Computers in Human Behavior, 23,* 1777–1791.

Little, T. D., Jones, S. M., Henrich, C. C., & Hawley, P. H. (2003). Disentangling the "whys" from the "whats" of aggressive behaviour. *International Journal of Behavioural Development, 27,* 122–133.

Lochman, J. E., & Wells, K. C. (2002). Contextual social-cognitive mediators and child outcome: A test of the theoretical model in the coping power program. *Development and Psychopathology, 14,* 945–967.

Lynam, D. R., Caspi, A., Moffitt, T. E., Loeber, R., & Stouthamer-Loeber, M. (2007). Longitudinal evidence that psychopathy scores in early adolescence predict adult psychopathy. *Journal of Abnormal Psychology, 116,* 155–165.

Lynch, M., & Cicchetti, D. (1998). An ecological-transactional analysis of children and contexts: The longitudinal interplay among child maltreatment, community violence and children's symptomatology. *Development and Psychopathology, 10,* 235–257.

Marsh, R., Gerber, A. J., & Peterson, B. S. (2008). Neuroimaging studies of normal brain development and their relevance for understanding childhood neuropsychiatric disorders. *Journal of the American Academy of Child and Adolescent Psychiatry, 47*(11), 1233–1251.

McCabe, K. M., Lucchini, S. E., Hough, R. L., Yeh, M., & Hazen, A. (2005). The relation between violence exposure and conduct problems among adolescents: A prospective study. *American Journal of Orthopsychiatry, 75*(4), 575–584.

Moffitt, T. E. (1993). The neuropsychology of conduct disorder. *Development and Psychopathology*, 5(1–2), 135–151.

Mishna, F., Saini, M., & Solomon, S. (2009). Ongoing and online: Children and youth's perceptions of cyber bullying. *Children and Youth Services Review*, 31, 1222–1228.

Offord, D. R., Boyle, M. G., Szatmari, P., Rae-Grant, N. I., Links, P. S., & Cadman, D. T. (1987). Ontario child health study II: Six-month prevalence of disorder and rates of service utilization. *Archives of General Psychiatry*, 44, 832–836.

Olweus, D. (1993). *Bullying at school: What we know and what we can do*. Oxford: Blackwell.

Olweus, D. (1995). Bullying or peer abuse at school: Facts and interventions. *Current Directions in Psychological Science*, 4(6), 196–200.

Patterson, G. R., Capaldi, D., & Bank, L. (1991). An early starter model for predicting delinquency. In D. Pepler & K. H. Rubin (Eds.), *The development and treatment of childhood aggression* (pp. 139–168). Hillsdale, NJ: Erlbaum.

Patterson, G. R., Reid, J., & Dishion, T. J. (1992). *A social learning approach*, vol. 4, *Antisocial boys*. Eugene, OR: Castaglia.

Patterson, G. R., Shaw, D. S., Snyder, J. J., & Yoerger, K. (2005). Changes in maternal ratings of children's overt and covert antisocial behavior. *Aggressive Behavior*, 31, 473–484.

Petty, C. R., Monteaux, M., Mick, E., Hughes, S., Small, J., & Faraone, S. V. (2009). Parsing the familiality of oppositional defiant disorder from that of conduct disorder: A familial risk analysis. *Journal of Psychiatric Research*, 43, 345–352.

Preddy, T. M., & Fite, P. J. (2012). Differential associations between relational and overt aggression and children's psychosocial adjustment. *Journal of Psychopathology and Behavioral Assessment*. doi:10.1007/s10862-011-9274-1

Putallaz, M., Grimes, C. L., Foster, K. J., Kupersmidt, J. B., Coie, J. D., & Dearing, K. (2007). Overt and relational aggression and victimization: Multiple perspectives within the school setting. *Journal of School Psychology*, 45, 523–547.

Quay, H. C. (1986). Conduct disorders. In H. C. Quay & J. S. Werry (Eds.), *Psychopathological disorders of childhood* (3rd ed.) (pp. 1–34). New York: John Wiley & Sons, Ltd.

Resnick, M. D., Bearman, P. S., Blum, R. W., Bauman, K. E., Harris, K. M., Jones, J. J.,... Udry, J. R. (1997). Protecting adolescents from harm. *Journal of the American Medical Association*, 278(10), 823–832.

Reebye, P. N., Moretti, M. M., & Gulliver, L. (1995). Conduct disorder and substance use disorder. Comorbidity in a clinical sample of preadolescents and adolescents. *Canadian Journal of Psychiatry*, 40, 313–319.

Rey, J. M. (1993). Opposition defiant disorder. *American Journal of Psychiatry*, 150, 1769–1777.

Rigby, K., & Slee, P. (1999). Suicidal ideation among adolescent school children, involvement in bully-victim problems, and perceived social support. *Suicide and Life-Threatening Behavior*, 29, 119–130.

Rothon, C., Head, J., Klineberg, E., & Stansfeld, S. (2011). Can social support protect bullied adolescents from adverse outcomes? A prospective study on the effects of bullying on the educational achievement and mental health of adolescents at secondary schools in East London. *Journal of Adolescence*, 34, 579–588.

Rutter, M. (1979). Protective factors in children's responses to stress and disadvantage. In M. Whalen & J. E. Rolf (Eds.), *Primary prevention of psychopathology: Vol. 3. Social competence in children* (pp. 49–79). Hanover, NH: University Press of New England.

Rydell, A., Berlin, L., & Bohlin, G. (2003). Emotionality, emotion regulation and adaptation among 5- to 8-year old children. *Emotion*, 3, 30–47.

Scheepers, F. E., Buitelaar, J. K., & Matthys, W. (2011). Conduct disorder and the specifier callous and unemotional traits in the DSM-5. *European Child and Adolescent Psychiatry*, 20, 89–93.

Schoenwald, S., Borduin, C. H., & Henggeler, S. W. (1998). Multisystemic therapy: Changing the natural and service ecologies of adolescents and families. In M. Epstein, K. Kutash, & A. Duchnowski (Eds.), *Outcomes for children and youth with emotional and behavioral disorders and their families: Programs and evaluation best practices* (pp. 485–511). Austin, TX: PRO-ED.

Schoffstall, C. L., & Cohen, R. (2011). Cyber aggression: The relation between online offenders and offline social competence. *Social Development, 20*(3), 587–604.

Stormshak, E. A., Bierman, K. L., McMahon, R. J., Lengua, L., & The Conduct Problems Prevention Research Group. (2000). Parenting practices and child disruptive behavior problems in early elementary school. *Journal of Clinical Child Psychology, 29*, 17–29.

Stranger, C., Achenbach, T. M., & Verhulst, F. C. (1997). Accelerated longitudinal comparisons of aggressive versus delinquent syndromes. *Development and Psychopathology, 9*, 43–58.

Teichner, G., Golden, C. J., Crum, T. A., Azrin, N. H., Donohue, B., & Van Hasselt, V. B. (2000). Identification of neuropsychological subtypes in a sample of delinquent adolescents. *Journal of Psychiatric Research, 34*, 129–132.

Tremblay, R. E., Japel, C., Perusse, D., McDuff, P., Boivin, M., Zoccolillo, M., & Montplaisir, J. (1999). The search for the age of "onset" of physical aggression: Rousseau and Bandura revisited. *Criminal Behavior and Mental Health, 9*, 8–23.

Tremblay, R., Nagin, D. S., Séguin, J. R., Zoccolillo, M., Zelazo, P. D., Boivin, M., . . . Japel, C. (2004). Physical aggression during early childhood: Trajectories and predictors. *Pediatrics, 114*, e43–e50.

Van Zeijl, J., Mesman, J., Stolk, M. N., Alink, L. R., van IJzendoorn, M. H., Bakermans-Kranenburg, M. J. . . . Koot, H. M. (2006). Terrible ones? Assessment of externalizing behaviors in infancy with the Child Behavior Checklist. *Journal of Child Psychology and Psychiatry, 47*, 801–810.

Viding, E., Blair, R. J. R., Moffitt, T. E., & Plomin, R. (2005). Evidence for substantial genetic risk for psychopathy in 7-year-olds. *Journal of Child Psychology and Psychiatry, 46*, 592–597.

Viding, E., Jones, A. P., Frick, P. J., Moffitt, T. E., & Plomin, R. (2008). Heritability of antisocial behaviour at 9: Do callous-unemotional traits matter? *Developmental Science, 11*, 17–22.

Vitaro, F., Barker, E. D., Boivin, M., Brendgen, M., & Tremblay, R. E. (2006). Do early difficult temperament and harsh parenting differentially predict reactive and proactive aggression? *Journal of Abnormal Child Psychology, 34*, 685–695.

Vitaro, F., Gendreau, P. L., Tremblay, R. E., & Oligny, P. (1998). Reactive and proactive aggression differentially predict later conduct problems. *Journal of Child Psychology and Psychiatry, 39*, 377–385.

Webster-Stratton, C. (1994). Advancing videotape parent training: A comparison study. *Journal of Consulting and Clinical Psychology, 62*, 583–593.

Widom, C. S. (1989). The cycle of violence. *Science, 244*(4901), 160–166.

Williams, K., & Guerra, N. (2007). Prevalence and predictors of internet bullying. *Journal of Adolescent Health, 41*(6), 514–521.

Wilmshurst, L. (2002). Treatment programs for youth with emotional and behavioral disorders: An outcomes study of two alternate approaches. *Mental Health Services Research, 4*, 85–96.

Wolak, J., Mitchell, K. J., & Finkelhorn, D. (2007). Accelerated longitudinal comparisons of aggressive versus delinquent syndromes. *Development and Psychopathology, 9*, 43–58.

World Health Organization (WHO). (1992). *The ICD-10 classification of mental and behavioural disorders. Clinical descriptions and diagnostic guidelines.* Geneva: Author.

Xu, Y., Farver, J. A., & Zhang, Z. (2009). Temperament, harsh and indulgent parenting, and Chinese children's proactive and reactive aggression. *Child Development, 80*, 244–258.

10

Internalizing Problems and Anxiety, Mood, and Somatic Disorders

Clinical and Educational Child Psychology, First Edition. Linda Wilmshurst.
© 2013 John Wiley & Sons, Ltd. Published 2013 by John Wiley & Sons, Ltd.

Chapter preview and learning objectives

Children and adolescents can express a wide range of emotional responses to distressing circumstances that can be transitory, and appropriate to their developmental level, or represent reactions that are more intense, severe, persistent, and beyond what would be normally anticipated. The objectives of this chapter include enhanced understanding of:

- internalizing problems evident in children and adolescents who respond to distressing circumstances by avoidance and overly controlled emotions. Responses often include worries, fears, phobias, anxieties, fluctuations in mood, or somatic complaints;
- the continuum in severity for any of the above difficulties, based on the intensity, severity, and duration of the problem, given developmental expectations;
- similarities and differences in criteria for determining whether problems are considered to be within the abnormal range and thereby considered to be disorders of childhood and adolescence, and how these disorders are conceptualized by the two different systems of classification.

There are several different types of anxiety disorder that can present with a wide variety of symptoms, including: specific phobias, separation anxiety disorder, generalized anxiety disorder, obsessive compulsive disorder, social phobia, and panic disorder (with or without agoraphobia). Although post-traumatic stress disorder (PTSD) and acute stress disorder have been listed in the category of anxiety disorders in the DSM, it is likely that these disorders will be reclassified under the category of stress disorders in the future, and for our purposes will be discussed under trauma in *Chapter 13*.

Internalizing problems: an overview

Internalizing problems result from behaviors that are "**overcontrolled.**" Achenbach and Rescorla (2001, p. 93) describe internalizing behaviors as "problems within the self, such as anxiety, depression, and somatic complaints," without known medical cause, which result in withdrawal from social contact.

What are the internalizing problems?

Anxiety disorders (anxious and inhibited responses), **mood disorders** (both unipolar depression and bipolar depression), and the **somatoform disorders** (emotional distress manifesting as physical discomfort) all share symptoms that are internally oriented.

Negative affectivity

Anxiety and depression often occur together in young children with a comorbidity rate as high as 60–70%. Developmentally, anxiety is a precursor to depression (Kovacs & Devlin, 1998); however, in young children, symptoms of generalized anxiety and depression often occur together as anxious-depressed symptoms before they become more differentiated (Ebesutani, Smith, Bernstein, & Chorpita, et al., 2011). Ebesutani et al. (2011, p. 679) describe **negative affectivity** as "a broad temperamental factor of emotional distress that is related to mood states such as sadness, fear, guilt, and anger," as opposed to **positive affectivity** which refers to a mood state that reflects a sense of enthusiasm. The concept of negative affectivity is derived from the tripartite model (Watson, Clark, & Carey, 1988) developed to explain the similarities and differences between anxiety and depression. Within this model, depression is recognized as a unique state of low positive affect (**anhedonia**); however, depression shares the state of negative affectivity with anxiety (Chorpita, 2002; Chorpita, Plummer, & Moffit, 2000).

The Anxious/Depressed scale of the Achenbach System of Empirically Based Behaviors (ASEBA) is a scale that measures negative affectivity, while the Withdrawn/Depressed Scale is a measure of low positive affect (Achenbach & Rescorla, 1996). It has been suggested that temperament may influence a child's responses to novel or challenging situations, in such a way that some children are predisposed to respond to challenging situations with high levels of negative affectivity evident in displays of anger, frustration, fear, irritability, or sadness (Putnam, Ellis, & Rothbart, 2001). High levels of negative affectivity have been associated with problems in self-regulation, poor social competence, and both externalizing and internalizing problems (Calkins, 2002). Although a child's temperament was once thought to be a relatively stable factor during early development (Buss & Plomin, 1984), it is now recognized that as children mature and face new challenges in different contexts and settings (such as transitions to school), their temperaments may change as they incorporate new self-regulatory behaviors into their repertoire. For example, Blandon, Calkins, Keane, and O'Brien (2008) reported that increases in young children's self-regulatory behaviors were accompanied by decreases in negative affectivity. Furthermore, Blandon et al. (2008) found that parenting practices could serve to moderate behavior in children who demonstrated higher biological reactivity. If the parent was warm and responsive, children exhibited a decline in negative emotions; however, if the parent was overly controlling and paid minimal attention to the child's goals and behaviors, children responded with increased negative affectivity.

Table 10.1   Common fears experienced at different developmental levels

Developmental stage	Common fears
Toddler stage (1–2 years)	Strangers, toileting activities, personal injury
Preschool (3–6 years)	Imaginary creatures, monsters, the dark, animals
Early school (6–10 years)	Small animals, the dark, environmental factors such as lightning and thunder, threats to personal safety

Source: Adapted from Barrios and Hartmann (1977).

Worries, fears, and rituals

The majority of children experience a wide variety of fears at various developmental levels. The most common fears for children at the preschool and primary level are presented in Table 10.1.

In their study of developmental trends in fears, worries, and ritualistic behaviors, Laing, Fernyhough, Turner, and Freeston (2009) distinguish between children's fears, "a concern regarding danger or threat to survival," and worries, "concern regarding possible social or cognitive discomfort" (p. 352). Fears and worries both tend to peak around seven years of age. However, while fears tend to dissipate after this age, the prevalence of worries increases dramatically, with 80% of children admitting to worrying after seven years of age (Muris, Merckelbach, Gadet, & Moulaert, 2000). Fears evolve from an earlier focus on imaginary creatures to more realistic concerns related to physical danger/bodily injury and ultimately to feared social or medical situations (Ollendick, Yule, & Ollier, 1991). Although common worries can be experienced by most children and adolescents at some stage (potential harm of a loved one, school performance, social groups), as children get older, there is more emphasis on worrying about performance issues and social evaluation (Laing et al., 2009). Girls report more fears (Ollendick et al., 1991) than boys at all ages, and also report more worries overall (Ollendick, 2001).

Engaging in ritualistic and repetitive behaviors is common in childhood, particularly between the ages of two and seven (Evans et al., 1997; Leonard, Goldberger, & Rapoport, 1990; Zohar & Felz, 2001). The most common rituals include: perfectionism (having to be "just right"), ordering and arranging objects in precise, prescribed ways; hoarding; and concerns about dirt (Evans et al., 1997; Leonard et al., 1990), or rituals embedded in common activities such as eating or bedtime routines (such as insisting that a parent read the same book over and over in a particular manner).

Why perform rituals?

Rituals can increase feelings of security and reduce anxious feelings related to fears about contamination, injury, and strangers (Evans, Gray, & Leckman, 1999).

Developmentally, preschoolers tend to dwell on a sense of "sameness," repetition, and constancy, while older children are more likely to demonstrate rigid adherence to complex rules that define games, or engage in behaviors intended to "undo" potential negative consequences (Laing et al., 2009). Although it has been suggested that ritualistic behaviors may initially (at four to seven years of age) fill an adaptive function by providing a sense of personal control, rituals may become increasingly maladaptive after this time. Laing et al. (2009) suggest that since worry and obsessions involve similar negative and potentially uncontrollable and intrusive thoughts, ritualistic behaviors may become increasingly associated with relieving tension and anxiety, setting the stage for the later development of obsessive compulsive disorder (OCD) which will be discussed later in this chapter.

Anxiety disorders

There are eight anxiety disorders currently listed in the DSM (APA, 2000), although two of the disorders (post-traumatic stress disorder and acute stress disorder) will most likely be reclassified under stress disorders in the future. For the purposes of this book, the anxiety disorders will be introduced according to developmental onset (earlier to later onset disorders), while the stress disorders will be covered in the final chapter on trauma. The eight anxiety disorders include: specific phobias, separation anxiety disorder, general anxiety disorder, obsessive compulsive disorder, social phobia, and panic disorder.

Specific phobias

A **specific phobia** is a persistent **unreasonable** fear of specific events or objects causing extreme anxiety (lasting at least six months). Although adolescents and adults recognize that the fear is unreasonable, children may not. Given the distress caused, there is a persistent tendency to avoid the feared object/situation.

Nature and course The most common specific phobias include: natural type (e.g., heights, storms), animal type, blood-injection type, situational type (e.g., elevators, bridges, enclosed spaces), and other specific fears (e.g., fear of clowns). Fear of animals is a common form of phobia with childhood onset, while one of the most common sources of phobias in middle childhood (nine to 13 years) is a fear of spiders (Muris, Merckelbach, Meesters, & Van Lier, 1997).

Etiology and prevalence Phobias develop and are maintained by a combination of biological factors (genetics, temperament), behavioral factors (modeling, operant or classical conditioning), cognitive factors and situational factors (e.g., fear of all dogs after being bitten, parenting practices). The prevalence rate for specific phobias in children is approximately 5%; however, they may be evident in 15% of children who are referred for other anxiety-related issues (Ollendick, King, & Muris, 2002).

Assessment and treatment Behavior rating scales, as discussed in *Chapter 5*, can be helpful in providing information about general symptoms of anxiety in children and adolescence. Semistructured interviews, such as the *Anxiety Disorders Interview Schedule for the DSM-IV: Child and Parent Versions* (ADIS for DSM-IV; Silverman & Albano, 1996; Silverman, Saavedra, & Pina, 2001), and affective scales, such as the *Revised Manifest Anxiety Scale-2* (RCMAS-2; Reynolds & Richmond, 2008) can be particularly helpful in the identification of anxious children.

Exposure treatments such as **participant modeling** and **reinforced practice** are two well-established treatments for phobic disorders in children (Ollendick & King,

1998). Adults or peers can serve as models and the procedure can take place in reality (**in vivo**), through media (e.g., video viewing) or by imagination, allowing the opportunity for children to experience positive and non-fearful reactions through **observational learning**. In vivo participation is the most successful of these methods.

Phobias and classical conditioning

In *Chapter 2*, we discussed how Little Albert was conditioned to fear a rat. The classical conditioning paradigm can be used to explain how Sally acquires her fear of flying, through a strong negative emotional association:

Flying (neutral stimulus) → means of travel (neutral response)
Turbulent flight (unconditioned stimulus) → fear (unconditioned response)
Flying (conditioned stimulus) → fear (conditioned response)

Sally is now fearful of flying which may even generalize to all airborne activities, such as parasailing and balloon riding, through **stimulus generalization**.

One important exposure technique, **systematic desensitization** (Wolpe, 1958) is based on principles of **successive approximation**, as an individual is gradually exposed to the feared object, while in a relaxed state. Desensitization requires three important steps:

1. development of a **fear hierarchy** (steps from the least to most feared aspect of the phobia);
2. training in deep relaxation;
3. pairing the feared object/event with deep relaxation at each step, until the fear is eventually mastered.

Using the previous example of fear of flying, the therapist would construct a fear hierarchy (lowest to highest fear associated with flying) based on Sally's **subjective units of distress** (SUDs). The program might begin with reading travel brochures, packing to go away, driving to the airport, and picking up the ticket. At each step, Sally would be instructed to do her relaxation exercises, until that step no longer elicited an anxious response. Ultimately, the final step would be to board the plane and take off.

Fear and emotive imagery

Lazarus and Abramowitz (1962) developed a systematic desensitization program for children substituting **emotive imagery** for relaxation training. The researchers had children face their fears by creating stories whereby their favorite hero conquered the fear. In this case, **child mastery** became the antidote for fear.

Table 10.2   Symptoms of separation anxiety disorder (SAD)

Separation anxiety disorder (SAD): intense worries about separation from the caregiver, evident in at least three of the following:

- Unrealistic, persistent worry about the caregiver succumbing to accident or harm, or not returning
- Preoccupation and worry that some future event (being lost, kidnapped) will result in separation from the caregiver
- Persistent reluctance to attend school or school refusal
- Reluctance to sleep alone, without caregiver
- Reluctance or refusal to sleep away from home
- Inappropriate fear of being alone without the caregiver
- Repeated nightmares about separation
- Persistent physical complaints (such as nausea, stomachache, headache)

If time is of the essence, then an exposure treatment called **flooding** is a possibility. Sally would immediately accompany the model on board the airplane, face her fear, and realize that all flights are not turbulent.

Separation anxiety disorder (SAD)

Children with SAD experience intense worries about separation from the caregiver, and are often consumed with fears of harm befalling a caregiver, which underlies the need to stay close to the caregiver.

Nature and course   Symptoms of SAD are very similar in both classification systems, with the exception that the ICD suggests onset prior to six years of age, compared to onset prior to 18 years in the DSM. Both systems require symptoms to be present for at least four weeks.

Children with SAD experience intense worries about separation from the caregiver evident in at least three symptoms presented in Table 10.2. It is not uncommon for children to become physically ill or to experience panic attacks when forced to leave the caregiver.

School refusal

The most common symptom of SAD is **school refusal**. However, while 75% of those with SAD refuse to attend school, only one-third of all children who demonstrate school refusal have SAD (Black, 1995). Other causes of school refusal include fear (bullying and victimization) or reluctance to return after a legitimate absence (illness).

Etiology and prevalence   The exact cause of SAD is unknown, although it has been suggested that temperament (*inhibited/wary*) and attachment patterns (*insecure/anxious*) interact in the wake of threats of separation to evoke **habitual stress**

responses (Ollendick, 1998). **Parent overprotectiveness** may reinforce a child's avoidant behaviors and increase a child's dependency on the caregiver (Hudson & Rapee, 2000). Approximately 4% of children and adolescents experience SAD, although among clinical populations the prevalence rate is more than double that (10%) of the population at large (APA, 2000). Once diagnosed with the disorder, children may re-experience symptoms if faced with stressful situations in the future, such as school transitions.

Treatment   Cognitive behavioral therapy (CBT) has been successful in treating SAD, general anxiety disorder (GAD), and social phobia (see Ollendick & King, 1998, for a review). The **Coping Cat Program** has been successful for a wide range of ages (seven to 16 years) and can be adapted for individuals (Kendall, 1994; Kendall & Southam-Gerow, 1996) or groups (Flannery-Schroeder & Kendall, 2000). Two shorter versions, Coping Koala and Coping Bear, have also been successful in the treatment of SAD, GAD, and social phobia, for individuals (Barrett, 1998) and groups (Muris, Meesters, & van Melick, 2002).

Coping Cat Program

The program consists of 16 to 18 sessions with approximately half of the sessions devoted to developing coping skills and the remainder to applying the skills in vivo and imagined conditions. The key stages in the process are represented by the FEAR acronym:

F   Feel frightened (physical symptom recognition).
E   Expect the worse (awareness of negative mental set).
A   Attitude/Actions can help (practice positive coping statements).
R   Results and Rewards (monitor, evaluate, and self-reward).

General anxiety disorder (GAD) or overanxious disorder

GAD is a condition of excessive worry and anxiety, where the individual is unable to control the worry, even if he or she is aware that the worry is unreasonable.

Nature and course   Both classification systems present a similar clinical picture for GAD with minor variations: the ICD requires evidence of three symptoms, while the DSM requires three symptoms for adults but only one symptom for children. In addition, the ICD requires that multiple symptoms *must* prevail across at least two situations. While the DSM acknowledges that worries about performance *may* be pervasive across academic and other activities, such as sports, this is not a requirement for diagnosis.

    Symptoms are consistent with "free-floating anxiety" and may include: excessive need for reassurance, marked tension (problems concentrating, sleeping, irritability), recurrent somatic complaints, or excessive concerns regarding performance, physical health, or other potential negative outcomes. The DSM cautions about over-diagnosis of children with GAD because many of the symptoms overlap with other disorders (e.g., ADHD, PTSD, mood disorders).

Etiology and prevalence   There is high heritability for GAD; if one twin has the disorder, there is a 30–40% likelihood the other twin will also have the disorder (Eley, 1999). The neurotransmitter **GABA** (*gamma-aminobutyric acid*) is responsible for sending a message to inhibit excitability and anxiety levels; however, a malfunction (too little GABA, or too few receptors) causes the anxiety loop to continue to fire (Lloyd, Fletcher, & Minuchin, 1992). From a cognitive behavioral perspective, heightened perceptions of threat drive an avoidant coping style which is negatively reinforced by reduced anxiety (Lengua & Long, 2002). Parents who are overprotective and anxious can actually exacerbate the problem by encouraging avoidant behaviors in their children (Dadds, Barrett, Rapee, & Ryan, 1996). Lifetime prevalence rate for GAD is between 2% and 5%, with likely child onset between eight and 10 years of age (Last, Perrin, Hersen, & Kazdin, 1992). Females are twice as likely to be diagnosed with GAD (APA, 2000).

Anxiety and attachment

Children who demonstrate anxious attachment patterns as infants are twice as likely to develop an anxiety disorder compared to peers who are securely attached (Warren, Huston, Egeland, & Sroufe, 2005).

Treatment   The Coping Cat Program discussed earlier (for SAD) is also appropriate for GAD. Although CBT can be successful for children with GAD, researchers have found that if the parents are also anxious, unless parents are simultaneously enrolled in a parent anxiety management program, the children do not benefit from CBT (Cobham, Dadds, & Spence, 1998).

Obsessive compulsive disorder (OCD)

The essential features of **obsessive compulsive disorder** (**OCD**) are recurrent and intrusive **obsessions** (thoughts) and/or persistent ritualistic **compulsions** (behaviors). Both systems of classification require the disorder to cause significant distress, and the recognition that the obsessions or compulsions are unreasonable, although the DSM suggests that children may not be aware that the obsessions and compulsions are unreasonable. Conceptually the two classification systems differ regarding symptom duration. While the ICD requires that symptoms exist for two consecutive weeks, the DSM focuses on the length of time engaged in the OCD rituals on a daily basis (e.g., more than an hour a day).

Nature and course   In children and youth, obsessions (irrational thoughts) and compulsions (stereotypical and uncontrollable behaviors) often represent a number of

Table 10.3   Common obsessions and compulsions in children and youth

Obsession	Compulsion
Contamination	Hand washing, excessive cleaning, showering, teeth brushing
Safety	Checking doors, windows, locks, appliances (turned off)
Orderliness/symmetry	Aligning, arranging
Repetitive rituals	Counting, tapping, touching, repetitive phrases
Hoarding	Collecting useless items (rubber bands, paper clips)
List making	Making lists, checking lists

recurring themes and preoccupations, the most common of which are presented in Table 10.3.

Although ritualistic behaviors are common and peak in the preschool years (two to four years of age), children with OCD demonstrate a pattern of increasing rituals and compulsions in middle and secondary school (Zohar & Bruno, 1997). In the youngest children, compulsive rituals are often not accompanied by obsessional thoughts (Geller et al., 1998).

In their study of 70 children and youth with OCD, Swedo, Rapoport, Leonard, Leanane, and Cheslow (1989) found that 85% engaged in compulsive hand washing resulting from fears of contamination, while almost half (46%) demonstrated checking rituals. Aggressive and violent images, including thoughts of self-harm, were evident in almost one-third (30–38%) of youth in another study, while somatic obsessions were evident in 38% of youth (Riddle et al., 1990). Rituals may go undetected if performed in secrecy and students may be misdiagnosed as "slow" due to problems completing work resulting from competing rituals (repeating words to themselves, tapping and counting, or the need to be perfect). They may also feel the need to hide their secret from family and peers (Wever & Phillips, 1994).

Etiology and prevalence   Biological, behavioral, cognitive, and parenting models have all suggested possible etiologies for OCD. Genetically, the risk for OCD is higher in first degree relatives with OCD or Tourette's disorder, and onset of OCD in childhood is associated with having a tic disorder, being male, and having multiple OCD symptoms (Tucker, Leckman, & Scahill, 1996). Since antidepressants (SSRIs) have been successful in treating cases of OCD, low levels of the neurotransmitter **serotonin** have been linked to the disorder. The **orbital region** of the frontal cortex and the **caudate nuclei** (in basal ganglia) are involved in turning thoughts into actions; specifically, the caudate nuclei is responsible for filtering primitive impulses (aggressive thoughts and images) prior to sending the messages to the **thalamus**. In individuals with OCD, PET scans have detected overactivity in these regions of the brain (Saxena, Brody, & Maidment, 1999).

Streptococcal infection and OCD

PANDAS "is an acronym for Pediatric Autoimmune Neuropsychiatric Disorders Associated with Streptococcal infection. As defined, the criteria include prepubertal children with either a tic or obsessive-compulsive disorder in whom a Group A beta-hemolytic streptococcal infection (GABHS) triggers the abrupt onset or exacerbation of tics/obsessive-compulsive behaviors" (Singer & Loiselle, 2003, p. 31). Murphy and Pichichero (2002) monitored 12 youth who developed abrupt onset of OCD or tic disorder after acquiring PANDAS. Murphy and Pichichero (2002) reported that severe OCD symptoms (hand washing and fear of contamination) disappeared when the throat infection was treated with antibiotics, but re-occurred in half the youth when the throat infection relapsed. However, re-introduction of the antibiotic caused OCD symptoms to disappear.

From a *behavioral* perspective, theorists have speculated that compulsions can be serendipitously reinforced, causing the behavior to be repeated (*I am nervous and wash my hands, which relieves my anxiety, then I am more likely to repeat this behavior*). *Family-based models* have investigated the influence of communication patterns, especially **expressed emotion** (**EE**), on the development of OCD. Valleni-Basile et al. (1995) found that 82% of youth with OCD had families that were high in EE (overly involved and high levels of criticism). Cooper (1996) investigated the impact of having a child with OCD on the family and found that over half the families (60%) complained of detrimental effects on marital harmony, siblings, and feelings of manipulation (youth often engage family members in the rituals). The *cognitive behavioral model* focuses on the role of maladaptive thinking in OCD behaviors and suggests that it is the detrimental combination of both feeling unable to control the thoughts or impulses and the need to engage in the repetitive behaviors (undoing) that is at the core of the disorder (Rachman, 1993).

Prevalence rates for OCD are between 2% and 4% of children and youth, with male onset at 6 to 15 years, earlier than for females at 20 to 29 years (Martini, 1995).

Treatment   Selective serotonin reuptake inhibitors (SSRIs) have been effective in the treatment of OCD in children and adolescents (McClellan & Werry, 2003). Although the tricyclic clomipramine is highly effective, adverse side effects suggest the medication should only be used in severe cases that do not respond to SSRIs (Geller, Biederman, & Stewart, 2003). Rachman's (1993) approach to the treatment of OCD, **exposure and response prevention** (**ERP**), uses behavioral principles of *exposure* to the anxiety provoking situation (e.g., dirty floor) and then blocking the compulsive *response* (cleaning). Repeated exposures, in the presence of blocked responses, take place in a gradual systematic way. ERP has been proven to be as successful as medication in reducing OCD symptoms in children and youth (March, Frances, Carpenter, & Kahn, 1997). Barrett, Healy-Farrell, and March (2004) investigated a **family-based cognitive behavioral treatment** (**CBFT**), called the **Focus Program** (**F**reedom from **O**bsessions and **C**ompulsions **U**sing **S**pecial tools), a 14-week program using principles of CBT and ERP, and engaging youth and family members in the treatment. The program is designed to increase awareness of the disorder, and has a built-in relapse prevention component. Results revealed clinically significant reduction in OCD symptoms.

Social phobia

Social phobia as an unreasonable and persistent fear of scrutiny by others, or fear of extreme embarrassment in social situations, resulting in an avoidance of situations that may produce a panic attack if confronted.

Social anxiety disorder of childhood

In addition to social phobia, the ICD also recognizes **social anxiety disorder of childhood** which has onset prior to age six and is a persistent or recurrent fear and/or avoidance of strangers which may occur with adults, peers, or both, in the presence of normal selective attachment. There is no equivalent category for this disorder in the DSM.

Nature and course   Social phobia must be present for six months for a diagnosis. Symptoms of the disorder in children must occur in peer settings as well as adult settings, and exposure may result in crying, tantrums, or freezing; children may not recognize the fear as unreasonable (APA, 2000). It is not surprising to find that onset is common in adolescence, as worries of social evaluation increase (Muris, Luermans, Merckelbach, & Mayer, 2000). Social phobias can relate to a generalized fear of embarrassment and humiliation in social situations (generalized social phobia) or can be more situation-specific, such as: fear of eating, writing, or speaking in public (APA, 2000).

Etiology and prevalence   The **behavioral inhibition system** (**BIS**), the brain system that alerts individuals to potential threat, has been linked to increased anxiety and avoidant responses, especially in children with OCD (Biederman et al., 1993; Gray, 1991). An inhibited temperament (wariness), behavioral inhibition (shy demeanor), and a tendency to approach new situations with avoidance and distress have all been implicated, and increased rates of social phobia have been found among children that are behaviorally inhibited (Biederman et al., 1993).

Although the lifetime prevalence for social phobia is between 3% and 13%, onset in childhood has been considered rare with only approximately 1–2% prevalence. However, among children with a history of GAD or SAD, more than one-quarter (27%) of those with GAD and 5% of those with SAD will also develop a social phobia (Bernstein & Borchardt, 1991).

Is selective mutism an early precursor to social phobia?

Based on your understanding of social phobia, do you think that selective mutism, which was discussed in Chapter 8, could be an early version of social phobia?

Treatment   Techniques that are helpful for specific phobias (exposure therapies, such as systematic desensitization) can also be successfully applied to social phobias. Inclusion of a social skills training component can also be valuable to increase confidence in social groups (LeCroy, 1994).

Panic attacks and panic disorder

Individuals with panic attacks experience an intense and overwhelming set of somatic, emotional, and cognitive symptoms. Although the attacks last approximately 10 minutes, a severe attack can resemble a heart attack.

Nature and course   The clinical features of panic attacks (panic episodes) are similar for the DSM and ICD, although the DSM requires a specified number of symptoms (four) to meet criteria:

- palpitations;
- sweating;
- trembling;
- shortness of breath;
- chest pain;
- feelings of smothering, dying;
- dizziness;
- a strong urge to escape;
- feelings of loss of control;
- fear of going crazy;
- sense of depersonalization.

Individuals who experience panic attacks often develop a **panic disorder**, which is a fear of having panic attacks. Individuals who develop a panic disorder may try to avoid going into public places (shops, crowds, buses, trains), especially alone, which places them at risk for developing panic disorder with **agoraphobia**, which may literally result in the individual becoming housebound.

Agoraphobia

The word "agoraphobia" is Greek for "fear of the marketplace" and is used to describe a fear that can accompany panic disorder.

The DSM does not recognize agoraphobia as a disorder in its own right, but uses the term as a specifier for panic disorder. However, the ICD recognizes agoraphobia as a disorder in and of itself and is diagnosed when anxiety is restricted to "at least two of the following situations: crowds, public places, travelling away from home, and travelling alone" and involves avoidance of the phobic situation (WHO, 1992, p. 113).

Etiology and prevalence   Youth who experience early onset panic disorder (prior to the age of 20) are 20 times more likely to have a first degree relative with the disorder. The **locus ceruleus**, rich in the neurotransmitter **norepinephrine**, has been linked to the onset of panic attacks, sending messages to the **amygdale**, responsible for triggering emotional responsiveness (Redmond, 1981). Cognitive theorists have suggested that panic attacks can be caused by tendencies to overact and misinterpret bodily signals (Gray, 1995).

Lifetime prevalence for panic disorder is 3.5% with the most likely onset from late teens to early 30s. Females are twice as likely as males to suffer from the disorder (APA, 2000).

Treatment   Antidepressant medications (SSRIs) can be successful in restoring norepinephrine to normal levels (Renaud, Birmaher, Wassick, & Bridge, 1999). However, if panic disorder is accompanied by agoraphobia, *exposure techniques* are also recommended.

The **Panic Control Treatment for Adolescents (PCT-A**; Hoffman & Mattis, 2000) has been successful in teaching adolescents awareness about the disorder and methods that can be used to reduce panic symptoms. The program uses cognitive behavioral techniques to correct faulty thought patterns, alleviate fear and anxiety, and increase feelings of self-efficacy.

Mood disorders: an overview

Although Bleuler initially wrote of childhood depression in 1934, and Spitz (1946) described **anaclitic depression** in infants in institutional care, many adhered to the psychodynamic belief that young children could not experience depression, since they lacked a well-defined ego. The term "depression" can be used to refer to a symptom, syndrome, or disorder (Angold, 1988).

Depressed mood   The transitory state of irritability and upset that a child experiences in response to a life adjustment (**adjustment disorder with depressed mood**) or disappointment are examples of a **depressed mood**. Children may become clingy or sulk, while others may act out aggressively. The nature of symptoms will reflect the circumstances and the child's developmental level.

Depressed syndrome   The ASEBA scales include two examples of depressed syndrome: *anxious/depressed syndrome* (characterized by a combination of negative emotions) and *depressed/withdrawn syndrome* (characterized by low positive affect and social withdrawal).

Depressive disorders   Mood disorders are classified according to the duration, severity, and nature of symptoms. **Unipolar depression** can exist in a chronic but milder form of **dysthymia**, requiring fewer symptoms, but longer duration (at least two years in adults, and one year in children), or an acute but more serious form of **major depressive disorder**, a severe depressive episode lasting at least two weeks. **Bipolar disorder** contains both episodes of depression (sadness) and mania (elation).

The discussion will begin with unipolar depression (major depressive disorder and dysthymia) and then consider bipolar disorder.

Major depressive disorder (MDD) and dysthymia

Major depressive disorder (MDD)   Individuals diagnosed with MDD meet criteria for a **major depressive episode**, which includes a pervasive depressed mood or loss of interest in pleasure, lasting at least two weeks, accompanied by five of a possible nine symptoms:

- significant weight loss/gain (children fail to meet weight/height ratios);
- insomnia;
- feelings of worthlessness/self-blame;
- problems concentrating;
- suicidal ideation;
- agitation or retardation;
- fatigue/loss of energy.

Depending on the number of symptoms, individuals may be diagnosed with mild, moderate, or severe forms of the disorder. Depressed mood can appear as irritable mood in children who may also fail to meet normal height/weight expectations (APA, 2000).

Depression and symptom clusters

Symptoms can also be divided into categories based on similar features: **vegetative symptoms** (appetite/sleep disturbance), **cognitive/affective symptoms** (worthlessness and guilt, concentration problems, suicidal ideation), and **behavioral/psychomotor symptoms** (agitation or retardation, fatigue/loss of energy).

Dysthymia: recurrent depression   Children (and teens) who evidence depressed mood (irritability) for a period of one year may be diagnosed with dysthymia, although for adults, the disorder must exist over a two-year period without an absence of symptoms for more than a two-month period. Individuals with dysthymia do not meet criteria for a major depressive episode, and a diagnosis requires at least two symptoms from the list of symptoms for major depressive episode.

Nature and course

Toddlers and preschool children   Luby et al. (2002, 2004, 2006) have isolated two forms of depression in preschoolers: **hedonic depression** (reactive depression) and **anhedonic depression** (loss of pleasure or joy associated with melancholia). Anhedonic depression, the more severe variant, includes: a genetic predisposition (family history of depression), more neurovegetative symptoms, and higher elevations of cortisol. Those with the hedonic form are more influenced by situational variables, such as poverty and living in a stressful environment.

Other depressive characteristics in preschoolers include: delay or regression in milestones, nightmares or night terrors, agitated expressions such as head-banging and rocking (Luby et al., 2004), and disorganized play (Mol Lous, de Wit, De Bruyn, & Riuksen-Walraven, 2002).

Primary school-age children   Contrary to findings by Luby et al., traditionally, research has found that the majority of children develop depression in response to environmental situations, with genetic factors playing a greater role in adolescent depression (Eley, Deater-Deckard, Fombonne, & Fulker, 1998; Thapar, Harold, & McGuffin, 1998).

Middle childhood to adolescence   Youth who suffer from depression may do so for a wide variety of reasons, including many of the stressors that were discussed in *Chapter 6*. Symptoms may also be difficult to distinguish from "adolescent moodiness," but may be evident in:

- vague somatic complaints (headaches, body aches);
- school absenteeism, poor school performance;
- over-sensitivity to criticism;
- reckless behavior, increased risk taking;
- loss of interest in social contact, withdrawal;
- complaints of boredom;
- irritable outbursts;
- easily upset, tearful;
- talk of running away;
- substance use or abuse;
- repeated comments that no one cares;
- difficulty in relationships. (NIMH Fact Sheet on Depression, 2011)

Etiology and prevalence   Significantly more research has focused on adult depression than depression in adolescents, and even fewer studies have investigated depression in childhood. Biological models have found low levels of the neurotransmitters serotonin and norepinephrine in adult cases of depression, and evidence of a neuroendocrine imbalance (hormone cortisol) in adults and recently preschoolers with depression (Luby et al., 2002).

Cognitive behavioral models have suggested that **negative thinking** (a bias to interpret events negatively; Beck, 1997) and **learned helplessness** (giving up in the face of repeated failures; Seligman, 1975) were root causes of depression due to maladaptive thinking. For Beck, thought patterns that emphasize the negative and minimize the positive produce a feedback loop called the **negative triad**, which results in feelings of *hopelessness*, *helplessness*, and *worthlessness*. Today, **attribution theory** has expanded Seligman's theory, integrating the nature of *global* (versus specific), *stable* (versus inconsistent), and *internal* (versus external) factors into the model. For example, if I interpret a negative event as global (having far-reaching consequences), stable (always happening), and internal (my fault), then I am far worse off than had I interpreted it as specific, inconsistent, and external.

Attribution theory and the stress generation hypothesis

Attribution theory can be applied to the stress-generation hypothesis (Hammen, 2006) discussed in *Chapter 6*. Stressful interpersonal events that are interpreted as global, stable and internal can set the stage for the perpetuation of stressful environmental conditions.

As has been discussed previously, family influences and parenting practices can be supportive to youth in distress. However, an adversarial family climate (high stress/low support) can increase the risk for depression. Sheeber, Hops, and Davis (2001) suggest that there is increased risk for depression in adolescents if the family negatively reinforces the depression (through attention and negative thinking) or provides little direction for enhancing emotion regulation.

Cicchetti and Toth (1998) developed an ecological transaction model to explain how skills and adaptations acquired or not acquired over the course of development can increase the risk or provide protection against the development of depressive disorders later on. For instance, a mother's ability to soothe an infant in distress can be instrumental in the maturation of brain networks to inhibit negative arousal levels and assist in the development of self-regulation in the child. Children who are unable to self-soothe can be in a perpetual state of distress.

Interpersonal problems that cause increased risk for developing depression include: family conflict, parenting style, and rejection by peers. Child temperament has also been implicated as a moderating factor. Children with **positive emotionality** tend to engage in more social activity and are much less prone to depression than their peers who demonstrate **negative emotionality** (fearfulness, irritability) and less positive social contact (Rothbart & Bates, 1998). Children with depression may evidence low frustration tolerance, vacillate between anger and sadness, and evidence poor academic and social outcomes (Yorbik, Birmaher, Axelson, Williamson, & Ryan, 2004).

The prevalence of depression more than doubles from childhood (2%) to adolescence (4–7%) (Costello et al., 2002). Higher rates of the **melancholic subtype (anhedonic)** are evident in adolescent populations. Characteristics of depression in adolescence most likely also include psychomotor retardation (hypersomnia, e.g., over-sleeping) and delusions (auditory hallucinations). In adolescence, there are significant tendencies for depression to be a comorbid feature of several other disorders, including: behavior disorders, ADHD, anxiety disorders, substance disorders, and eating disorders (APA, 2000). Although rates for depression are similar for younger boys and girls, by 16 years of age twice as many females suffer from depression than males (Hankin & Abramson, 2001).

Assessment and treatment

Assessment   Behavioral rating scales discussed in *Chapter 5* can provide a general sense of whether a child's or adolescent's level of depression is outside normal expectations. Affect rating scales, such as the *Beck Youth Inventories* (Beck, Beck, & Jolly,

2005), include a specific scale for student self-ratings for depression (thoughts related to self, life, and future expectations).

Treatment   Medication has been far less successful in the treatment of depression in children. Currently, in the United States, only fluoxetine (Prozac) is approved for use with children eight years of age and older, although other medications have been prescribed on an **off-label basis**. Close monitoring is required, since the medication can worsen the depression and pose a suicide risk. Most of the successful treatment programs involve CBT, which may not be developmentally appropriate for very young children. Commonly used therapeutic techniques for very young children involve art therapy and play therapy, although empirical support is often lacking for these programs.

Medical management of depression in children and youth has been highly controversial for several reasons. Approximately 30–40% of children fail to improve and many antidepressants (Prozac, Zoloft, Paxil) carry high risks for increased depression and suicide attempts (Emslie et al., 1997). However, after an extensive review of pediatric medication trials, Bridge et al. (2007) suggest that the benefits of antidepressant medications far outweigh the risks. CBT is the most frequent treatment for depression in adolescents (67%), with youth-focused treatment far more common than family-focused treatment (Weisz, Doss, & Hawley, 2005). Specific programs that have achieved success include a cognitive behavioral treatment program developed by Lewinsohn, Clarke, Rhode, Hops, and Seeley (1996), and a 12-week interpersonal therapy program for adolescents developed by Mufson, Dorta, Moreau, and Weissman (2005).

Bipolar disorder (BD)

While unipolar depression is associated with low positive affect (anhedonia), bipolar depression involves both a depressed mood and an **elated mood** of which there are three versions: **mania**, **hypomania**, or **mixed episodes**. The following discussion will focus on cases of bipolar disorder that evidence moods of mania (Bipolar I) or hypomania (Bipolar II).

Nature and course   Individuals with BD vacillate between moods of depression and elation. Manic episodes are less enduring than depressive episodes, with episodes often triggered by some stressful event. Manic episodes last for at least one week, and include an elevated, expansive mood, likely to include a number of the following symptoms (at least three, according to the DSM):

- inflated self-esteem/grandiosity;
- pressured speech;
- decreased need for sleep;
- distractibility/poor attention;
- flight of ideas;
- increased goal-directed and motor activity;
- engagement in high-risk behaviors (sexual, financial).

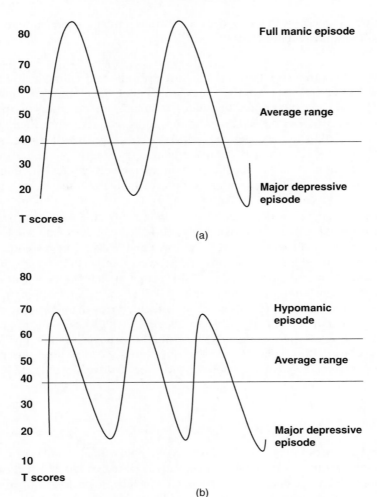

Figure 10.1   (a) Bipolar I. (b) Bipolar II.

Variations and types of BD   Severity of BD is related to the nature of the manic episode. **Bipolar I** meets criteria for a major depressive episode (MDE) and a manic episode, resulting in marked impairment in functioning, while **Bipolar II** meets criteria for MDE and a hypomanic episode (elevated mood, lasting for at least four days, accompanied by three symptoms of less severe impact), without causing marked dysfunction.

A third type of disorder that has both depressed and elated moods is **cyclothymic disorder**, a chronic condition (like dysthymia), lasting for years and vacillating between periods of hypomania and depression which does not meet criteria for MDE. Adults who experience four cycles within one year are considered to be **rapid cycling**. Bipolar with mania and hypomania are displayed in Figure 10.1.

Issues in the diagnosis of BD in young children   BD is a chronic psychiatric disorder that is highly heritable. Until recently, BD was thought to have its earliest onset in late adolescence or only to exist in adults (Loranger & Levine, 1979). Recent investigations suggest that cases of adult BD have prepubertal onset (Geller, Zimerman, Williams, Bolhofner, & Craney, 2001).

BD in adolescence   In their research on BD, Masi et al. (2006, p. 682) asked two very important questions:

1.   Is BD in childhood the same clinical disorder in adolescence?
2.   Are there variations in symptom presentation at these developmental levels?

Research suggests that although the disorder remains stable across the lifespan (Biederman et al., 2005), the symptom presentation manifests differently across the lifespan. Characteristics which distinguish adolescent onset from childhood onset include the following:

- Adolescent onset is marked by more frequent displays of elated moods/euphoria. Adolescents can appear irritable in a manic state and demonstrate chronic mixed mania episodes.
- Adolescents with BD also meet criteria for depression, ADHD, disruptive behavior disorders, psychosis, and anxiety disorders.
- Adolescents with BD are more equally distributed by gender.
- Adolescent moods are more chronic than episodic compared to adults (Masi et al., 2006).
- Adolescent onset is associated with higher risk for separation anxiety disorder and obsessive compulsive disorder (Lewinsohn, Klein, & Seeley, 2000).
- Adolescents with BD are at greater risk for substance use disorders, as well as drug and alcohol use (Wilens et al., 2007).

Adolescent onset BD is associated with significant deterioration in function, academically (especially mathematics), and in interpersonal relationships.

Stress, BD, and adolescence

An increase in stressors (family, romantic relationships, peers) can cause increased mood deterioration in adolescents with BD (Kim, Miklowitz, Biukians, & Mullen, 2007). Although 85% of adolescents with unipolar depression graduate from secondary school on time, only 58% with BD graduate on schedule (Kutcher, 2005).

Etiology and prevalence   According to the biological model, BD is a highly heritable condition; if one parent has the disorder there is a 30–40% risk of a diagnosis in offspring (Levine, 1999). Low levels of serotonin and high levels of norepinephrine have been linked to BD (Shastry, 2005), as have low glutamate levels in adults and children (Goff et al., 2002). The antipsychotic drug, risperidone, has met with some success in treating BD in children. Amygdale (emotional processing center) volume irregularities have been found in adults and adolescents with BD but not in children with BD (Chang et al., 2005). Executive functioning is also impaired in youth with the disorder, including sustained attention, working memory, and processing speed (Doyle et al., 2005).

When is the likely onset for BD?

In an investigation of the continuity between adult and pediatric BD, Chang et al. (2005) report that 50% of adults indicate onset prior to 19 years of age, while 15–28% report onset before 13 years of age. Earlier onset is associated with the most severe, chronic, forms of BD with higher rates of comorbidity (Perlis et al., 2004).

Internationally, prevalence rates for adult BD are similar; however, "there is considerable transatlantic debate and European skepticism over the high prevalence of pediatric BD in the United States" (Soutullo et al., 2005, p. 498). In the United Kingdom, not a single case of pre-adolescent mania was reported in either a large epidemiological study (Taylor, Dopfner, & Sergeant, 2004) or a clinical sample of 2500 children (10 years of age or younger), who were seen at a psychiatric facility in Manchester over a 10-year period (Meltzer, Gatward, Goodman, & Ford, 2000). However, in the United States, rates of BD in children have been escalating. Brotman et al. (2007) compared discharge rates for children, adolescents, and adults from a psychiatric facility between 1996 and 2004. Although BD was the least frequent diagnosis for children in 1996, by 2004 BD had become the most common diagnosis, with a 53.2% increase in children and a 58.5% increase in adolescents, compared to a 3.5% increase in adults. Possible reasons for the increase were suggested as increased practitioner sensitivity to the disorder in children and adolescents, or "rebranding' children and youth with BD who had previously been diagnosed with other disorders.

Why is it so difficult to diagnose BD in children?

Diagnosis of BD in children is difficult for many reasons, including shared symptoms with ADHD (38.7%) and oppositional defiant disorder (35.9%), and symptoms of a chronic irritable subtype that differs from symptoms of BD in adolescence or adulthood (Masi et al., 2006).

Childhood onset is significantly more prevalent in males and manic symptoms can be evident at five years of age or younger (Biederman et al., 2005). A predominant feature of childhood BD is a severe form of irritability often associated with aggressive and out-of-control behavior (Wozniak et al., 1995). Geller et al. (2001) found that 85% of their sample with BD (with an average age of seven years) had **rapid cycling**, often evident in rapid mood shifts on a daily basis. Wilens et al. (2003) modified the symptoms of the DSM to better suit diagnostic impressions for preschool and primary school-age children. The adapted symptom list is available in Table 10.4.

Table 10.4   Wilens et al.'s modified DSM-IV-TR criteria for BD in preschool and primary school-age children

---

"Mania: A severely impairing episode, lasting for a week or longer", with elevated symptoms of "giddy, goofy, drunk-like" or "severely irritable mood with frequent temper tantrums," including at least three of the following symptoms:

- Grandiosity (feeling superior, trying to complete tasks well beyond ability level)
- Insomnia
- Pressured speech (may be unintelligible)
- Flight of ideas (resulting in confusion)
- Increased distractibility
- Extreme goal-oriented behavior (high risk, perseverative behaviors)
- Engaging in excessive pleasurable activities (e.g., masturbation)

Source: Wilens et al. (2003, p. 497).

Treatment   Medical management of the disorder is the first line of defense. In addition to risperidone, lithium (a mood stabilizer) has also been successful in treating BD in children. However, unpleasant side effects from lithium (stomach upset, nausea, weight gain) often can result in poor compliance with a medical regime (Tueth, Murphy, & Evans, 1998), and high relapse rates (90%) for those who do not comply (Strober, Morrell, Lampert, & Burroughs, 1990). The American Academy of Child and Adolescent Psychiatry (AACAP, 2007) recommends a multimodal treatment plan combining medical management and psychotherapeutic interventions.

Diagnosis and medical management

Youth with BD who are given an antidepressant without a mood stabilizer may produce a manic state. Misdiagnosis of BD as ADHD and subsequent placement on stimulant medication can cause excessive manic symptoms and high levels of aggression (NIMH Fact Sheet: Child and Adolescent Bipolar Disorder, n.d.).

Suicide and suicide prevention

In a global study of suicide rates among adolescents from 90 countries (aged 15 to 19 years), suicide accounted for 9.1% of all deaths (7.4 per 100,000) with more than twice the rate in males (10.5 per 100,000) than females (4.1 per 100,000), placing suicide as the fourth leading cause of death in young males, and the third leading cause of death in young females (Wasserman, Cheng, & Jiang, 2005). A study of suicide patterns among Finnish youth found that shooting was the most common method of suicide and, while adult suicides were most prevalent in the spring, youth suicides peaked in autumn, corresponding with the start of the school year (Lahti et al., 2006). Currently, suicide rates in the United States and Canada are among the highest in the industrialized world (Johnson, Krug, & Potter, 2000).

   Although suicide is rare in childhood, rates become increasingly common after 14 years of age. Approximately 2000 teens commit suicide annually in the United States, although as many as 500,000 are estimated to make unsuccessful suicide attempts (Goldman & Beardslee, 1999). Youth with depressive disorders account for one-third to one-half of all suicide attempts (Beautrais, 1998).

Not all suicidal thoughts (**suicidal ideation**) will result in a **suicide attempt** or **completed suicide**. However, warning signs of a potential suicide attempt may include:

- oversensitivity to criticism;
- preoccupation with death (drawings, stories);
- social withdrawal, loneliness, self-criticism;
- running away;
- temper tantrums;
- low frustration tolerance. (Papolos, Hennen, & Cockerham, 2005)

Risks for suicide   High levels of neuroticism, novelty seeking, and low self-esteem have all been associated with increased risk for suicide, as has a family history of a suicide attempt (Fergusson, Beautrais, & Horwood, 2003). Association with deviant peers increases the risk for suicide, possibly due to accompanying alcohol abuse (Brent, 2001). The three factors most strongly related to completed suicides are a previous suicide attempt, substance/alcohol abuse, and having a mood disorder. Suicide attempts most often are precipitated by a stressful incident, including: teen pregnancy, physical or sexual abuse, trouble with school or the law, family discord, exposure to suicide (contagion effect), and a recent relocation (Shaffer et al., 1996). Dave and Rashaad (2009) found that body dissatisfaction (perception of being overweight) in adolescent girls increased the risk of suicidal ideation by 6%, and suicide attempts by 3.6%.

Protective factors   Absence of a family history of suicide (Fergusson et al., 2003), family cohesion, and family connectedness (Borowsky, Ireland, & Resnick, 2001) are protective factors in the home. Having a cohesive support group of peers reduces the risk for girls, while sharing activities with friends reduces the risk for boys (Bearman & Moody, 2004).

Etiology   Having a relative who was suicidal increases the risk for suicide over 30% (Gould, Shaffer, & Davies, 1990). Low serotonin levels can increase the risk for another suicide attempt tenfold (Roy, Rylander, & Sarchiapone, 1997). There is speculation that aggressive males have lower serotonin levels which makes them more likely to act on suicidal impulses (Mann, Brent, & Arango, 2001).

Treatment and prevention   Treatment for depressed mood often involves some combination of CBT and medication. School-based suicide screening and prevention programs are common, but most have met with disappointing results and possibly even **iatrogenic effects** (when treatments harm). For example, in one study, students who were most in need reported feeling even more distressed and hopeless after participating in the program (Overholser, Hemstreet, Spirito, & Vyse, 1989). One very successful program that has empirically demonstrated a 40% reduction in suicide attempts is the **Signs of Suicide (SOS) Prevention Program** (Aseltine, 2003; Aseltine & DiMartino, 2004; Aseltine, James, Schilling, & Glanovsky, 2007). As of 2004–2005, the program had been launched in 675 schools across the United States. The program focuses on treating suicidal ideation as a medical emergency, and trains secondary school students to recognize the warning signs and provide an immediate response (**ACT**: *Acknowledge the suicide signs of others and take them seriously; let them know you* **C**are, *and you want to tell; and* **T**ell *a responsible adult*). SOS is a comprehensive curriculum-based program that instructs students in recognizing suicidal ideation and provides an opportunity to complete a self-administered screening device (currently the program uses the *Brief Screen for Adolescent Depression* (BSAD); Lucas et al., 2001) to indicate whether they score above a level that indicates the need for immediate help. Part of the curriculum is delivered through a short film called *Friends for Life* to assist in the recognition of and response to suicidal ideation in peers.

Somatic complaints and problems

Adults with **somatoform disorders** express mental distress through physical symptoms, in the absence of any organic cause. There are two major types: **hysterical disorders** (accompanied by actual loss or change of physical function) or **preoccupation disorders** (excessive concern regarding physical well-being or status). However, adult symptom criteria are often difficult to apply to children due to the nature of the symptoms required. A descriptive summary of hysterical and preoccupation disorders is presented in Table 10.5.

Table 10.5   Somatoform disorders

Hysterical disorders	*Actual loss or change in physical functioning*
Somatization disorder	Long-standing, recurring, and causing significant distress and impaired functioning: Pattern of multiple somatic complaints located in *four different bodily regions* (e.g., head, back, joints, stomach, chest, etc.); Evidence of at least *eight different pain symptoms, including: gastrointestinal (2 symptoms) sexual (1 symptom) pseudoneurological (1 symptom, e.g., paralysis, conversion symptoms, problems swallowing, amnesia, fainting, etc.)*
Undifferentiated somatization disorder	One or more physical complaints *(fatigue, loss of appetite, gastrointestinal problems, etc.)* that endure for *at least six months*, are without medical cause, and cause significant distress and impaired functioning
Conversion disorder	Loss of function *(motor or sensory, e.g., hand paralysis, issues swallowing, blindness, deafness, problems with balance)* without medical basis; criteria state that a psychosocial stressor or psychological factor must be linked to the onset of the disorder
Pain disorder	Significant pain in the absence of medical reasons
Preoccupation disorders	*Excessive concern about physical status or well-being*
Hypochondriasis	Preoccupation with the belief that one has a serious disease, causing significant distress and dysfunction
Body dysmorphic disorder	Preoccupation with an imagined or exaggerated defect in physical appearance, causing significant distress and dysfunction

The diagnostic criteria for **somatization disorder** preclude a diagnosis in childhood, since one of the symptoms is pain related to sexual function. As a result some studies have used undifferentiated somatization disorder as an alternative. **Conversion disorder** is one of the most researched somatoform disorders due to its dramatic nature, and disabling symptoms, such as paralysis, blindness, or seizures, without any organic basis. **Pain disorder**, especially **recurrent abdominal pain** (**RAP**), is a high incidence disorder that can be a chronic and long-term condition. Little is known about **hypochondriasis** and **body dysmorphic disorder** (**BDD**) in pediatric populations, although BDD often has onset in adolescence. Since, there is limited information about these disorders in children and adolescents, the following discussion will briefly describe how children and adolescents manifest internalizing problems through physical and somatic complaints.

Nature and course   There is relatively little documentation of developmental trends in somatic complaints despite the fact that at least one study found that 20% of children who visit physicians with somatic complaints have no verifiable cause (Robinson, Greene, & Walker, 1988), while another revealed that health services use peaked for children during times of increased stress and school transitions (Schor, 1986). Headaches (25%), low energy (21%), sore muscles (21%), and abdominal pain or discomfort (17%) are the four commonest symptom complaints, with younger children reporting a predominant symptom (headache, stomachache), and older children citing multiple symptoms, including: pain in the extremities, muscle aches, and neurological symptoms (Garber, Walker, & Seman, 1991; Walker, Garber, & Greene, 1993).

Etiology and prevalence

Somatization disorder   Although symptom requirements for somatization disorder often preclude a diagnosis in children, using the criteria for undifferentiated somatization disorder, Essau, Conradt, and Petermann (2000) sampled 1035 German adolescents (aged 12 to 17), and found that two-thirds met criteria for undifferentiated somatoform disorder. In this study, the most commonly reported symptoms were headaches (15.5%), a lump in the throat (14.4%), and abdominal pain (12.4%). Females reported more symptoms than males (Garber et al., 1991) and 10–20% of females with the disorder have a close relative with the disorder (APA, 2000).

Conversion disorder   Conversion disorder is rarely diagnosed in children under 10 years of age, and more likely to be diagnosed in later childhood or early adulthood. In childhood, the most likely symptoms are seizures and loss of balance (APA, 2000), with a 10-year study in Australia reporting that 69% of children presented with abnormal gait (Grattan-Smith, Fairley, & Procopis, 1988). It is not uncommon for preschool children to develop pseudoparesis or a limp, lasting hours or days, following a minor injury (Fritz, Fritsch, & Hagino, 1997). In their study of 194 Australian children with conversion disorder, Kozlowska et al. (2007) found that 55% presented with multiple conversion symptoms, the most common of which included: disturbances of motor function (64%) and sensory function (24%), pseudoseizure (23%), and respiratory problems (14%). High rates of comorbidity were found with anxiety, depression, and symptoms of fatigue and pain.

Little is known about the etiology of the disorder; however, some studies suggest that symptoms are related to errors in emotional information processing (Kozlowska, 2005), while maintenance of a conversion disorder might result from the reinforcement the condition receives. At least one study has found that 90% of children who developed conversion disorder had experienced a significant stressor at home or at school prior to developing the disorder (Siegel & Barthel, 1986), while a more recent study by Kozlowska et al. (2007) emphasizes the need to consider more commonplace stressors for children such as family conflict or loss/separation from attachment figures.

Pain disorder   The most common form of **pain disorder** among young children is **recurrent abdominal pain (RAP).** Between 10% and 30% of young children (Garber, Walker, & Seman, 1991) presenting with symptoms of **(RAP)** report that the pain occurs three or more times within a three-month period, causing significant distress, but without any organic physical basis.

Children who report RAP at four years of age have a threefold risk of reoccurrence six years later (Borge, Nordhagen, Botten, & Bakketeig, 1994).

Body dysmorphic disorder (BDD)   In adolescence, negative body image and body dissatisfaction can have a significant impact on feelings of self-worth (Rudiger, Cash, Roehrig, & Thompson, 2007) and can place teenagers at increased risk for depression, anxiety, and disorders related to body image, such as eating disorders and BDD (Greenberg et al., 2010; Phillips, 2005). It is not surprising to find that onset of BDD often occurs in adolescence (Phillips et al., 2005). Youth with BDD are severely distressed and impaired by imagined flaws that distort their self-view, causing them to spend excessive time (more than one hour, and often three to eight hours) in front of a mirror checking or grooming defects, the most common of which relate to skin (acne, scarring, blotches), hair, or stomach (Phillips et al., 2006). Time devoted to dwelling on their imperfections can cause significant dysfunction in other parts of their lives (homework, schoolwork, peer relationships) and places them at risk for increased isolation (Hadley, Greenberg, & Hollander, 2002).

Assessment and treatment   There are few assessment instruments that address somatic complaints. However, two of the most popular are the Somatic Complaints syndrome scale (ASEBA; Achenbach & Rescorla, 2001), and the Somatic Concerns scale of the Personality Inventory for Youth (PIY; Lachar & Gruber, 1995).

Limited information is available about the causes and treatment of somatoform disorders in young children, although approximately 90% of onsets are associated with significant stressors in the home or school (Fritz, Fritsch, & Hagino, 1997). Initially, children are likely to be seen by the medical profession and may go undiagnosed for a lengthy period of time.

At least one study has demonstrated success with adolescents using a cognitive behavioral program and SSRIs for the treatment of BDD (Albertini, Phillips, & Guevremont, 1996), while a more recent case study reported clinically significant improvement (77.8% reduction in symptoms of BDD) after 12 individual sessions of CBT, with parent involvement, over an eight-week period. Several different techniques were involved in the program, including: reframing maladaptive and self-defeating thought patterns, development of a reward program with parent involvement, and exposure and response prevention (Greenberg et al., 2010).

References

Achenbach, T. M., & Rescorla, L. A. (2001). *Manual for the ASEBA school-age forms and profiles.* Burlington, VT: University of Vermont, Research Center for Children, Youth and Families.

Albertini, R. S., Phillips, K. A., & Guevremont, D. (1996). Body dysmorphic disorder. *Journal of the American Academy of Child and Adolescent Psychiatry, 35*, 1425–1426.

American Academy of Child and Adolescent Psychiatry (AACAP). (2007). Practice parameter for the assessment and treatment of children and adolescents with bipolar disorder. *Journal of the American Academy of Child and Adolescent Psychiatry, 46*, 107–125.

American Psychiatric Association (APA). (2000). *Diagnostic and statistical manual of mental disorders* (4th ed., text revision). Washington, DC: Author.

Angold, A. (1988). Childhood and adolescent depression. I. Epidemiological and etiological aspects. *British Journal of Psychiatry, 152*, 601–617.

Aseltine, R. H. (2003). Evaluation of a school based suicide prevention program. *Adolescent and Family Health, 3*, 81–88.

Aseltine, R. H., & Di Martino, R. (2004). An outcome evaluation of the SOS suicide prevention program. *American Journal of Public Health, 94*, 446–451.

Aseltine, R. H., James, A., Schilling, E. A., & Glanovsky, J. (2007). Evaluating the SOS suicide prevention program: A replication and extension. *BMC Public Health*. Retrieved from http://www.biomedcentral.com/1471-2458/7/161

Barrett, P. M. (1998). Evaluation of cognitive-behavioral group treatments for childhood anxiety disorders. *Journal of Clinical Child Psychology, 27*, 459–468.

Barrett, P. M., Healy-Farrell, L., & March, J. S. (2004). Cognitive-behavioral family treatment of childhood obsessive-compulsive disorder: A controlled trial. *Journal of the American Academy of Child and Adolescent Psychiatry, 43*(1), 46–62.

Barrios, B. A., & Hartmann, D. P. (1997). Fears and anxieties. In E. Mash & L. Terdal (Eds.), *Assessment of childhood disorders* (3rd ed.) (pp. 230–327). New York: Guilford Press.

Bearman, P. S., & Moody, J. (2004). Suicide and friendships among American adolescents. *American Journal of Public Health, 94*, 89–95.

Beautrais, A. L. (1998). Risk factors for serious suicide and attempted suicide among young people: A case-control study. In R. J. Klosky, H. S. Eshkevari, R. D. Godney, & R. Hassan (Eds.), *Suicide prevention: The global context* (pp. 167–181). New York: Plenum.

Beck, A. T. (1997). Cognitive therapy: Reflections. In J. K. Zeig (Ed.), *The evolution of psychotherapy: The third conference* (pp. 55–64). New York: Brunner/Mazel.

Beck, A., Beck, J., & Jolly, J. (2005). *The Beck Youth Inventories of Emotional and Social Impairment (BYI).* San Antonio, TX: Psychological Corporation.

Bernstein, G. A., & Borchardt, C. M. (1991). Anxiety disorders of childhood and adolescence: A critical review. *Journal of the American Academy of Child and Adolescent Psychiatry, 30*, 519–532.

Biederman, J., Faraone, S., Wozniak, J., Mick, E., Kwon, A., & Cayton, G. (2005). Clinical correlates of bipolar disorder in a large, referred sample of children and adolescents. *Journal of Psychiatric Research, 39*, 611–622.

Biederman, J., Rosenbaum, J. F., Boldue-Murphy, E. A., Faraone, S. V., Chaloff, J., & Hirshfeld, D. R. (1993). A 3-year follow-up of children with and without behavioral inhibition. *Journal of the American Academy of Child and Adolescent Psychiatry, 32*, 814–821.

Black, B. (1995). Separation anxiety disorder and panic disorder. In J. S. March (Ed.), *Anxiety disorders in children and adolescents* (pp. 212–234). New York: Guilford.

Blandon, A. Y., Calkins, S. D., Keane, S. P., & O'Brien, M. (2008). Contributions of child's physiology and maternal behavior on children's trajectories of temperamental reactivity. *Developmental Psychology, 40* (5), 1089–1102.

Bleuler, E. (1934). *Textbook of psychiatry.* New York: Macmillan.

Borge, A., Nordhagen, B., Botten, G., & Bakketeig, L. S. (1994). Prevalence and persistence of stomach ache and headache among children: Follow-up of a cohort of Norwegian children from 4 to 10 years of age. *Acta Pediatrics, 83*, 433–437.

Borowsky, I., Ireland, M., & Resnick, M. D. (2001). Adolescent suicide attempts: Risks and protectors. *Pediatrics, 107*, 485–493.

Brent, D. A. (2001). Assessment and treatment of the youthful suicidal patient. In H. Hendin & J. J. Mann (Eds.), *The clinical science of suicide prevention*, vol. *932* (pp. 106–131). New York: Annals of the New York Academy of Sciences.

Bridge, J. A., Iyengar, S., Salary, C. B., Barbe, R. P., Birmaher, B., & Pincus, H. A. (2007). Clinical response and risk for reported suicidal ideation and suicide attempts in pediatric antidepressant treatment: A meta-analysis of randomized controlled trials. *Journal of the American Medical Association, 297*, 1683–1696.

Brotman, M. A., Rich, B. A., Schmajuk, M., Reising, M., Monk, C. S., & Dickstein, D. P. (2007). Attention bias to threat faces in children with bipolar disorder and comorbid lifetime anxiety disorders. *Biological Psychiatry, 61*, 819–821.

Buss, A. H., & Plomin, R. (1984). *Temperament: Early developing personality traits*. Hillsdale, NJ: Erlbaum.

Calkins, S. D. (2002). Does aversive behavior during toddlerhood matter? The effects of difficult temperament on maternal perceptions and behavior. *Infant Mental Health Journal, 23*, 381–402.

Chang, K., Karchemskly, R., Barnea-Goraly, A., Garrett, A., Simeonova, D., & Reiss, A. (2005). Reduced amygdalar gray matter volume in familiar pediatric bipolar disorder. *Journal of the American Academy of Child and Adolescent Psychiatry, 44*, 565–573.

Chorpita, B. F. (2002). The tripartite model and dimensions of anxiety and depression: An examination of structure in a large school sample. *Journal of Abnormal Psychology, 30*, 177–190.

Chorpita, B. F., Plummer, C. P., & Moffitt, C. (2000). Relations of tripartite dimensions of emotion to childhood anxiety and mood disorders. *Journal of Abnormal Child Psychology, 28*, 299–310.

Cicchetti, D., & Toth, S. L. (1998). The development of depression in children and adolescents. *American Psychologist, 53*(2), 221–241.

Cobham, V.E., Dadds, M. R., & Spence, S. H. (1998). The role of parental anxiety in the treatment of childhood anxiety. *Journal of Consulting and Clinical Psychology, 66*, 893–905.

Cooper, M. (1996). Obsessive compulsive disorder: Effects on family members. *American Journal of Orthopsychiatry, 66*, 296–304.

Costello, J., Pine, D., Hammen, C., March, J., Plotsky, P. M., Weissman, M., . . . Leckman, J. F. (2002). Development and natural history of mood disorders. *Biological Psychiatry, 52*(6), 529–542.

Dadds, M., Barrett, P. M., Rapee, R. M., & Ryan, S. (1996). Family process and child anxiety and aggression: An observational analysis. *Journal of Abnormal Child Psychology, 24*, 715–734.

Dave, D., & Rashad, I. (2009). Overweight status, self-perception, and suicidal behaviours among adolescents. *Social Science and Medicine, 68*, 1685–1691.

Doyle, A. E., Wilens, T. E., Kwon, A., Seidman, L. J., Faraone, S. V., Fried, R., . . . Biederman, J. (2005). Neuropsychological functioning in youth with bipolar disorder. *Biological Psychiatry, 58*, 540–548.

Ebesutani, C., Smith, A., Bernstein, A., & Chorpita, B. F. (2011). A bifactor model of negative affectivity: Fear and distress components among younger and older youth. *Psychological Assessment, 23*, 679–691.

Eley, T. C. (1999). Behavioral genetics as a tool for developmental psychology: Anxiety and depression in children and adolescents. *Clinical Child and Family Psychology Review, 2*, 21–36.

Eley, T. C., Deater-Deckard, K., Fombonne, E., & Fulker, D. W. (1998). An adoption study of depressive symptoms in middle childhood. *Journal of Child Psychology and Psychiatry and Allied Disciplines, 39*, 337–345.

Emslie, G. J., Rush, A. J., Weinberg, W. A., Kowatch, R. A., Hughes, C., Carmody, T., & Rintelmann, J. (1997). A double-blind, randomized, placebo-controlled trial of fluoxetine in children and adolescents with depression. *Archives of General Psychiatry, 54*, 1031–1037.

Essau, C. A., Conradt, J., & Petermann, F. (2000). Frequency, comorbidity and psychosocial impairment of specific phobia in adolescents. *Journal of Clinical Child Psychology, 29*, 221–232.

Evans, D. W., Gray, F. L., & Leckman, J. F. (1999). The rituals, fears and phobias of young children: Insights from development, psychopathology and neurobiology. *Child Psychiatry and Human Development, 29*, 261–276.

Evans, D. W., Leckman, J. F., Carter, A., Reznick, J. S., Henshaw, D., King, R. A., & Pauls, D. (1997). Ritual, habit and perfectionism: The prevalence and development of compulsive-like behavior in normal young children. *Child Development, 68*, 58–68.

Fergusson, D. M., Beautrais, A. L., & Horwood, L. J. (2003). Vulnerability and resiliency to suicidal behaviors in young people. *Psychological Medicine, 33*, 61–73.

Flannery-Schroeder, E., & Kendall, P. C. (2000). Group and individual cognitive-behavioral treatments for youth with anxiety disorders: A randomized clinical trial. *Cognitive Therapy and Research, 24*, 251–278.

Fritz, G. K., Fritsch, S., & Hagino, O. (1997). Somatoform disorders in children and adolescents: A review of the last ten years. *Journal of the American Academy of Child and Adolescent Psychiatry, 36*, 1329–1338.

Garber, J., Walker, L. S., & Seman, J. (1991). Somatization symptoms in a community sample of children and adolescents: Further validation of the Children's Somatization Inventory. *Journal of Consulting and Clinical Psychology, 199*, 588–595.

Geller, D. A., Biederman, J., Jones, J., Park, K., Schwartz, S., Shapiro, S., & Cofey, B. (1998). Is juvenile obsessive-compulsive disorder a developmental subtype of disorder? A review of the pediatric literature. *Journal of the American Academy of Child and Adolescent Psychiatry, 37*, 420–427.

Geller, D. A., Biederman, J., & Stewart, S. E. (2003). Impact of comorbidity on treatment response to paroxetine in pediatric obsessive-compulsive disorder: Is the use of exclusion criteria empirically supported in randomized clinical trials? *Journal of Child and Adolescent Psychopharmacology, 13*(2, supplement), S19–S29.

Geller, B., Zimerman, B., Williams, M., Bolhofner, K., & Craney, J. L. (2001). Bipolar disorder at prospective follow-up of adults who had prepubertal major depressive disorder. *American Journal of Psychiatry, 158*(1), 125–127.

Goff, D. C., Hennen, J., Lyoo, I. K., Tsai, G., Wald, L., & Evins, A. (2002). Modulation of brain and serum glutamatergic concentrations following a switch from conventional neuroleptics to olanzapine. *Biological Psychiatry, 51*, 493–497.

Goldman, S., & Beardslee, W. R. (1999). Suicide in children and adolescents. In D. G. Jacobs (Ed.), *The Harvard medical school guide to suicide assessment and intervention* (pp. 417–422). San Francisco: Jossey Bass.

Gould, M. S., Shaffer, D., & Davies, M. (1990). Truncated pathways from childhood to adulthood: Attrition in follow-up studies due to death. In L. Robins & M. Rutter (Eds.), *Straight and devious pathways from childhood to adulthood* (pp. 3–9). Cambridge: Cambridge University Press.

Grattan-Smith, P., Fairley, M., & Procopis, P. (1988). Clinical features of conversion disorder. *Archives of Disabilities and Children, 63*, 408–414.

Gray, J. A. (1991). The neuropsychology of temperament. In J. Strelau & A. Angleiter (Eds.), *Explorations in temperament: International perspectives in theory and measurement* (pp. 105–128). New York: Plenum.

Gray, J. A. (1995). Neural systems, emotion and personality. In J. Madden, S. Matthysse, & J. Barchas (Eds.), *Adaptation, learning and affect*. New York: Raven Press.

Greenberg, J. L., Markowitz, S., Peteronko, M., Taylor, C. E., Wilhelm, S., & Wilson, G. T. R. (2010). Cognitive-behavioral therapy for adolescent body dysmorphic disorder. *Cognitive and Behavioral Practice, 17*, 248–258.

Hadley, S. J., Greenberg, J., & Hollander, E. (2002). Diagnosing and treatment of body dysmorphic disorder in adolescents. *Current Psychiatry Reports, 4*, 108–113.

Hammen, C. (2006). Stress generation in depression: Reflections on origins, research and future directions. *Journal of Clinical Psychology, 62*, 1065–1082.

Hankin, B. L., & Abramson, L. Y. (2001). Development of gender differences in depression: An elaborated cognitive vulnerability–transactional stress theory. *Psychological Bulletin, 127*, 773–796.

Hoffman, E. C., & Mattis, S. G. (2000). A developmental adaptation of panic control treatment for panic disorder in adolescence. *Cognitive and Behavioral Practice, 7*, 253–261.

Hudson, J. L., & Rapee, R. M. (2000). The origins of social phobia. *Behavior Modification, 24*, 102–129.

Johnson, G. R., Krug, E. G., & Potter, L. B. (2000). Suicide among adolescents and young adults: a cross national comparison of 34 countries. *Suicide and Life Threatening-Behavior, 30*, 74–82.

Kendall, P. C. (1994). Treating anxiety disorders in children: Results of a randomized clinical trial. *Journal of Consulting and Clinical Psychology, 62*, 100–110.

Kendall, P. C., & Southam-Gerow, M. (1996). Long-term follow-up of a cognitive-behavioral therapy for anxiety disordered youths. *Journal of Consulting and Clinical Psychology, 64*, 724–730.

Kim, E. Y., Miklowitz, D., Biukians, A., & Mullen, K. (2007). Life stress and the course of early-onset bipolar disorder. *Journal of Affective Disorders, 99*, 37–44.

Kovacs, M., & Devlin, B. (1998). Internalizing disorders in childhood. *Journal of Child Psychology and Psychiatry and AlliedDisciplines, 39*, 47–63.

Kozlowska, K. (2005). Healing the disembodied mind: Contemporary models of conversion disorder. *Harvard Review of Psychiatry, 13*, 1–13.

Kozlowska, K., Nunn, K. P., Rose, D., Morris, A., Ouvrier, R. A., & Varghese, J. (2007). Conversion disorder in Australian pediatric practice. *Journal of the American Academy of Child and Adolescent Psychiatry, 46*, 68–75.

Kutcher, S. (2005). ADHD/bipolar children and academic outcomes. *Directions in Psychiatry, 25*, 111–117.

Lachar, D., & Gruber, C. P. (1995). *Personality Inventory for Youth (PIY). Manual*. Los Angeles: Western Psychological Services.

Lahti, A., Rasanen, P., Karoven, K., Sarkioja, T., Meyer-Rochow, B., & Hakko, H. (2006). Autumn peak in shooting suicides of children and adolescents from Northern Finland. *Neuropsychobiology, 54*, 140–146.

Laing, S. V., Fernyhough, C., Turner, M., & Freeston, M. H. (2009). Fear, worry, and ritualistic behaviour in childhood: Developmental trends and interrelations. *Infant and Child Development, 18*, 351–366.

Last, C. G., Perrin, S., Hersen, M., & Kazdin, A. E. (1992). DSM-III-R anxiety disorders in children. Sociodemographic and clinical characteristics. *Journal of the American Academy of Child and Adolescent Psychiatry, 31*, 1070–1076.

Lazarus, A. A., & Abramowitz, A. (1962). The use of emotive imagery in the treatment of children's phobias. *Journal of Mental Science, 108*, 191–195.

LeCroy, C. W. (1994). Social skills training. In C. W. LeCroy (Ed.), *Handbook of child and adolescent treatment manuals* (pp. 126–169). New York: Lexington.

Lengua, L. J., & Long, A. C. (2002). The role of emotionality and self-regulation in the appraisal-coping process: Tests of direct and moderating effects. *Journal of Applied Developmental Psychology, 23*, 471–493.

Leonard, H., Goldberger, E., & Rapoport, J. L. (1990). Childhood rituals: Normal development or obsessive compulsive symptoms? *Journal of the American Academy of Child and Adolescent Psychiatry, 21*, 17–23.

Levine, M. (1999). How can we differentiate between ADHD, bipolar disorder in children? *Brown University Child and Adolescent Psychopharmacology Update, 8*, 4–5.

Lewinsohn, P. M., Clarke, G. N., Rhode, P., Hops, H., & Seeley, J. (1996). A course in coping: A cognitive-behavioral approach to the treatment of adolescent depression. In E. D. Hibbs & P. S. Jensen (Eds.), *Psychosocial treatments for child and adolescent disorders: Empirically based strategies for clinical practice* (pp. 109–135). Washington, DC: APA.

Lewinsohn, P. M., Klein, D. N., & Seeley, J. R. (2000). Bipolar disorder during adolescence and young adulthood in a community sample. *Bipolar Disorder, 3*, 281–293.

Lloyd, G. K., Fletcher, A., & Minuchin, M.C.W. (1992). GABA agonists as potential anxiolytics. In G. D. Burrows, S. M. Roth, & R. Noyes, Jr. (Eds.), *Handbook of anxiety*, vol. 5. Oxford: Elsevier.

Loranger, A. W., & Levine, P. M. (1979). Age of onset of bipolar affective illness. *Archives of General Psychiatry, 35*, 1345–1348.

Luby, J. L., Heffelfinger, A., Mrakotsky, C., Hessler, M., Brown, K., & Hildebrand, T. (2002). Preschool major depressive disorder: Preliminary validation for developmentally modified DSM–IV criteria. *Journal of the American Academy of Child and Adolescent Psychiatry, 41*, 928–937.

Luby, J. L., Mrakotsky, C., Heffelfinger, A., Brown, K., & Spitznagel, E. (2004). Characteristics of depressed preschoolers with and without anhedonia: Evidence for a melancholic depressive subtype in young children. *American Journal of Psychiatry, 161*, 1998–2005.

Luby, J. L., Sullivan, J., Belden, A., Stalets, M., Blankenship, S., & Spitznagel, E. (2006). An observational analysis of behavior in depressed preschoolers: Further validation of early onset depression. *Journal of the American Academy of Child and Adolescent Psychiatry, 45*, 203–212.

Lucas, C. P., Zhang, H., Fisher, P., Shaffer, D., Regier, D. A., Narrow, W. E., . . . Friman, P. (2001). The DISC Predictive Scales (DPS): efficiently screening for diagnoses. *Journal of the American Academy of Child and Adolescent Psychiatry, 40*, 443–449.

Mann, J. J., Brent, D., & Arango, V. (2001). The neurobiology and genetics of suicide and attempted suicide: A focus on the serotonergic system. *Neuropsychopharmacology, 24*, 467–477.

March, J., Frances, A., Carpenter, D., & Kahn, D. (1997). Expert consensus guidelines: Treatment of obsessive-compulsive disorder. *Journal of Clinical Psychology, 58*, suppl. 4.

Martini, D. R. (1995). Common anxiety disorders in children and adolescents. *Current Problems in Pediatrics, 25*, 271–280.

Masi, G., Perugi, G., Millepiedi, S., Mucci, M., Toni, C., & Bertini, N. (2006). Developmental differences according to age at onset in juvenile bipolar disorder. *Journal of Child and Adolescent Psychopharmacology, 16*, 679–685.

McClellan, J. M., & Werry, J. (2003). Evidence-based treatments in child and adolescent psychiatry: An inventory. *Journal of the American Academy of Child and Adolescent Psychiatry, 42*(12), 1388–1400.

Meltzer, H., Gatward, R., Goodman, R., & Ford, T. (2000). *Mental health of children and adolescents in Great Britain*. London: Stationery Office.

Mol Lous, A., de Wit, C., De Bruyn, D., & Riuksen-Walraven, J. M. (2002). Depression markers in young children's play: A comparison between depressed and nondepressed 3- to-6-year-olds in various play situations. *Journal of Child Psychology and Psychiatry, 43*, 1029–1038.

Mufson, L. D., Dorta, K. P., Moreau, D., & Weissman, M. M. (2005). Efficacy to effectiveness: Adaptations of interpersonal psychotherapy for adolescent depression. In E. D. Hibbs &

P. S. Jensen (Eds.), *Psychosocial treatments for child and adolescent disorders: Empirically based strategies for clinical practice* (2nd ed.) (pp. 165–186). Washington, DC: APA.

Muris, P., Luermans, J., Merckelbach, E., & Mayer, R. (2000). "Danger is lurking everywhere": The relation between anxiety and threat perception abnormalities in normal children. *Journal of Behavior Therapy and Experimental Psychiatry, 31,* 123–136.

Muris, P., Meesters, C., & van Melick, M. (2002). Treatment of childhood anxiety disorders: A preliminary comparison between cognitive-behavioral group therapy and a psychological placebo intervention. *Journal of Behavior Therapy and Experimental Psychiatry, 33,* 143–158.

Muris, P., Merckelbach, H., Gadet, B., & Moulaert, V. (2000). Fears, worries and scary dreams in 4–12 year old children: Their content, developmental pattern and origins. *Journal of Clinical Child Psychology, 29,* 43–52.

Muris, P., Merckelbach, H., Meesters, C., & Van Lier, P. (1997). What do children fear most often? *Journal of Behavior Therapy and Experimental Psychiatry, 28*(4), 263–267.

Murphy, M. I., & Pichichero, M. E. (2002). Prospective identification and treatment of children with pediatric autoimmune neuropsychatric disorder associated with Group A streptococcal infection (PANDAS). *Archives of Pediatric and Adolescent Medicine, 156,* 356–361.

National Institute on Mental Health (NIMH). (n.d.). Fact sheet on bipolar disorder in children and adolescents. Retrieved from http://www.nimh.nih.gov/health/publications/bipolar-disorder-in-children-and-adolescents/index.shtml

National Institute on Mental Health (NIMH). (2011). Fact sheet on depression. Retrieved from http://www.nimh.nih.gov/health/publications/depression-in-children-and-adolescents/index.shtml

Ollendick, T. H. (1998). Panic disorder in children and adolescents: New developments, new directions. *Journal of Clinical Child Psychology, 27,* 234–245.

Ollendick, T. H. (2001). Self-reported anxiety in children and adolescents: a three-year follow-up study. *Journal of Genetic Psychology, 162,* 5–19.

Ollendick, T. H., & King, N. J. (1998). Empirically supported treatment for children with phobic and anxiety disorders: Current status. *Journal of Clinical Child Psychology, 27,* 156–167.

Ollendick, T. H., King, N. J., & Muris, P. (2002). Fears and phobias in children: Phenomenology, epidemiology, and aetiology. *Child and Adolescent Mental Health, 7,* 98–106.

Ollendick, T. H., Yule, W., & Ollier, K. (1991). Fears in British children and their relationship to anxiety and depression. *Journal of Child Psychology and Psychiatry, 32,* 321–331.

Overholser, J., Hemstreet, A. H., Spirito, A., & Vyse, S. (1989). Suicide awareness programs in the schools: Effects of gender and personal experience. *Journal of the American Academy of Child and Adolescent Psychiatry, 28,* 925–930.

Papolos, D., Hennen, J., & Cockerham, M. S. (2005). Factors associated with parent-reported suicide threats by children and adolescents with community-diagnosed bipolar disorder. *Journal of Affective Disorders, 86,* 267–275.

Perlis, R. H., Miyahara, S., Marangell, L., Wisniewski, S. R., Ostacher, M., DelBello, M., ... STEP-BD Investigators (2004). Long-term implications of early onset in bipolar disorder: Data from the first 1000 participants in the systematic treatment enhancement program for bipolar disorder (STEP:BD). *Biological Psychiatry, 55,* 875–881.

Phillips, K. A. (2005). *The broken mirror: Understanding and treating body dysmorphic disorder –Revised and expanded edition.* Oxford: Oxford University Press.

Phillips, K. A., Coles, M. E., Menard, W., Yen, S., Fay, C., & Weisberg, R. B. (2005). Suicidal ideation and suicide attempts in body dysmorphic disorder. *Journal of Clinical Psychiatry, 66,* 717–725.

Phillips, K. A., Didie, E. R., Menard, W., Pagano, M. E., Fay, C., & Weisberg, R. B. (2006). Clinical features of body dysmorphic disorder in adolescents and adults. *Psychiatry Research, 141,* 306–314.

Putnam, S. P., Ellis, L., & Rothbart, M. K. (2001). The structure of temperament from infancy through adolescence. In A. Elisaz & A. Angleitner (Eds.), *Advances in research on temperament* (pp. 165–182). Lengerich: Pabst-Science.

Rachman, S. (1993). Obsessions, responsibility, and guilt. *Behaviour Research and Therapy, 31,* 149–154.

Redmond, D. E. (1981). Clonidine and the primate locus coeruleus: Evidence suggesting anxiolytic and anti-withdrawal effects. *Progress in Clinical & Biological Research, 71,* 147–163.

Renaud, J., Birmaher, B., Wassick, C. C., & Bridge, J. (1999). Use of selective serotonin reuptake inhibitors for the treatment of childhood panic disorder: A pilot study. *Journal of Child and Adolescent Psychopharmacology, 9,* 73–83.

Reynolds, C. R., & Richmond, B. O. (2008). *Revised Child Manifest Anxiety Scale-2.* Los Angeles: Western Psychological Services.

Riddle, M. A., Scahill, L., King, R., Hardin, M. T., Toublin, K. E., & Ort, S. I. (1990). Obsessive-compulsive disorder in children and adolescents. Phenomenology and family history. *Journal of the American Academy of Child and Adolescent Psychiatry, 29,* 766–772.

Robinson, D. P., Greene, J. W., & Walker, L. S. (1988). Functional somatic complaints in adolescents: Relationship to negative life events, self concept, and family characteristics. *Journal of Pediatrics, 113,* 588–593.

Rothbart, M. K., & Bates, J. E. (1998). Temperament. In N. Eisenberg (Ed.), *Handbook of child psychology: Vol. 3. Social, emotional and personality development* (5th ed., series Ed. W. Damon) (pp. 105–176). New York: John Wiley & Sons, Ltd.

Roy, A., Rylander, G., & Sarchiapone, M. (1997). Genetics of suicide. Family studies and molecular genetics. *Annals of the New York Academy of Sciences, 836,* 135–157.

Rudiger, J. A., Cash, T. F., Roehrig, M., & Thompson, J. K. (2007). Day-to-day body image states: Prospective predictors of intra-individual level and variability. *Body Image, 4,* 1–9.

Saxena, S., Brody, A. L., & Maidment, K. M. (1999). Localized orbitofrontal and subcortical metabolic changes and predictors of response to paroxetine treatment in obsessive-compulsive disorder. *Neuropsychopharmacology, 21*(6), 683–693.

Schor, E. (1986). Use of health care services by children and diagnoses received during presumably stressful life transitions. *Pediatrics, 77,* 835–841.

Seligman, M. E. P. (1975). *Helplessness.* San Francisco: W. H. Freeman.

Shaffer, D., Gould, M. S., Fisher, P., Trautment, P., Moreau, D., Kleinman, M., & Flory, M. (1996). Psychiatric diagnoses in child and adolescent suicide. *Archives of General Psychiatry, 53,* 339–348.

Shastry, B. S. (2005). Bipolar disorder: An update. *Neurochemistry International, 46,* 273–279.

Sheeber, L., Hops, H., & Davis, B. (2001). Family processes in adolescent depression. *Clinical Child and Family Psychology Review, 4,* 19–35.

Siegel, M., & Barthel, R. (1986). Conversion disorders on a child psychiatry consultation service. *Psychosomatics: Journal of Consultation Liaison Psychiatry, 27*(3), 201–204.

Silverman, W. K., & Albano, A. M. (1996). *Anxiety Disorders Interview Schedule for Children for DSM –IV (Child and Parent Versions).* San Antonio, TX: Psychological Corporation.

Silverman, W. K., Saavedra, L. M., & Pina, A. A. (2001). Test-retest reliability of anxiety symptoms and diagnoses using the Anxiety Disorders Interview Schedule for DSM–IV: Child and parent versions (ADIS for DSM–IV:C/P). *Journal of the American Academy of Child and Adolescent Psychiatry, 40,* 937–944.

Singer, H. S., & Loiselle, C. (2003). PANDAS: A commentary. *Journal of Psychosomatic Research, 55*(1), 31–39.

Soutullo, C. A., Chang, K. D., Diez-Suarez, A., Figueroa-Quntana, A., Escamilla-Canales, I., Rapado-Castro, M., & Ortuno, F. (2005). Bipolar disorder in children and adolescents: International perspective on epidemiology and phenomenology. *Bipolar Disorders, 7,* 497–506.

Spitz, R. A. (1946). Anaclitic depression. *Psychoanalytic Study of the Child, 2,* 313–342.

Strober, M., Morrell, W., Lampert, C., & Burroughs, J. (1990). Relapse following discontinuation of lithium maintenance therapy in adolescents with bipolar illness: A naturalistic study. *American Journal of Psychiatry, 147,* 457–461.

Swedo, S. E., Rapoport, J. L., Leonard, H., Leanane, M., & Cheslow, D. (1989). Obsessive-compulsive disorder in children and adolescents: Clinical phenomenology of 70 consecutive cases. *Archives of General Psychiatry, 46,* 335–341.

Taylor, E., Dopfner, M., & Sergeant, J. (2004). European clinical guidelines for hyperkinetic disorder-first upgrade. *European Child and Adolescent Psychiatry, 13,* 7–30.

Thapar, A., Harold, G., & McGuffin, P. (1998). Life events and depressive symptoms in childhood – shared genes or shared adversity? A research note. *Journal of Child Psychology and Psychiatry, 39,* 1153–1158.

Tucker, D. M., Leckman, J. F., & Scahill, L. A. (1996). A putative poststreptococcal case of OCD with chronic tic disorder, not otherwise specified. *Journal of the American Academy of Child and Adolescent Psychiatry, 35*(12), 1684–1691.

Tueth, M., Murphy, T. K., & Evans, D. L. (1998). Special considerations: Use of lithium in children, adolescents and elderly populations. *Journal of Clinical Psychiatry, 59,* 66–73.

Valleni-Basile, L. A., Garrison, C. Z., Jackson, K., Waller, J., McKeown, R. E., & Addy, C. (1995). Family and psychosocial predictors of obsessive-compulsive disorder in a community sample of young adolescents. *Journal of Child and Family Studies, 4,* 193–206.

Walker, L. S., Garber, J., & Greene, J. W. (1993). Psychosocial correlates of recurrent childhood pain: A comparison of pediatric patients with recurrent abdominal pain, organic illness and psychiatric disorders. *Journal of Abnormal Child Psychology, 102,* 248–258.

Warren, S. L., Huston, L., Egeland, B., & Sroufe, L. A. (1997). Child and adolescent anxiety disorders and early attachment. *Journal of the American Academy of Child and Adolescent Psychiatry, 36,* 637–644.

Wasserman, D., Cheng, Q., & Jiang, G. (2005). Global suicide rates among young people aged 15–19. *World Psychiatry, 4,* 114–120.

Watson, D., Clark, L. A., & Carey, G. (1988). Positive and negative affectivity and their relation to anxiety and depressive disorders. *Journal of Abnormal Psychology, 97,* 346–353.

Weisz, J. R., Doss, A. J., & Hawley, K. M. (2005). Youth psychotherapy outcome research: A review and critique of the evidence base. *Annual Review of Psychology, 56,* 337–363.

Wever, C., & Phillips, N. (1994). *The secret problem.* Sydney: Shrink-Rap Press.

Wilens, T., Biederman, J., Forkner, P., Ditterline, J., Morris, M., & Moore, H. (2003). Patterns of comorbidity and dysfunction in clinically referred preschool and school-age children with bipolar disorder. *Journal of Child and Adolescent Psychopharmacology, 13,* 495–505.

Wilens, T., Biederman, J., Adamson, J., Monuteaux, M., Henin, A., & Sgambati, S. (2007). Association of bipolar substance use disorders in parents of adolescents with bipolar disorder. *Biological Psychiatry, 62,* 129–134.

Wolpe, J. (1958). *Psychotherapy by reciprocal inhibition.* Stanford, CA: Stanford University Press.

World Health Organization (WHO). (1992). *The ICD-10 classification of mental and behavioral disorders. Clinical descriptions and diagnostic guidelines.* Geneva: Author.

Wozniak, J., Biederman, J., Kiely, K., Ablon, S., Faraone, S., Mundy, E., & Mennin, D. (1995). Mania-like symptoms suggestive of childhood onset bipolar disorder in clinically referred children. *Journal of the American Academy of Child and Adolescent Psychiatry, 34,* 867–876.

Yorbik, O., Birmaher, B., Axelson, D., Williamson, D., & Ryan, N. (2004). Clinical characteristics of depressive symptoms in children and adolescents with major depressive disorder. *Journal of Clinical Psychiatry, 65,* 1654–1659.

Zohar, A. H., & Bruno, R. (1997). Normative and pathological obsessive-compulsive behavior and ideation in childhood: A question of timing. *Journal of Child Psychology and Psychiatry, 38,* 993–999.

Zohar, A. H., & Felz, L. (2001). Ritualistic behavior in young children. *Journal of Abnormal Child Psychology, 29*(2), 121–128.

11

Later Onset Problems: Eating Disorders and Substance Use/Abuse

Chapter preview and learning objectives

There is increasing concern, worldwide, regarding adolescents who in the midst of significant physical, cognitive, emotional, and social changes are at increased risk for developing eating disorders and substance use/abuse problems. In this chapter, discussion will focus on issues and concerns about the appropriateness of the ICD and DSM criteria for these disorders in children and youth, and the challenges that prevention programs face in trying to reduce the onset of these problems.

In this chapter, readers will gain an increased understanding of:

- the similarities and differences between anorexia nervosa (AN) and bulimia nervosa (BN), and binge eating disorder (BED);
- developmental features of the eating disorders and probable causes as to why the disorders occur;
- treatment options for eating disorders and the status of prevention program development;
- worldwide trends in youth substance use over the past 15 years;
- prevalence rates for four of the most commonly used substances: alcohol, tobacco, cannabis, and inhalants;
- gateway drugs;
- treatment challenges, and programs for substance use in youth;
- global prevention programs aimed at resistance to initiation of drug use and reducing drug use.

Eating disorders: an introduction

Body dissatisfaction can develop in youth who try to measure up to the thin ideal portrayed in the media, placing them at increased risk for developing eating disorders, the third leading cause of chronic illness among young women 15 to 19 years of age (Rosen, 2003). In this chapter, the question addressed is: *When does disordered eating become an eating disorder?* The ICD and the DSM recognize two important eating disorder syndromes that share a preoccupation with body weight or shape (morbid fear of fatness) and deliberate attempts to control and sustain weight loss: **anorexia nervosa (AN)** and **bulimia nervosa (BN)**. Approximately 80 to 90% of those with eating disorders engage in self-induced vomiting, while one-third misuse laxatives (APA, 2000). In addition to the main eating disorder categories, the classification systems also recognize atypical eating disorders. In the category of eating disorders not otherwise specified (EDNOS), the DSM includes such atypical variants as *binge eating disorder (BED)*, which refers to out of control eating, or binge eating, consuming an excessive amount of food without the compensatory behaviors found in bulimia nervosa.

Anorexia nervosa (AN)

Nature and course   The two classification systems are in agreement that a diagnosis of AN must include a body weight maintained at less than 85% of that expected, or Quetelet's **body-mass index (BMI)** of 17.5 or less (the ICD recommends using BMI for individuals aged 16 years or over). In prepubertal patients, failure to meet expected gain during growth may be evident.

$$BMI = \frac{Weight\ (lb) \times 703}{Height^2\ (in^2)}$$

$$BMI = \frac{Weight\ (kg)}{Height^2\ (m^2)}$$

BMI is defined as the individual's body weight divided by the square of his or her height. Although the ranges may vary by country, the normal range is approximately 18.5 to 25. A score of 25+ is considered to be overweight, while a score below 18.5 is considered to be underweight.

In addition, several other criteria are required for a diagnosis of AN. Symptoms are very similar in both classification systems, although the ICD focuses more on physical side effects (problems of metabolism, endocrine system, electrolyte imbalance), while the DSM focuses more on the behavioral patterns and the identification of subtypes within the disorder. Other criteria include:

- intense fear of gaining weight or becoming fat;
- body image distortion/disturbance in perception of body weight;
- endocrine system malfunction, loss of menstrual cycles in females (amenorrhea), or loss in sexual interest/potency in males.

In addition to the above criteria, the DSM specifies two types of AN: the restricting type (which has an absence of binge-eating or purging), and the binge eating/purging type (engaging in binge eating followed by purging behaviors (self-induced vomiting, misuse of laxatives or diuretics).

According to the DSM, the **restricting subtype** is evident in approximately half of those diagnosed with AN who maintain their low weight through restraint and self-deprivation. Fasting and excess exercise may characterize this subtype. Those with the **binge eating/purging subtype** engage in acts to purge the body of calories associated with food intake, on a regular (weekly) basis. Herzog et al. (1999) found that individuals with the binge eating/purging subtype had less overall life satisfaction and poorer scores on global functioning than those with the restricting subtype. The restricting subtype can become trapped in an **anorexic cycle** which is displayed in Figure 11.1.

The categories of **atypical anorexia nervosa** (ICD) and **EDNOS** (DSM) can be used to classify individuals who have all the symptoms to a mild degree, or who are missing some of the key features of AN (e.g., they do not meet the criteria for significant weight loss, or **amenorrhea** is absent). Individuals with AN can develop physiological side effects resulting from chronic starvation and weight loss which can place them at risk for succumbing to severe dehydration and electrolyte imbalance that could result in hospitalization. One out of 10 with AN who are hospitalized will die, either from physical complications or suicide (APA, 2000, p. 588).

Although the disorder is primarily associated with adolescent girls and young women, it is also possible to diagnose the disorder in adolescent boys, young men, children approaching puberty, and older women. While it was once thought that the typical onset for AN was 14 to 18 years of age, studies are showing evidence of eating

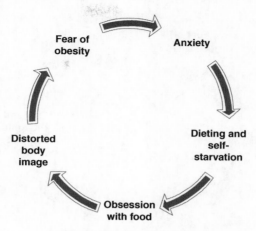

Figure 11.1 Anorexic cycle.

disorders (ED) at younger and younger ages (six to 12 years of age), with more boys having ED than previously thought, and in trends that are recognized internationally (Cumella, 2005; Favaro, Caregaro, Tenconi, Bosell, & Santonastaso, 2009; Pinhas, Morris, Crosby, & Katzman, 2011). Until recently, the disorder was primarily seen in Western and developed, industrialized societies (APA, 2000).

Where in the world?

AN is found most frequently in the United States, Canada, Europe, Australia, Japan, New Zealand, and South Africa. Prevalence rates drop significantly in countries where women have less say in the decision-making process (Miller & Pumariega, 1999).

Developmental features   Symptoms may appear different in young adolescents compared to adults. Typical behaviors may include: the wearing of baggy clothes to hide thin physique, self-induced vomiting, food restriction, avoiding eating with others, preoccupation with food or food preparation, and low self-esteem. Children may restrict fluids as well as solids, resulting in serious medical outcomes (Nicholls, 2005). Onset prior to puberty has been associated with more disordered eating habits, greater need for social desirability, and higher scores on measures of internal locus of control (Arnow, Sanders, & Steiner, 1999).

Who is in control?

Rotter's (1966) **locus of control (LOC) theory** suggests that individuals can take responsibility for their own actions (**internal locus of control**) or place control in the hands of others; for example, luck or fate (**external locus of control**). It is not surprising to find that adolescents with AN score higher on internal LOC.

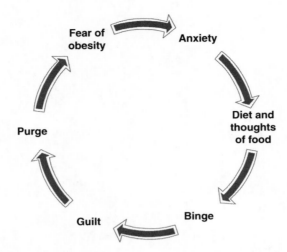

Figure 11.2   Bulimia nervosa: the binge–purge cycle.

Bulimia nervosa (BN)

Nature and course   Although BN and AN share common features, BN is typically characterized by repeated patterns of **bingeing** (overindulgence and overeating) followed by guilt-induced **purging** patterns (vomiting, laxatives). Criteria for BN are similar in both the DSM and the ICD, and include:

- persistent preoccupation with eating, and succumbing to overeating, consuming large quantities of food in an concentrated period of time;
- overeating followed by compensatory behavior, such as self-induced vomiting, drugs (appetite suppressants, diuretics).

However, while the ICD does not specifically state any duration or frequency criteria, the DSM is more stringent, stating specific times related to the *duration* of overeating (e.g., two hours) and the *frequency* with which binge-purge episodes occur (twice weekly, for at least three months). In addition the DSM also includes two specifiers for BN: a **purging type of BN** (where individuals engage in immediate compensatory behaviors to remove food from the system, such as self-induced vomiting, enemas, laxatives, or diuretics) and a **non-purging type of BN** (where individuals engage in other forms of compensatory behaviors, such as excess exercise or fasting).

Repeated self-induced vomiting can cause excess stomach acids that deteriorate the esophagus and teeth enamel. Vomiting can actually increase appetite, leading to another binge–purge episode (Wooley & Wooley, 1985). As is evident in Figure 11.2, the **binge–purge cycle** is a self-perpetuating and self-defeating practice of guilt and shame for overeating, resulting in purging to remove the food.

Strategies to avoid detection can include: eating in several different restaurants over the course of a binge; buying food in different locations; and hiding in a private location (bedroom) to indulge in privacy. As might be anticipated, these activities only serve to increase emotional discomfort, self-loathing, and shame.

Developmental features   Impulsivity and loss of control can increase the risk for alcohol and drug use/abuse. High school students with BN are at increased risk for substance use, sexual activity, suicide attempts, and theft (Conason & Sher, 2006). Piran and Robinson (2006) suggest that individuals with BN may be drawn to illicit drugs such as stimulants and cocaine, since these drugs suppress appetite and increased metabolism, both of which could enhance weight loss. Symptoms of bingeing, purging, and dieting in middle school and secondary school have been linked to marijuana use, tobacco use, and alcohol consumption (Field et al., 2002). Johnson, Cohen, Kasen, & Brook, (2002) found that adolescents with BN are at higher risk for major depression and substance abuse, while Stice, Burton, and Shaw (2004) found a bidirectional relationship between BN and depression, such that each disorder carried an increased risk for the other disorder.

AN and BN: a comparative look

AN and BN share a morbid fear of obesity, a distorted perception of body shape and weight, and preoccupation with thinness and food. In addition, both can have onset after an intense period of dieting. The main distinction between these two disorders is weight: individuals with AN maintain a body weight less than 85% of the ideal; individuals with BN have fluctuating weight loss/gain. When features of the *classic restricting type of AN* are viewed in relation to features of the *classic purging type of BN*, differences are evident in several areas (see Table 11.1).

Personality differences are also evident in different eating disorder types. For example, those with AN tend to be more withdrawn and perfectionist, and can be obsessional in their thinking. Comorbidity with obsessive compulsive disorder has been noted for individuals with AN (Anderluh, Tchanturia, & Rabe-Hesketh, 2003). Individuals with BN can engage in more risk-taking behavior and tend to come from families that are more negative, emotive, and chaotic.

Issues in classification: a developmental perspective   Appropriateness of the current diagnostic criteria for eating disorders in children and youth is the subject of debate (Bryant-Waugh & Lask, 1995; Nicholls, Chater, & Lask, 2000). In a sample of 81 children aged seven to 16 years, Nicholls et al. (2000) compared the reliability of diagnostic criteria for eating disorders for the ICD, DSM, and the Great Ormond Street classification system which was developed specifically for children (GOS; Bryant-Waugh & Lask, 1995; Lask & Bryant-Waugh, 2000). Inter-rater reliability was lowest for ICD (likely due to the large number of categories) and substantial for DSM, with the exception of the EDNOS category which was broad enough to apply to over half their sample (51.2%). The highest inter-rater reliability was for the GOS, which the authors attribute to appropriateness of the criteria for child populations and the inclusion of "characteristics that must be absent for the diagnosis to be made" (Nicholls et al., 2000, p. 322), which greatly assisted diagnostic decision making.

The GOS identifies five eating disorders: anorexia nervosa, bulimia nervosa, food avoidance emotional disorder, selective eating, and pervasive refusal (See Table 11.2 for criteria).

Based on the GOS categories, 26% of children were diagnosed with "food avoidance with emotional disorder" while 13.7% were diagnosed with "selective eating" (13.7%). Differential diagnoses using the three classification systems for AN were 28% (ICD),

Table 11.1   A comparison of characteristics of AN and BN

Anorexia nervosa: restricting type	Bulimia nervosa: purging type
• Onset 14 to 18 years	• Onset 15 to 21 years
• Menstrual cycles cease (three months)	• Menstrual cycles may be irregular but do not cease
• Refusal to maintain body weight within 85% of average	• Fluctuation in body weight, low to high
• Greater severity of medical complications, including: Low body temperature; low blood pressure Reduced bone density Slow heart rate Metabolic and electrolyte imbalance Dry skin, hair loss **Lanugo** (fine down-like covering on face, extremities, and trunk)	• Less medical complications and risk, with the following possible complications: Esophagus and teeth damage Chronic diarrhea (laxative misuse) Potassium deficiencies Kidney disease
• More obsessive qualities	• More sexually experienced, more concerned about pleasing others and having relationships
• Families tend to be enmeshed, rigid, overprotective, deny conflict	• Families have more psychopathology, expressed emotion, hostility, and confrontation
• Personality withdrawn, rigid, perfectionist, and obsessive	• Personality impulsive, loss of control, outgoing and social

Sources: DSM-IV-TR (APA, 2000); Birmingham & Beumont (2004); Halmi (2002); Striegel-Moore, Silberstein, & Rodin (1993).

32.1% (DSM), and 49.6% (GOS); for BN, the respective rates were 4% (ICD), 2.5% (DSM), and 4.1% (GOS).

Recently, in the wake of revisions to the DSM and ICD, and research evidence of increased prevalence rates and decreased ages of onset for eating disorders, there has been a resurgence in advocacy for revising current criteria "to characterize developmentally sensitive alterations in symptom expression seen in children and adolescents" (Bravender et al., 2010, p. 81).

Bravender et al. (2010) suggest several flaws in the current criteria which are not conducive to child applications, because they do not recognize developmental limitations that compromise their suitability for children, including: cognitive criteria inherent in concepts of endorsing *a fear of fatness, risk appraisal of weight loss*, and *relating self-concept to body image*; physical criteria, such as *amenorrhea* which is not applicable to prepubertal girls or males; and *weight lost criteria* which are not appropriate developmentally, since wide variability exists in individual growth patterns in children. Instead, the authors recommend that for children behavioral indicators should replace "cognitive" criteria, that a parent should assist in providing symptom descriptions, and that in the case of bulimia and binge episodes, the threshold of symptom frequency and duration should be lowered to one "out of control" eating episode in three months. Finally, Bravender et al. (2010, p. 86) suggest that loss of control eating can be operationalized for children under 12 years of age by the use of such

Table 11.2 The Great Ormond Street (GOS) criteria for eating disorders in children

Eating disorder	Criteria
Anorexia nervosa	• Determined weight loss • Abnormal cognitions regarding weight/shape • Morbid preoccupation with weight/shape
Bulimia nervosa	• Recurrent binges and purges • Sense of lack of control • Morbid preoccupation with weight/ shape
Food avoidance emotional disorder	• Food avoidance (not related to primary affective disorder) • Weight loss • Mood disturbance (not meeting criteria for affective disorder) • No abnormal cognitions (weight/shape) • No morbid preoccupation (weight/shape) • No organic brain disease (psychosis)
Selective eating	• Narrow range of foods (for at least two years) • Unwillingness to try new foods • No abnormal cognitions (weight/shape) • No fear of choking/vomiting • Weight can vary (low, normal, high)
Pervasive refusal syndrome	• Profound refusal to eat, drink, walk, talk • Resistance to assistance
Functional dysphagia	• Food avoidance • Fear of choking/vomiting • No abnormal cognitions • No morbid preoccupation • No organ brain disease (psychosis)

behavioral identifiers as "secretive eating, food seeking in response to negative affect and food hoarding."

There is much empirical support for the criticisms made by Bravender et al. For example, Madden, Morris, Zurynski, Kohn, & Elliot (2009) found that when the DSM-IV diagnostic criteria for eating disorders were applied to children hospitalized with early onset eating disorders (EOEDs), only 38% met the criteria for anorexia nervosa. There were also inconsistencies, in that although 67% met both psychological criteria, only 51% met the weight criteria, despite the fact that 61% had evidence of life-threatening complications of malnutrition. Similarly, in another study, Pinhas et al. (2011) found that although 47% required hospitalization, only 62% met DSM criteria for anorexia nervosa, while many, although medically compromised, did not meet criteria.

The importance of early diagnosis and intervention is crucial for children and youth whose bodies and brains are still in the process of development. As was discussed in *Chapter 2*, although the young adolescent's brain is highly sensitive to risky and emotive situations, neural development of areas of cognitive control are not mature until the end of adolescence and early adulthood. Therefore, malnutrition can seriously compromise brain development, and can also threaten physical and emotional responses. From a physical perspective, loss of bone density can compromise future growth trajectories, while other physical changes, such as metabolism and thyroid levels, can cause the bodily system to malfunction, in an attempt to compensate for malnutrition (Hamilton, 2007).

Prevalence of eating disorders A recent survey of over 10,000 adolescents in the United States revealed lifetime prevalence rates for anorexia nervosa (0.3%), bulimia nervosa (0.9%), and binge eating disorder (1.6%), and while the majority sought treatment of some form, only a small portion actually received specific treatment for their eating disorder (Swanson, Crow, LeGrange, Swendsen, & Merikangas, 2011). A surveillance study in Canada targeting children five to 12 years of age found the incidence of early onset restrictive eating to be evident in 2.6 cases per 100,000 cases seen by pediatricians, over a two-year period. In this sample of 2453 children, the ratio of girls to boys was 6:1, although boys demonstrated more growth delay (54.5%) than girls (47.2%) resulting from their restricted eating habits (Pinhas et al., 2011). A surveillance study conducted in Britain, collecting data on 0–9-year-olds, over a 14-month period, found an overall incidence rate of 3.01 per 100,000 cases: 37% met criteria for anorexia nervosa; 1.4% for bulimia nervosa; and 43% for EDNOS. Of those that met criteria for a diagnosis, approximately half were hospitalized (Nicholls, Lynn, & Viner, 2011). An Australian study of early onset eating disorders in children five to 12 years of age found national incidence to be 1.4 per 100 000 children. In this study, the authors defined an eating disorder as "determined food avoidance plus weight loss or a failure to gain weight during a period of growth, in the absence of any identifiable organic cause" based on their review of criteria from the DSM, ICD, and GOS (Madden et al., 2009, p. 410). In a sample of 44 Japanese patients (nine to 14 years of age) diagnosed with early onset eating disorders, 50% met criteria for restricting type anorexia nervosa; 15.9% for binge eating type anorexia nervosa; and 18.2% for bulimia nervosa of the purging type (Denda et al., 2002).

The medical complications of eating disorders cannot be over-stated. Unfortunately, only one in 10 with the disorder will achieve a complete recovery, while approximately 50% will experience partial recovery (Herzog et al., 1999). The vast majority (90%) with AN are female (Pate, Pumariega, Hester, & Garner, 1992), although over the past several decades disorders of body image have grown increasingly common among men in Western societies (Pope, Phillips, & Olivardia, 2000).

Lifetime prevalence for BN is between 1% and 3% and is significantly higher in females than males (ratio of 10:1). Onset was once thought to occur in late adolescence or early adulthood; however, research is pointing to earlier onset, and many individuals with BN can go undiagnosed.

Etiology, treatment, and prevention of eating disorders

Etiology of eating disorders Eating disorders often begin with patterns of disordered eating that can progress to dysfunction and distress. Between 9 and 11.3% of youth demonstrate symptoms of AN or BN (Stice, Killen, Hayward, & Taylor, 1998). Causes of **eating disorders** (**ED**) can be related to interactions among many characteristics of a bio-psycho-social nature.

Biological model Having a relative with ED increases the risk sixfold (Strober, Freeman, Lampert, Diamond, & Kaye, 2000). For a monozygotic twin with BN, there is a 23% chance that the other twin will develop the disorder (Walters & Kendler, 1995). High rates of comorbidity of ED and depression are likely explained by low levels of serotonin associated with ED and depression.

Cognitive and behavioral models   Often self-defeating thought patterns can be negatively reinforcing and self-perpetuating. Negative self-appraisals, maladaptive thoughts about body shape/weight, and preoccupation with food are intricately involved.

Parenting and family models   Research has linked AN to overprotective families that have rigid boundaries and deny underlying conflict (Minuchin, Rosman, & Baker, 1978). Within these confines, the adolescent simultaneously asserts her *independence* by refusing to eat, while at the same time ensures her *dependence*, by thwarting future growth and development (cessation or delaying of menstruation). By contrast, BN often occurs in families that exhibit lack of control, open conflict, and hostility (Fairburn, Welch, Doll, Davies, & O'Connor, 1997).

Sociocultural models   The media, peer pressure, and the "thin ideal" have led to increased body dissatisfaction among youth (Ricciardelli & McCabe, 2001). With increasing emphasis on the Anglo-European model of beauty on television, in movies, in magazines, and the on internet, the line between disordered eating and eating disorders becomes increasingly difficult to distinguish (Herzog & Delinsky, 2001).

Athletic performers, especially in "elite sports" or "aesthetic sports" (diving, figure skating, gymnastics), also feel increased pressure to be thin. Sundgot-Borgen and Torstveit (2004) compared 1500 Norwegian elite athletes and controls and found that 10.5% of the athletes had ED compared to only 3.2% of the controls. The rates among those with ED included 45% with EDNOS, 36% with BN, and 11% with AN.

Treatment for AN   Treatment for AN can be challenging, with the patient trying to regain control at a time when they have likely been coerced into treatment (Patel, Pratt, & Greydanus, 2003). Treatment often occurs in response to a crisis, as significant weight loss results in acute or chronic medical complications (Comerci & Greydanus, 1997; Mehler & Andersen, 1999). Programs specifically designed to treat AN include three main stages:

- restore patients' nutritional and metabolic state to normal;
- multifaceted therapy (individual, group, family psychotherapy), nutritional counseling, and exercise management;
- focus on long-term remission, rehabilitation and recovery. (Comerci & Greydanus, 1997)

Medical interventions   Although the goal is to deliver service in outpatient settings as much as possible (Pyle, 1999), the location of the treatment (hospital, out-patient) will depend upon the severity and the extent of medical intervention required (feeding tubes, restoring electrolyte balance).

Behavioral interventions   During the acute phase of AN, behavior modification, contingency management, and activity management are the most appropriate behavioral interventions that support a return to normalization and stabilization (Patel, Pratt, & Greydanus, 2003).

Cognitive behavioral therapy (CBT)   There is increased understanding of the need to correct maladaptive thinking patterns in youth with AN (King, 2001). CBT programs often target the need for control and reframe attempts to gain independence in more positive ways (Robin, Siegel, & Moye, 1995). In their combined cognitive and family therapy program, Robin, Bedway, Siegel, and Gilroy (1996) achieved a 64% success rate (i.e., teens reached their ideal body weight) after 16 months of treatment, which was maintained (by 82% of them) one year later.

Treatment for BN

Medical interventions   Less than 5% of those with BN require inpatient treatment (Phillips, Greydanus, Pratt, & Patel, 2003). However, medication management is becoming more prevalent as antidepressants are increasingly prescribed for individuals with BN (Caruso & Klein, 1998; Freeman, 1998; McGilley & Pryor, 1998). Antidepressants (SSRIs, such as fluoxetine (Prozac)) can assist 25–40% of those diagnosed with BN (Mitchell et al., 2002).

Cognitive behavioral therapy (CBT)   CBT is the most widely researched treatment for BN and has demonstrated long-term success (Agras & Apple, 1997; Wilson & Fairburn, 1993). Agras and Apple (1997) reviewed more than 30 controlled studies and found approximately 50% of clients eliminate bingeing and purging after treatment, with five-year follow-up studies indicating that improvements remain stable in the long term. Although some of the participants in these studies report a periodic relapse of bingeing and purging, the success rate is significant.

Interpersonal psychotherapy (IPT)   IPT has also proven successful in the treatment of BN (Fairburn, 1993). Rather than focusing on the eating disorder, IPT targets the client's interpersonal relationships and focuses on ways to make these more satisfactory (Agras & Apple, 1997; Fairburn, 1993).

Family interventions   Until recently, well-controlled studies of family intervention for BN were lacking. There has been some recent evidence of the potential feasibility of family therapy in the treatment of adolescents with BN, although most studies are restricted to small sizes (Dodge, Hodes, Eisler, & Dare, 1995). Two contemporary studies employing randomized clinical trials have demonstrated that family treatment can benefit some adolescents with BN (Le Grange, Crosby, Rathouz, & Leventhal, 2007; Schmidt et al., 2007). Le Grange and Lock (2007) demonstrated the successful implementation of a manualized program proved superior to generic individual therapy, while Schmidt et al. (2007) found family therapy was superior to CBT for adolescents, but that more of the adolescents refused to participate in the family therapy program. Clearly more research is warranted in this area.

Prevention of eating disorders   The majority of prevention programs have targeted young females in mid- to late adolescence, and have met with limited success (Striegel-Moore, Jacobson, & Rees, 1997). Several researchers have reviewed primary prevention programs that have focused on education (healthy weight management, adverse effects of dieting) and/or assertiveness skills (resistance to societal pressures). The consensus is that these programs increase the participants' knowledge levels but have either no effect on changing attitudes towards dieting, or limited impact at best (Carter, Stewart, Dunn, & Fairburn, 1997; Piran, 1997).

Primary and secondary prevention

Recall that programs focusing on **primary prevention** target reducing the risks and increasing the protective factors for developing ED in the population at large. On the other hand, **secondary prevention** programs focus on early identification of symptoms of ED (e.g., body dissatisfaction) with the intent of reducing the risk.

Pratt and Woolfenden (2006) reviewed 12 prevention programs matched for strict inclusion criteria (randomization, control group), the majority of which (nine out of 12) were school-based. Their review yielded only one procedure that was successful in reducing the risk of ED, namely, discussions and critical evaluations of media messages regarding body image (Kusel, 1999; Neumark-Sztainer, Sherwood, Coller, & Hannon, 2000).

Substance use and abuse

The term **substance** is used to refer to a drug of abuse, medication, or a toxin. Although many different types of substances exist, there are three major categories that substances can be grouped into: **depressants** (which slow down the activity of the central nervous system (CNS)), **stimulants** (which increase CNS activity), and **hallucinogens** (which alter perceptions and sensations).

Nature and course The DSM and ICD provide similar diagnostic criteria for two substance disorders:

1. substance dependence;
2. substance abuse.

The classification systems also provide substance-specific symptoms for **intoxication** and **withdrawal.**

Substance dependence occurs if there is a compulsive reliance on a substance, and three out of the following seven symptoms are present within a 12-month period: *tolerance, withdrawal symptoms, increased use and increased amounts, unsuccessful attempts to quit, extensive time in procuring the substance, forgoing important activities, and continued use despite adverse consequences.*

Tolerance

Tolerance occurs when more of a substance is required to obtain the same effect. For example, a novice may show signs of intoxication with very little of a substance (one beer); however, an individual who has built a tolerance may require several beers to achieve the same effect.

Substance abuse or **harmful use** is evident when *recurrent and adverse conse-quences* are caused by the substance use, and one or more of the following is present over a 12-month period: *failure to fulfill a major obligation, engaging in high-risk behaviors, legal problems, and/or significant relationship problems.* The disorders are considered to be mutually exclusive, and cannot co-occur. If symptoms are met for both, then substance abuse or harmful use (the more serious of the two disorders) is diagnosed.

Issues in classification: a developmental perspective There is concern that criteria derived for adults are not appropriate for youth. Harrison, Fulkerson, and Beebe (1998, p. 487) argue that terms such as "tolerance" and "impaired control" are prob-lematic when applied to adolescents, since "many adolescents initiate substance use with out of control use," while "withdrawal syndromes" may take years to develop. Since experimentation with substances is somewhat anticipated in adolescence, the severity of the problem may be unclear (Burrow-Sanchez, 2006). Winters (2001) recommends a continuum rather than a categorical approach for evaluating substance use in youth. A proposed continuum could be based on the following hierarchy of involvement with substances:

- abstinence;
- experimental use;
- early abuse;
- abuse;
- dependence;
- recovery.

Winters considers the continuum to be fluid, with the possibility of relapse after recovery, returning to initial stages and working through the process again, until recovery is complete.

Adolescent substance use: an international perspective

The tendency for youth to engage in risky behavior is not a new phenomenon; however, the nature of the risk can shift across generations. Drug use can place youth at significant risk for negative outcomes in mental, physical, and emotional health. Studies of experimentation and initial substance use have found increased risk in youth that have a parent or older sibling who uses drugs (Brook, Whiteman, Gordon, & Brook, 1990). Early exposure to alcohol or tobacco places youth at three times the risk for later cannabis use (Wagner & Anthony, 2002).

Overall trends in drug usage There has been a concentrated worldwide effort to increase understanding of trends in substance use. In the United States, *Monitoring the Future* (MTF; Johnston, O'Malley, Bachman, & Schulenberg, 2008c) has collected data on youth drug habits for over 30 years, and currently surveys students in Grade 8 (13 to 14 years of age), Grade 10 (15 to 16 years of age), and Grade 12 (17 to 18 years of age). In Europe, the *European School Survey Project on Alcohol and Other Drugs* (ESPAD; Hibell et al., 2009) has been collecting data for the past 12 years and currently has information on drug usage in 15- to 16-year-olds (equivalent to Grade

Table 11.3   Prevalence rates in percentages for substance use among youth in the United States and Europe

Substance	United States (2007) Grade 8	United States (2007) Grade 10	United States (2007) Grade 12	Europe (2007) 15–16 years
Tobacco (lifetime)	22.1	34.6	46.2	58
Tobacco (past 30 days)	7.1	14.0	21.6	29
Alcohol (lifetime)	38.9	61.7	72.2	66
Alcohol (report being "drunk," intoxicated in the last 12 months)	12.6	34.4	46.1	39
Binge drinking or heavy episodic drinking*	10.3	21.9	25.9	43
Any illicit drug other than cannabis (lifetime)**	11.1	18.2	25.5	7
Cannabis (lifetime)	14.2	31	41.8	19
Steroids (lifetime)	1.5	1.8	2.2	1
Inhalants (lifetime)	15.6	13.6	10.5	9
Tranquillizers, sedatives, non-prescription use (lifetime)	Tranquillizers: 3.9 Sedatives: NA	Tranquillizers: 7.4 Sedatives: NA	Tranquillizers: 9.5 Sedatives: 9.3	Total = 6

Notes: *Five or more drinks in a row on the same occasion: in last two weeks (US sample), or in last 30 days (European sample).

**** Illicit drugs other than cannabis included:**

US sample: Grade 12 group: LSD, other hallucinogens, crack, other cocaine, or heroin; or any use of other narcotics, amphetamines, sedatives (barbiturates), or tranquilizers not under a doctor's orders. For eighth and tenth graders only: the use of other narcotics and sedatives (barbiturates) has been excluded since these groups tend to over-respond (misinterpreting it as any prescribed medications).

European sample: amphetamines, cocaine, crack, ecstasy, LSD and heroin.

Sources: Johnston, O'Malley, Bachman, & Schulenberg (2008a, 2008b); Hibell et al. (2009).

10 in the US sample) from 35 countries. A comparison of reported drug usage for 2007 is available in Table 11.3.

Prevalence rates

Prevalence rates can provide information about the rate of occurrence of an event over the span of one's lifetime (**lifetime prevalence**), or various other time periods (e.g., annual prevalence, 30 days, two weeks, etc.).

The highest lifetime prevalence rates reported by American students enrolled in Grade 10 include: alcohol (61.7%), tobacco (34.6%), cannabis (31%), any illicit drug other than cannabis (18.2%), and inhalants (13.6%). Among European youth (15 to 16 years of age), the highest lifetime prevalence rates were reported for: alcohol (66%), tobacco (58%), cannabis, (19%) and inhalants (9%). Compared to similar-aged American peers, European youth report significantly higher rates of tobacco use, and significantly lower rates of cannabis use and illicit drug use. MTF collects data on sedatives only for senior students (Grade 12); however, use of tranquillizers in Grade 10 (7.4%) is still higher than the combined use of tranquillizers and sedatives in European youth (6%).

Trends in the United States In the United States, trends show a decline in drug usage and stabilization for the majority of areas assessed, with the exception of **MDMA (ecstasy)**, which had been declining significantly since 2000. Rates now show a gradual increase in use in the upper grades, with increased approval ratings among eighth graders, signs that researchers suggest may predict that the drug is making a "comeback."

Trends in Europe The ESPAD survey reports the most stable trends (no further increases) are evident in the United Kingdom, Finland, Iceland, Ireland, and Sweden, while increased substance usage trends are evident in the Czech and Slovak republics.

Alcohol Lifetime prevalence for alcohol was the highest reported substance in the ESPAD (Hibell et al., 2009) and MTF (Johnston et al., 2008c) surveys. MTF rates show increased consumption with age, from eighth grade (38.9%) to tenth grade (61.7%) to twelfth grade (72.2%). Half of the ESPAD sample reported being intoxicated over their lifetime, while 39% were intoxicated within the last 12 months. The MTF reports 12.6% of eighth graders, 34.4% of tenth graders, and almost half of twelfth graders were intoxicated within the previous year. Data were also collected on **binge drinking** or **heavy episodic drinking** (consuming five or more drinks on a single occasion). The MTF survey reports that overall use of alcohol has declined over the years and remains relatively stable, with the greatest decline from previous surveys in eighth graders who also reported experiencing more difficulty with the *availability* of alcohol.

   Although the ESPAD survey found the majority of prevalence rates for alcohol consumption were unchanged from previous surveys, heavy episodic drinking indicated a small but continuous increase, especially in girls, who went from 35% (2003) to 42% (2007).

Outcomes of alcohol use Intoxication is associated with increased risk for accidents, injury, violence, and suicide attempts. In their study of over 1400 youth (14 to 18 years of age), Spirito, Jelalian, Rasile, Rohrbeck, & Vinnick (2000) found that 21% of males and 15% of females had had at least one alcohol-related injury. Student reports (Hibell et al., 2009) of alcohol-related problems include: serious parent conflict (15%), poor school performance (13%), serious problems with friends (higher among girls), and getting into physical fights or having problems with the police (higher among boys).

Risks for alcohol use Bahr, Hoffmann, and Yang (2005) found that increased risk for alcohol consumption was related to parent tolerance (80%) and sibling drinking (71%), while risk for binge drinking doubled as the number of close friends who also drank increased.

Tobacco Since 2001, tobacco use in children and youth in the eighth and tenth grades has been declining (Johnston et al., 2008c). However, the *National Survey on Drug Use and Health* (SAMHSA, 2008) reports that tobacco use increases dramatically between 12 (8.5%) and 19 years of age (68.7%). The ESPAD survey reports that 58% of students had reported smoking at least once, while 29% had had a cigarette within the past month. About 7% said they started smoking at 13 years of age or younger. Rates for early onset smoking were highest for the Czech Republic, Estonia, Latvia, and the Slovak Republic (about 13%), and least common in Greece and Romania (about 3%). Despite significantly higher rates of smoking than in the United States, the ESPAD data revealed a decline in smoking in the majority of countries relative to previous surveys.

Hawkins, Hill, Guo, & Battin-Pearson (2002) found that lower risk of tobacco initiation was associated with stronger maternal bonding, while higher risk was related to acceptance of smoking in the child's peer group.

Cannabis (marijuana) **Cannabis** is derived from the cannabis plant which is dried and rolled into cigarettes; **hashish oil** is a more concentrated form. The chemical most active in cannabis is **THC** (delta-9-tetrahydrocannabinol), the potency of which has increased significantly, from concentrations of 1–5% in the 1960s to current levels of 10–15% (DSM-IV-TR; APA, 2000, p. 235).

Cannabis use among youth

The *World Youth Report* (UN, 2003, p. 159) states that in several countries (Australia, Canada, France, Ireland, the United Kingdom, and the United States) cannabis use has been *normalized* with over 25% of secondary school students reporting use in the past year.

Cannabis is the most prevalent *illicit drug* used by youth (Hibell et al., 2009; Johnston et al., 2008c). Wide variation in cannabis use was found among countries participating in ESPAD. The highest prevalence rates were in western Europe, with the Czech Republic and the Isle of Man reporting that one out of six students had used cannabis within the previous 30 days. Lifetime prevalence rates among American youth 15 to 16 years of age (31%) were significantly higher than the overall average for their European peers (19%), while rates for 17- to 18-year-old American youth were even higher (41.8%), yet rates show a gradual decline for all ages since 1996 (Johnston et al., 2008c). Cannabis, alcohol, caffeine, and nicotine use are often evident early in adolescence and are linked to the development of dependency on other substances, which has led to speculation that cannabis may be a **gateway drug** for other substances (Hall & Lynskey, 2005).

Inhalants There are over 1000 different household and commercial products that can be abused by sniffing, **inhaling**, or "**huffing**" (inhaling through one's mouth) to produce an intoxicating effect. The majority of inhalants act as a depressant, slowing down the central nervous system, and can lead to unconsciousness or **Sudden Sniffing Death Syndrome** – especially associated with butane, propane, and aerosols. Table 11.4 presents a list of inhalants and prevalence rates for youth who initiated inhalant use in the previous 12 months, based on combined data for 2002 to 2006 collected by the *National Survey of Drug Use and Health* (*NSDUH*; SAMSHA, 2008).

Table 11.4 Category of inhalants and percentage usage for youth initiates aged 12 to 17 in the United States, 2002–2006

Category of inhalant	Types of inhalants	Percentage usage
Volatile solvents		
	Correction fluid, degreaser, or cleaning fluid	19.4
	Lacquer thinner or other paint solvents	12.5
Nitrites		
	Glue, shoe polish, toluene	29.6
	Amyl nitrite, "poppers," locker room odorizers, "rush"	15.3
Gases		
	Gasoline or lighter fluid	25.7
	Nitrous oxide or whippets	22.7
	Lighter gases, such as butane or propane	8.7
Aerosols (sprays)		
	Spray paints	24.4
	Other aerosol sprays	20.5

Source: SAMHSA (2002–2006).

There is worldwide concern regarding inhalant abuse, especially in poorer communities. In Africa, inhalants and cannabis appear to be the illicit substances most commonly used by youth, while a reported 24% of nine- to 18-year-olds living in poverty in São Paulo, Brazil, admit to using inhalants (UN, 2003).

Inhalant use among American eighth graders (13- to 14-year-olds) reached an all-time high (21.6%) in 1995, and has been declining since that time until a resurgence in 2005 (17.1%). In 2007, rates for tenth graders (who would have been in the eighth grade in 2005) increased to the highest rates for this age group since 2001 (15.2%). European youth (Hibell et al., 2009) from Cyprus, the Isle of Man, Malta, and Slovenia reported the highest prevalence rates for inhalant use in 2007 (16%), while the lowest rates were evident in Bulgaria, Lithuania, and the Ukraine (3%).

Gateway drugs   Researchers have questioned whether certain drugs act as a potential **gateway** (by initiating the user to other drugs). Drug use in the United States has for the most part revealed the trajectory from legal drugs (tobacco and alcohol) to illegal drugs (cannabis) and other illicit drugs (hallucinogens, club drugs) with the most serious drugs, heroin and cocaine, occurring latest (Kandel, 2002). Recent information about **inhalant use** suggests that this drug may be the first drug used by many due to ease of availability.

Generational forgetting

Johnston, O'Malley, and Bachman (2006) suggest that a new wave of drug users can rediscover drugs abandoned by previous generations due to adverse effects, a phenomenon they refer to as **generational forgetting.** The researchers suggest this phenomenon can explain increased inhalant use in 2005 and the recent increase in the use of MDMA (ecstasy).

Vulnerability and risk for drug use   The European Action Plan on Drugs lists several factors that increase the risk for drug abuse, including poor school achievement, lack of social and life skills, school exclusion and non-attendance, engaging in delinquent activities, self-destructive behaviors, aggression, and anxiety (EMCDDA, 2003).

A study of over 1500 Finnish adolescent twins revealed that early onset depressive disorders predicted daily smoking, smokeless tobacco use, frequent alcohol use, and recurrent intoxication (Sihovla et al., 2008).

Movies and alcohol use

Exposure to popular American movies that depict drinking is related to early onset teen alcohol use (Sargent, Willis, Stoolmiller, Gibson, & Gibbons, 2006).

Increases in substance use often coincide with the onset of other comorbid disorders (Ferdinand, Blum & Verhulst, 2001). Many disorders can place youth at risk for substance use, including: ADHD, depression, disruptive behavior disorders, eating disorders, and anxiety disorders (Kendler, Gallagher, Abelson, & Kessler, 1996; Loeber, Farrington, Stouthamer-Loeber, & Van Kammen, 1998).

Etiology, treatment, and prevention of substance use/abuse

Etiology   From a *biological* perspective, children of alcoholics have a higher risk for alcohol abuse and dependence compared to peers (Cadoret, Yates, Troughton, Woodworth, & Stewart, 1995). Many drugs impact dopamine which produces a pleasurable effect. An abnormal dopamine receptor (D2) has been found in most alcoholics and half of those addicted to cocaine (Lawford et al., 1997). From a *behavioral* perspective, drug usage can be self-rewarding and relieve tension, causing a greater tendency to **self-medicate** to reduce stress. From a *sociocultural* perspective, having a close friend who uses alcohol, tobacco, or cannabis, increases the risk for subsequent use (Maxwell, 2002).

Treatment programs   Group treatments are the most common approach for substance use problems (Khantzian, 2001); however, the concern of possible **iatrogenic effects** when aggregating youth with similar problems represents a serious treatment challenge (Dishion, McCord, & Poulin, 1999; MacGowan & Wagner, 2005).

The **12-step treatment models** developed by Alcoholics Anonymous (AA) and Narcotics Anonymous (NA) consider addiction as a progressive disease that requires abstinence. Youth who attend 12-step treatment programs have better outcomes than youth who do not seek treatment (Kassel & Jackson, 2001). Other forms of treatment that have been successful include CBT with a **relapse prevention component** (Liddle & Hogue, 2001) and CBT or multisystemic therapy (MST) programs that include family in the treatment process (Donohue & Azrin, 2001; Henggeler, Schoenwald, Borduin, Rowland, & Cunningham, 1998).

Prevention programs   **Primary prevention** or **universal prevention programs** provide "resistance training," promote well-being, and attempt to curtail or delay the onset of substance use. Most are school-based programs that provide information about the harmful effects of drugs, and how to be more assertive in resisting drugs when they are offered. However, despite the fact that federal funds have been available since 1994 for the use of empirically supported programs, 75% of schools in the United States continue to use programs that have not been supported by research (Ringwalt et al., 2002).

The DARE program

The most common "prevention program" used by schools in the United States is the *Drug Abuse Resistance Education Program (DARE)* which has been extensively researched, but found ineffective in the prevention of drug use and abuse (West & O'Neal, 2004).

Global Initiative Project　　Several worldwide initiatives have been aimed at the prevention of substance use in youth. The *Global Initiative Project on Primary Prevention of Substance Abuse* is a joint project of the United Nations Office on Drugs and Crime (UNODC) and the World Health Organization (WHO), which was implemented in eight countries between 1998 and 2003. The project involved community outreach in three regions: Southern Africa (South Africa, Tanzania, and Zambia); Central and Eastern Europe (Belarus and Russia), and South-east Asia (the Philippines, Thailand and Vietnam). The aim was to develop good practices in the area of primary prevention through community mobilization, working with local organizations, and providing them with training and financial and technical support. Readers can visit the website for additional information (http://www.who.int/substance_abuse/activities/global_initiative/en/).

The *World Youth Report* (United Nations, 2003) emphasizes incorporating an *interactive group process* as part of the prevention programs to engage youth in peer activities such as "role playing, simulations, service learning projects, brainstorming, cooperative learning and peer-to-peer discussions to promote active participation by youth" (p. 166) to provide opportunities for youth to clarify their beliefs, and to practice skills in conflict resolution, assertiveness, and communication.

The National Institute on Drug Abuse (NIDA) released the second edition of *Preventing Drug Use among Children and Adolescents: A Research-Based Guide* (NIDA, 2003). The document highlights important *family components* (drug awareness; parent skills training; increased monitoring and supervision; and the need for consistent discipline and limit-setting) and *school components*, such as the need to focus on increasing age-appropriate behaviors and reducing maladaptive behaviors. At the preschool level, the focus is on reduction of aggression and increases in self-control; elementary school students should acquire increased emotional awareness, social problem solving, communication, and academic skills; in secondary school emphasis should be on improved study habits, academic support, drug resistance skills, self-efficacy, and the development of anti-drug attitudes. The guidelines recommend combined family and school programs to enhance cohesiveness and a sense of belonging in the community.

Life Skills Training (LST)   LST has been implemented in 29 inner-city schools in New York and has successfully lowered rates of alcohol, cigarette, and inhalant abuse among at-risk minority students in the seventh grade who have poor academic performance and associations with substance-abusing peers (Botvin, Griffin, Diaz, & Ifill-Williams, 2001; Griffin, Botvin, Nichols, & Doyle, 2003). Fifteen lessons (45 minutes) are embedded into the regular curriculum and focus on the development of social skills, drug refusal, and personal management.

Best practices in prevention   Montoya, Atkinson, and McFaden (2003) reviewed school-based programs, family-based programs, and community-based programs over the past 20 years to identify best practices in prevention programs for youth. Six factors emerged that were key to successful programs:

- good parenting (strong family bonds, and parental involvement in school-based drug prevention programs);
- skill development (resistance skills, social skills) and normative education (awareness of faulty beliefs that drug use is acceptable and prevalent);
- counteracting peer influence to engage in substance-related activities;
- retention of program participants and prevention of drop-out from the program;
- anti-drug media campaigns;
- support of laws and policies for a drug-free environment.

The authors identified three important steps in prevention program development:

Step 1. Isolate the relevant risk factors.
Step 2. Select the necessary characteristics to overcome the risks.
Step 3. Determine the best environment (home, school, community) for conducting the program. (Montoya et al., 2003, p. 81)

References

Agras, W. S., & Apple, R. F. (1997). *Overcoming eating disorders.* San Antonio, TX: Graywind.

American Psychiatric Association (APA). (2000). *Diagnostic and statistical manual of mental disorders* (4th ed., text revision). Washington, DC: Author.

Anderluh, M., Tchanturia, K., & Rabe-Hesketh, S. (2003). Childhood obsessive-compulsive personality traits in adult women with eating disorders: Defining a broader eating disorder phenotype. *American Journal of Psychiatry, 160,* 242–247.

Arnow, B., Sanders, M. J., & Steiner, H. (1999). Premenarcheal versus postmenarcheal anorexia nervosa: A comparative study. *Clinical Child Psychology and Psychiatry, 4,* 403–414.

Bahr, S. J., Hoffmann, J. P., & Yang, X. (2005). Parental and peer influences on the risk of adolescent drug use. *Journal of Primary Prevention, 26,* 529–551.

Birmingham, C. L., & Beumont, P. (2004). *Medical management of eating disorders: A practical handbook for health care professionals.* New York: Cambridge University Press.

Botvin, G. J., Griffin, K. W., Diaz, T., & Ifill-Williams, M. (2001). Preventing binge drinking during early adolescence: One- and two-year followup of a school-based prevention intervention. *Psychology of Addictive Behaviors, 15,* 360–365.

Bravender, T., Bryant-Waugh, R., Herzog, D., Katzman, D., Kriepe, R. D., Lask, B., ... Zucher, N. (2010). Classification of eating disturbance in children and adolescents: Proposed changes for the DSM-V. *European Eating Disorders Review, 18,* 79–89.

Brook, J. S., Whiteman, M., Gordon, A. S., & Brook, D. W. (1990). The role of older brothers' drug use viewed in the context of parent and peer influences. *Journal of Genetic Psychology*, *151*, 59–75.

Bryant-Waugh, R., & Lask, B. (1995). Eating disorders in children. *Journal of Child Psychology and Psychiatry*, *36*, 191–202.

Burrow-Sanchez, J. (2006). Understanding adolescent substance abuse: Prevalence, risk factors and clinical implications. *Journal of Counseling and Development*, *84*, 283–290.

Cadoret, R., Yates, W. R., Troughton, E., Woodworth, G., & Stewart, M. A. (1995). Adoption study demonstrating two genetic pathways to drug abuse. *Archives of General Psychiatry*, *52*, 42–52.

Carter, J., Stewart, D., Dunn, V., & Fairburn, C. (1997). Primary prevention of eating disorders: Might it do more harm than good? *International Journal of Eating Disorders*, *22*, 167–172.

Caruso, D., & Klein, H. (1998). Diagnosis and treatment of bulimia nervosa. *Seminars in Gastrointestinal Disease*, *9*(4), 176–182.

Comerci, G. D., & Greydanus, D. E. (1997). Eating disorders: Anorexia nervosa and bulimia. In A. D. Hoffmann & D. E. Greydanus (Eds.), *Adolescent medicine* (3rd ed.) (pp. 683–699). Stamford, CT: Appleton and Lange.

Conason, A. H., & Sher, L. (2006). Alcohol use in adolescents with eating disorders. *International Journal of Adolescent Medicine and Health*, *18*(1), 31–36.

Cumella, E. J. (2005). Eating disorders across the lifespan. *Counselor*, *6*(4), 41–46.

Denda, K., Sunami, T., Inoue, S., Sasake, F., Sasake, Y., Asakura, S., . . . Kita, S. (2002). Clinical study of early-onset eating disorders. *Japanese Journal of Child and Adolescent Psychiatry*, *43*(1), 30–56.

Dishion, T. J., McCord, J., & Poulin, F. (1999). When interventions harm. Peer groups and problem behavior. *American Psychologist*, *54*, 755–764.

Dodge, E., Hodes, M., Eisler, I., & Dare, C. (1995). Family therapy for bulimia nervosa in adolescents: An exploratory study. *Journal of Family Therapy*, *17*, 59–77.

Donohue, B., & Azrin, N. (2001). Family behavior therapy. In E. F. Wagner & H. B. Eldron (Eds.), *Innovations in adolescent substance abuse interventions* (pp. 205–227). Oxford: Elsevier Science.

European Monitoring Centre for Drugs and Drug Addiction (EMCDDA). (2003). Drugs in focus. Retrieved from http://www.emcdda.europa.eu/publications/search results?action=list&typ=PUBLICATIONS&SERIES_PUB=w7

Fairburn, C. G. (1993). Interpersonal psychotherapy for bulimia nervosa. In G. L. Klerman & M. Weissman (Eds.), *New applications of interpersonal psychotherapy* (pp. 353–378). Washington, DC: APA.

Fairburn, C. G., Welch, S., Doll, H. A., Davies, B. A., & O'Connor, M. F. (1997). Risk factors for bulimia nervosa: A community-based case-control study. *Archives of General Psychiatry*, *54*, 509–517.

Favaro, A., Caregaro, L., Tenconi, E., Bosell, R., & Santonastaso, P. (2009). Time trends in age at onset of anorexia nervosa and bulimia nervosa. *Journal of Clinical Psychiatry*, *70*(12), 1715–1721.

Ferdinand, R. F., Blum, M., & Verhulst, F. C. (2001). Psychopathology in adolescence predicts substance use in young adulthood. *Addiction*, *96*, 861–870.

Field, A. E., Austin, S. B., Frazier, A. L., Gillman, M. W., Comargo, C. A. & Colditz, G. A. (2002). Smoking, getting drunk and engaging in bulimic behaviors: In which order are the behaviors adopted? *Journal of the American Academy of Child and Adolescent Psychiatry*, *41*, 846–853.

Freeman, C. (1998). Drug treatment for bulimia nervosa. *Neuropsychobiology*, *37*, 72–79.

Griffin, K. W., Botvin, G. J., Nichols, T. R., & Doyle, M. M. (2003). Effectiveness of a universal drug abuse prevention approach for you at high risk for substance use initiation. *Prevention Medicine*, *36*, 1–7.

Hall, W. D., & Lynskey, M. (2005). Is cannabis a gateway drug? Testing hypotheses about the relationship between cannabis use and the use of other illicit drugs. *Drug and Alcohol Review*, *24*, 39–48.

Halmi, K. A. (2002). Eating disorders. In A. Martin, L. Scahill, D. S. Charney, & J. F. Leckman (Eds.), *Pediatric psychopharmacology* (pp. 592–602). Oxford: Oxford University Press.

Hamilton, J. D. (2007). Eating disorders in pre-adolescent children. *Nurse Practitioner*, *32*, 44–48.

Harrison, P. A., Fulkerson, J. A., & Beebe, T. J. (1998). DSM-IV substance use disorder criteria for adolescents: A critical examination based on a statewide school survey. *American Journal of Psychiatry*, *155*, 486–492.

Hawkins, F. D., Hill, K. G., Guo, F., & Battin-Pearson, S. R. (2002). Substance use norms and transitions in substance use. In D. B. Kandel (Ed.), *Stages and pathways of drug involvement* (pp. 42–64). Cambridge: Cambridge University Press.

Henggeler, S. W., Schoenwald, S. K., Borduin, C. M., Rowland, M. D., & Cunningham, P. B. (1998). *Multisystemic treatment of antisocial behavior in youth*. New York: Guilford.

Herzog, D., & Delinsky, S. (2001). Classification of eating disorders. In R. H. Striegel-Moore & L. Smolak (Eds.), *Eating disorders: Innovative directions in research and practice* (pp. 32–50). Washington, DC: APA.

Herzog, D., Dorer, D., Keele, P. K., Selwyn, S. Ekeblad, E., Flores, A. T., Keller, . . . M. B. (1999). Recovery and relapse in anorexia and bulimia nervosa. *Journal of the American Academy of Child and Adolescent Psychiatry*, *38*, 829–837.

Hibell, B., Guttormsson, U., Ahlström, S., Balakireva, O., Bjarnason, T., Kokkevi, A. & Kraus, L. (2009). *The 2007 ESPAD Report. Substance use among students in 35 European countries*. Stockholm: Swedish Council for Information on Alcohol and Other Drugs.

Johnson, J. G., Cohen, P., Kasen, S., & Brook, J. S. (2002). Eating disorders during adolescence and the risk for physical and mental disorders during early adulthood. *Archives of General Psychiatry*, *59*, 545–552.

Johnston, L. D., O'Malley, P. M., & Bachman, J. G. (2006). *Monitoring the future: National survey results on adolescent drug use: Overview of key findings, 2005*. NIH Publication No. 06-5882. Bethesda, MD: National Institute on Drug Abuse.

Johnston, L. D., O'Malley, P. M., Bachman, J. G., & Schulenberg, J. E. (2008a). Various stimulant drugs show continuing gradual declines among teens in 2008, most illicit drugs hold steady. University of Michigan News Service, Ann Arbor, MI, December 11. Retrieved from http://www.monitoringthefuture.org

Johnston, L. D., O'Malley, P. M., Bachman, J. G., & Schulenberg, J. E. (2008b). More good news on teen smoking: Rates at or near record lows. University of Michigan News Service, Ann Arbor, MI, December 11. Retrieved from http://www.monitoringthefuture.org

Johnston, L. D., O'Malley, P. M., Bachman, J. G., & Schulenberg, J. E. (2008c). *Monitoring the future: National results on adolescent drug use: Overview of key findings, 2007*. NIH Publication No. 08-6418. Bethesda, MD: National Institute on Drug Abuse.

Kandel, D. B. (2002). Examining the gateway hypothesis. In D. B. Kandel (Ed.), *Stages and pathways of drug involvement* (pp. 3–15). Cambridge: Cambridge University Press.

Kassel, J. D., & Jackson, S. I. (2001). Twelve-step-based interventions for adolescents. In E. F. Wagner & H. B. Waldron (Eds.), *Innovations in adolescent substance abuse interventions* (pp. 329–342). Oxford: Elsevier Science.

Kendler, K. S., Gallagher, T. J., Abelson, J. M., & Kessler, R. C. (1996). Lifetime prevalence, demographic risk factors and diagnostic validity of nonaffective psychosis as assessed in a US community sample. The National Comorbidy Survey. *Archives of General Psychiatry*, *53*, 1022–1031.

Khantzian, E. (2001). Reflections on group treatments as corrective experiences for addictive vulnerability. *International Journal of Group Psychotherapy*, *51*, 11–20.

King, N. (2001). Young adult women: Reflections on recurring themes and a discussion of the treatment process and setting. In B. Kinoy (Ed.), *Eating disorders: New directions in treatment and recovery* (2nd ed.) (pp. 148–158). New York: Columbia University Press.

Kusel, A. B. (1999). Primary prevention of eating disorders through media literacy training of girls. *Dissertation Abstracts International B: The Sciences and Engineering, 60*(4–B), 1859.

Lask, B., & Bryant-Waugh, R. (2000). *Anorexia nervosa and related eating disorders in children and adolescents* (2nd ed.). Hove: Psychology Press.

Lawford, B. R., Young, R., Rowell, J. A., Gibson, J. N., Feeney, G. F. X., Ritchiee, T. L.,... Noble, E. P. (1997). Association of the D2 dopamine receptor A1 allele with alcoholism: Medical severity of alcoholism and type of controls. *Biology and Psychiatry, 41,* 386–393.

Le Grange, D., Crosby, R., Rathouz, P., & Leventhal, B. (2007). A randomized controlled comparison of family-based treatment and supportive psychotherapy for adolescent bulimia nervosa. *Archives of General Psychiatry, 64,* 1049–1056.

Le Grange, D., & Lock, J. (2007). *Treatment manual for bulimia nervosa: A family-based approach.* New York: Guilford.

Liddle, H. A., & Hogue, A. (2001). Multidimensional family therapy for adolescent substance abuse. In E. F. Wagner & H. B. Waldron (Eds.), *Innovations in adolescent substance abuse interventions* (pp. 229–261). Oxford: Elsevier Science.

Loeber, R., Farrington, D. P., Stouthamer-Loeber, M., & Van Kammen, W. B. (1998). Multiple risk factors for multiproblem boys: Co-occurrence of delinquency, substance use, attention deficit, conduct problems, physical aggression, covert behavior, depressed mood and shy/withdrawn behaviour. In R. Jessor (Ed.), *New perspectives on adolescent risk behavior* (pp. 90–149). New York: Cambridge University Press.

Macgowan, M. J., & Wagner, E. F. (2005). Iatrogenic effects of group treatment on adolescents with conduct and substance use problems: A review of the literature and a presentation of a model. In C. Hilarski (Ed.), *Addiction, assessment and treatment with adolescents, adults and families* (pp. 79–90). Birmingham, NY: Haworth Social Work Practice Press.

Madden, S., Morris, A., Zurynski, Y., Kohn, M. & Elliot, E. J. (2009). Burden of eating disorders in 5–13-year-old children in Australia. *Medical Journal of Australia, 190,* 410–414.

Maxwell, K. A. (2002). Friends: The role of peer influence across adolescent risk behaviors. *Journal of Youth and Adolescents, 31,* 267–277.

McGilley, B. M., & Pryor, T. L. (1998). Assessment and treatment of bulimia nervosa. *American Family Physician, 57,* 2743–2750.

Mehler, P. S., & Andersen, A. E. (1999). *Eating disorders: A guide to medical care and complications.* Baltimore, MD: Johns Hopkins University Press.

Miller, M. N., & Pumariega, B. (1999). Culture and eating disorders. *Psychiatric Times, XVI* (2). Retrieved from http://www.psychiatrictimes.com/p990238.html

Minuchin, S., Rosman, N. L., & Baker, L. (1978). *Psychosomatic families: Anorexia nervosa in context.* Cambridge, MA: Harvard University Press.

Mitchell, J. E., Halmi, K., Wilson, G. T., Agras, W., Kraemer, H., & Crow, S. (2002). A randomized secondary treatment study of women with bulimia nervosa who fail to respond to CBT. *International Journal of Eating Disorders, 32,* 271–281.

Montoya, I. D., Atkinson, J., & McFaden, W. C. (2003). Best characteristics of adolescent gateway drug prevention programs. *Journal of Addictions Nursing, 14,* 75–83.

National Institute on Drug Abuse (NIDA). (2003). *Preventing drug use among children and adolescents: A research-based guide.* Bethesda, MD: US Department of Health and Human Services.

Neumark-Sztainer, D., Sherwood, N., Coller, T., & Hannon, P. (2000). Primary prevention of disordered eating among preadolescent girls: Feasibility and short term effects of a community-based intervention. *Journal of the American Dietetic Association, 100,* 1466–1473.

Nicholls, D. (2005). Eating disorders in children. In C. Norring & B. Palmer (Eds.), *EDNOS: Eating Disorders Not Otherwise Specified* (pp. 241–265). Hove: Routledge.

Nicholls, D., Chater, R., & Lask, B. (2000). Children into DSM don't go: A comparison of classification systems for eating disorders in childhood and early adolescence. *International Journal of Eating Disorders, 28,* 317–324.

Nicholls, D., Lynn, R., & Viner, R. M. (2011). Childhood eating disorders: British national surveillance study. *British Journal of Psychiatry, 198*(4), 295–301.

Pate, J. E., Pumariega, A., Hester, C., & Garner, D. M. (1992). Cross-cultural patterns in eating disorders: A review. *Journal of the American Academy of Child and Adolescent Psychiatry, 31,* 802–808.

Patel, D. R., Pratt, H. D., & Greydanus, D. E. (2003). Treatment of adolescents with anorexia nervosa. *Journal of Adolescent Research, 18,* 244–260.

Phillips, E. L., Greydanus, D. E., Pratt, E. D., & Patel, D. R. (2003). Treatment of bulimia nervosa: Psychological and psychopharmacologic considerations. *Journal of Adolescent Research, 18,* 261–279.

Pinhas, L., Morris, A., Crosby, R. D., & Katzman, D. K. (2011). Incidence and age-specific presentation of restrictive eating disorders in children; A Canadian pediatric surveillance program study. *Archives of Pediatric and Adolescence Medicine, 165*(10), 895–899.

Piran, N. (1997). Prevention of eating disorders. *Psychopharmacology Bulletin, 33,* 419–423.

Piran, N., & Robinson, S. R. (2006). Associations between disordered eating behaviors and licit and illicit substance use and abuse in a university sample. *Addictive Behaviors, 31,* 1761–1775.

Pope, H. G., Phillips, K. A., & Olivardia, R. (2000). *The Adonis complex: The secret crisis of male body obsession.* New York: Free Press.

Pratt, B. M., & Woolfenden, S. R. (2006). Interventions for preventing eating disorders in children and adolescents. *Cochrane Database of Systematic Reviews.* doi:10.1002/14651858.CD002891

Pyle, R. L. (1999). Dynamic psychotherapy. In M. Hersen & A. S. Bellack (Eds.), *Handbook of comparative interventions for adult disorders* (2nd ed.) (pp. 465–490). Hoboken, NJ: John Wiley & Sons, Ltd.

Ricciardelli, L. A., & McCabe, M. P. (2001). Self-esteem and negative affect as moderators of sociocultural influences on body dissatisfaction, strategies to decrease weight and strategies to increase muscles among adolescent boys and girls. *Sex Roles, 44,* 189–207.

Ringwalt, C. L., Ennett, S., Vincus, A., Thorne, J., Rohrbach, L. A., & Simons-Rudolph, A. (2002). The prevalence of effective substance use prevention curricula in US middle schools. *Prevention Science, 3,* 257–265.

Robin, A. L., Bedway, M., Siegel, P. T., & Gilroy, M. (1996). Therapy for adolescent anorexia nervosa. Addressing cognitions, feelings and the family's role. In E. D. Hibbs & P. S. Jensen (Eds.), *Psychosocial treatments for child and adolescent disorders: Empirically-based strategies for clinical practice* (pp. 239–259). Washington, DC: APA.

Robin, A. L., Siegel, P. T., & Moye, A. (1995). Family versus individual therapy for anorexia: Impact on family conflict. Topical section: Treatment and therapeutic processes. *International Journal of Eating Disorders, 17,* 313–322.

Rosen, D. (2003). Eating disorders in children and young adolescents: Etiology, classification, clinical features, and treatment. *Adolescent Medicine – The Spectrum of Disordered Eating: Anorexia Nervosa, Bulimia Nervosa and Obesity: State of the Art Review, 14,* 49–59.

Rotter, J. B. (1966). Generalized expectancies for internal versus external control of reinforcements. *Psychological Monographs, 80*(609).

Sargent, J. D., Willis, T. A., Stoolmiller, M., Gibson, J. J., & Gibbons, R. X. (2006). Alcohol use in motion pictures and its relation with early-onset teen drinking. *Journal of Studies in Alcohol, 67,* 54–65.

Schmidt, U., Lee, S., Beecham, J., Perkins, S., Treasure, J. L., & Yi, I. A. (2007). Randomized controlled trial of family therapy and cognitive behavior therapy guided self-care for adolescents with bulimia nervosa and related conditions. *American Journal of Psychiatry,* *164,* 591–598.

Sihvola, E., Rose, R. J., Dick, D. M., Pulkkinen, L., Mauri Marttunen, M., & Kaprio, J. (2008). Early-onset depressive disorders predict the use of addictive substances in adolescence: A prospective study of adolescent Finnish twins. *Addiction Research Report, 103,* 2045–2053.

Spirito, A., Jelalian, E., Rasile, D., Rohrbeck, C. & Vinnick, L. (2000). Adolescent risk taking and self-reported injuries associated with substance use. *American Journal of Drug and Alcohol Abuse, 26*(1), 113–123.

Stice, E., Burton, E. M., & Shaw, H. (2004). Prospective relations between bulimic pathology, depression and substance abuse: Unpacking comorbidity in adolescent girls. *Journal of Consulting and Clinical Psychology, 72,* 61–72.

Stice, E., Killen, J. D., Hayward, C., & Taylor, C. B. (1998). Age of onset for binge eating and purging during late adolescence: A 4-year survival analysis. *Journal of Abnormal Psychology, 107,* 671–675.

Striegel-Moore, R. H., Jacobson, M. S., & Rees, J. M. (1997). Risk factors for eating disorders. In M. Jacobson, C. Irwin, N. H. Golden, & J. M. Rees (Eds.), *Adolescent nutritional disorders: Prevention and treatment* (pp. 98–109). New York: Academy of Sciences.

Striegel-Moore, R. H., Silberstein, L. R., & Rodin, J. (1993). The social self in bulimia nervosa: Public self-consciousnesses, social anxiety, and perceived fraudulence. *Journal of Abnormal Psychology, 102*(2), 297–303.

Strober, M., Freeman, R., Lampert, C., Diamond, J., & Kaye, W. (2000). Controlled family study of anorexia nervosa and bulimia nervosa: Evidence of shared liability and transmission of partial syndromes. *American Journal of Psychiatry, 157*(3), 393–401.

Substance Abuse and Mental Health Services Administration (SAMHSA). (2002–2006). Underage alcohol use: Findings from the 2002–2006 National Surveys on Drug Use and Health. Retrieved from http://www.samhsa.gov/data/underage2k8/Cover.htm

Substance Abuse and Mental Health Services Administration (SAMHSA). (2008). Results from the 2008 National Survey on Drug Use and Health: National findings. Retrieved from http://www.oas.samhsa.gov/nsduh/2k8nsduh/2k8Results.cfm

Sundgot-Borgen, J., & Torstveit, M. (2004). Prevalence of eating disorders in elite athletes is higher than in the general population. *Clinical Journal of Sport Medicine, 14,* 25–32.

Swanson, S., Crow, S., LeGrange, D., Swendsen, J., & Merikangas, K. R. (2011). Prevalence and correlates of eating disorders in adolescents: Results from the national comorbidity survey replication adolescent supplement. *Archives of General Psychiatry, 68*(7), 714–723.

United Nations (UN). (2003). World Youth Report. Retrieved from http://www.un.org/ esa/socdev/unyin/documents/worldyouthreport.pdf

Wagner, F. A., & Anthony, J. C. (2002). From first drug use to drug dependence: Developmental periods of risk for dependence upon marijuana, cocaine, and alcohol. *Neuropsychopharmacology, 26*(4), 479–488.

Walters, E. E., & Kendler, K. S. (1995). Anorexia nervosa and anorexia-syndromes in a population based female twin sample. *American Journal of Psychiatry, 152,* 64–71.

West, S. L., & O'Neal, K. K. (2004). Project D.A.R.E. outcome effectiveness revisited. *American Journal of Public Health, 94,* 1027–1029.

Wilson, G. T., & Fairburn, C. G. (1993). Cognitive treatments for eating disorders. *Journal of Consulting and Clinical Psychology, 61,* 261–269.

Winters, K. C. (2001). Assessing adolescent substance use problems and other areas of functioning: State of the art. In M. Monti, S. M. Colby, & T. A. O'Learly (Eds.), *Adolescents, alcohol, and substance abuse: Reaching teens through brief interventions* (pp. 80–108). New York: Guilford.

Wooley, S. C., & Wooley, O. W. (1985). Intense outpatient and residential treatment for bulimia. In D. M. Garner & P. E. Garfinkel (Eds.), *Handbook of psychotherapy for anorexia nervosa and bulimia* (pp. 303–320). New York: Guilford.

12

Child Maltreatment and Self-Injurious Behaviors

Clinical and Educational Child Psychology, First Edition. Linda Wilmshurst.
© 2013 John Wiley & Sons, Ltd. Published 2013 by John Wiley & Sons, Ltd.

Chapter preview and learning objectives

Historically, "child abuse" was primarily associated with thoughts of physical abuse or severe cases of child neglect; however, more contemporary views of child maltreatment focus on four primary sources of maltreatment: physical, sexual, emotional/psychological, and neglect. There are also frequent reports of multiple maltreatment, where a child is subjected to more than one form of abuse. The chapter has been placed in close proximity to the chapter on trauma, since many of the children suffering from abuse develop symptoms of post-traumatic stress disorder (PTSD) which will be address in *Chapter 13*. Categorically, although most countries agree on the four types of abuse, there is wide variation as to what constitutes abuse within those categories. For example, definitions of physical abuse differ significantly depending on the cultural practices of disciplining children that are acceptable. Due to these variations, the definitions for maltreatment in this chapter are derived from definitions found in the *World Report on Violence and Health* developed by the World Health Organization (WHO; Krug, Dahlberg, Mercy, Zwi, & Lozano, 2002). This chapter will provide readers with an increased understanding of:

- the nature and characteristics of different types of abuse and maltreatment;
- outcomes for children exposed to maltreatment;
- prevalence rates for the different types of abuse, internationally;
- initiatives in primary, secondary, and tertiary prevention.

Although not all children who engage in self-injurious behavior (self-inflicted injuries without suicidal intent) suffer from abuse, many do, and therefore information on this subject is also included within this chapter.

Child maltreatment

Definition and prevalence rates

Historical background   Prior to the nineteenth century, childhood was not considered to be a unique period of development (children were seen as miniature adults) and child-rearing was based on prevailing religious, cultural, and social influences dominated by theories of social control. Within this context, children were considered to be chattel; parents had sole ownership of them and could do as they pleased with them (Scannapieco & Connell-Carrick, 2005). However, by the fifteenth century, scholars and educators were beginning to see children in a different light, although this only benefitted children of privilege, since poor children were still in high demand for the labor force. Philosophers in Europe, in the seventeenth and eighteenth centuries, debated parents' role in child rearing, voicing opinions at the ends of two extremes. In England, John Locke was of the opinion that children were born into this world as a blank slate (*tabula rasa*), and it was the parents' duty to nurture and teach the child. In France, Jacques Rousseau pleaded with parents to let nature take its course, and let the children grow without interference (*laissez faire*). The nature nurture debate has continued since that time.

   With the arrival of the industrial revolution and child labor laws, advocates began to "save" the children from the hardship of the workforce; however, in the process, many were abandoned by their parents, because they were no longer of use and became a hindrance. Street children often ended up living in appalling conditions in "almshouses" or poorhouses, which were eventually replaced by orphanages and ultimately foster home placements (Scannapieco & Connell-Carrick, 2005).

Definitions of maltreatment today differ significantly from what was historically considered to be abuse or neglect, and definitions vary depending on culture, the prevailing social policy, and the jurisdiction, and among different professionals and organizations, which can often make it difficult for the workers involved (Giovannoni, 1989). Similarly, as will soon be addressed, lack of uniformity in definitions also causes problems in estimating prevalence rates for child maltreatment and in collating data across research studies for the purposes of conducting a meta-analysis.

Historically, the term "child abuse" was primarily associated with thoughts of physical abuse or severe cases of child neglect. One of the first speculations about the existence of emotional neglect was recorded by L. Emmett Holt in his book *The Diseases of Infancy and Childhood*, in which he described conditions of infant "wasting" and malnutrition that could be associated with clinical factors, a term he later referred to as "failure to thrive" in the tenth edition of his text which was published in the mid-1930s (Holt, as cited in Schwartz, 2000). Several years later, René Spitz (1946) drew attention to the consequences of emotional neglect when he wrote of his observations of institutionalized infants who seemed to waste away despite having their physical needs met, a condition referred to as **marasmus**. Spitz referred to the infants' listlessness and continual sobbing as an early form of depression which he labeled **anaclitic depression**.

Failure to thrive or "maternal deprivation syndrome" (later renamed "parental deprivation syndrome") was finally recognized by the American Psychiatric Association (APA) when "reactive attachment disorder" was officially entered into the third edition of the *Diagnostic and Statistical Manual of Mental Disorders* in the late 1960s (Schwartz, 2000). Also at this time, Kempe, Silverman, Steele, Droegemueller, and Silver (1962) published their renowned article on the "battered child syndrome" wherein they claimed that "physicians have a duty and responsibility to the child to require a full evaluation of the problem and to guarantee that no expected repetition of trauma will be permitted to occur" (p. 17).

It is now recognized that child maltreatment can occur as a result of acts of "commission," such as physical, sexual, or emotional abuse, or acts of "omission," such as cases of severe emotional, educational, or physical neglect that jeopardizes a child's health and well-being (Ronan, Canoy, & Burke, 2009).

Definition of child maltreatment   Despite differences in the exact wording of different definitions, most agree that maltreatment predominantly refers to acts of abuse that can occur in four ways: physical abuse, neglect, sexual abuse, and emotional abuse. However, what is considered to be subsumed under these categories may vary widely, as will soon become evident. Acts of maltreatment can be perpetrated by parents, caregivers, siblings, or other significant individuals in the child's life, and more often than not by individuals whom the child knows and trusts.

According to the APA (1996), children who experience maltreatment can be conflicted for several reasons, including: ambivalence between wanting to put an end to the violence but feeling a sense of loyalty and belongingness to the perpetrator; the abuse may be followed by reconciliation and affection which reinforces the child's hope that the situation has changed for the better; and abuse and power tend to increase over time, increasing the child's threshold for victimization.

According to the WHO, any definition of child maltreatment "must take into account the differing standards and expectations for parenting behaviour in the range of cultures around the world" and with this underlying premise in mind, the WHO drafted the following definition of child abuse and maltreatment:

> Child abuse or maltreatment constitutes all forms of physical and/or emotional ill-treatment, sexual abuse, neglect or negligent treatment or commercial or other exploitation, resulting in actual or potential harm to the child's health, survival, development or dignity in the context of a relationship of responsibility, trust or power.
>
> (Krug et al., 2002, p. 59)

Prevalence rates of child maltreatment

Problems in obtaining accurate prevalence rates   Accurate prevalence rates for maltreatment are difficult to obtain and compare for several reasons, including differences in: definitions of maltreatment; types of maltreatment included in studies; population sampled (socio-economic status, education level, community versus clinic); the type of statistics reported; the measures used to obtain the data; and whether prevalence rates are reported as annual or lifetime rates. In addition, the "accuracy" of estimates may be questionable since not all incidents of child abuse are reported to authorities (Feather & Ronan, 2009).

Some prevalence rate statistics   In the United States, it is estimated that 10 out of every 1000 children will experience some form of maltreatment (USDHHS, 2010). In the United Kingdom, using a broad definition of maltreatment which includes bullying as well as family-based violence, it was reported that about one million out of 13 million children are victims of maltreatment (Hobbs, 2005). In the United States and the United Kingdom, when data include information on non-family physical assault, such as bullying, approximately 20% of children and youth admit to being physically threatened (bullying) outside the family context (Cawson, Wattam, Brooker, & Kelly, 2000). However, based on data acquired in the United Kingdom, Cawson et al. (2000) report that despite elevated levels of bullying, children continue to be most at risk within the context of their own family, and that among the different forms of maltreatment, children are more at risk of physical and emotional abuse than sexual abuse.

In the Netherlands, adopting the methodology used to determine prevalence rates in the United States (National Incidence Studies (NISs), which will be discussed shortly), Euser, van IJzendoom, Prinzie, and Bakermans-Kranenburg (2010) gathered data about child maltreatment cases reported by professionals, as well as those cases registered with the Dutch Child Protection Services (CPS). The overall rate of maltreatment in the Netherlands was reported as 30 cases per 1000 children. Euser et al. (2010) report that one of the most disturbing findings in their study was that only 12.6% of the total number of maltreatment cases were ever reported to the CPS.

Hauser, Schmutzer, Brahler, Glaesmer, and Roseveare (2011) surveyed youth 14 years of age and older in a representative sample of over 2500 persons in Germany. Results revealed the following prevalence rates for different types of abuse:

Table 12.1   The Fourth National Incidence Study of Child Abuse and Neglect (NIS-4)

Total (Endangerment Standard) = 2,905,800 (almost 3 million)					
Abused 835,000			**Neglected 2,251,600**		
29%			77%		
476,600	302,600	180,500	1,192,200	1,173,800	360,500
Physical abuse	Emotional abuse	Sexual abuse	Physical neglect	Emotional neglect	Educational neglect
57%	36%	22%	53%	52%	16%

Source: Sedlak et al. (2010).

1.6% reported severe emotional abuse; 2.8% reported severe physical abuse; and 1.9% reported severe sexual abuse. In this study, neglect was subdivided into physical and emotional components, with 6.6% reporting severe emotional neglect and another 10.8% reporting severe physical neglect.

Comparing lifetime prevalence rates for the United States, the United Kingdom, and New Zealand reveals comparable rates, with average percentages for sexual abuse approximately 10% and physical abuse within the family context between 7% and 9% (Ronan, Canoy, & Burke, 2009).

The Fourth National Incidence Study of Child Abuse and Neglect   The most recent and comprehensive collection of data on child maltreatment in the United States is the Fourth National Incidence Study of Child Abuse and Neglect (NIS-4; Sedlak et al., 2010) which has recently completed analysis of data collected during 2005–2006, representing 6208 reports submitted by "sentinels" (designated staff in schools, day care centers, hospitals, etc.) and 10,667 forms completed by participating CPS agencies. For the purposes of data analysis, the NIS used a definition of maltreatment that satisfied one of two conditions: the **Harm Standard**, an objective measure of demonstrable harm of abuse or neglect; or the **Endangerment Standard**, which includes all children who meet criteria for the Harm Standard, but also includes children who, although "not yet harmed by abuse or neglect," are considered to be in danger of abuse or neglect. The latter standard also allows for inclusion of perpetrators other than parents in certain categories. The results of the latest data analysis are presented in Table 12.1.

The total number of children who were reported to have been abused, neglected, or endangered is almost three million, with a ratio of one out of every 25 children. These rates are not appreciably different from rates that were collected for the NIS-3 in 1993 (Sedlak & Broadhurst, 1996), although the distribution has changed, with categories of physical, sexual, and emotional abuse declining in percentage rates in the interim (29%, 47%, and 48%, respectively) and rates for emotional neglect more than doubling with an 83% increase in rate. The report suggests that increased rates may reflect the heightened awareness of emotional neglect since the previous report. However, increased research is required in this area to provide further insight. Based on results of this report, physical and emotional neglect surface as the predominant forms of maltreatment for children.

With respect to physical and emotional neglect, the NIS-4 (Sedlak et al., 2010) reports that prevalence rates were lowest for the oldest children (15- to 17-year-olds) and highest for children in the six- to eight-year-old category. In addition, compared to the NIS-3, researchers found increases in the reported rates of victimization for the youngest children (0–2 years of age) for sexual abuse (Harm Standard) and overall maltreatment (Endangerment Standard) although it is unclear, at this time, why this is so.

Types of maltreatment   The four major types of maltreatment are: physical, sexual, emotional/psychological, and neglect. Multiple maltreatment includes various combinations of the major areas. The following discussion will address some of the most common characteristics that have been identified with each form of abuse. However, it is important to emphasize that many studies do not distinguish between the different forms of abuse. For this reason, the concluding section on child maltreatment will provide an overview of risks and protective factors as they relate to child maltreatment in a generic sense, considering child and family characteristics in terms of cognitive, behavioral, social, medical, and psychiatric outcomes that have been associated with child and adolescent maltreatment.

Spare the rod and spoil the child

The WHO states that "corporal punishment of children – in the form of hitting, punching, kicking or beating" is socially accepted and is legal in at least 60 countries for juvenile offenders, and in at least 65 countries for use in schools and other institutions, and legally acceptable in the home in all but 11 countries. The WHO recognizes that corporal punishment continues to exist despite the United Nations Convention on the Rights of the Child which was developed to protect children from physical and mental violence and is incompatible with corporal punishment (Krug et al., 2002, p. 60).

Physical maltreatment

Definition and prevalence rates   The WHO defines physical abuse of a child as "those acts of commission by a caregiver that cause actual physical harm or have the potential to harm" (Krug et al., 2002, p. 60).

Philosophically, the use of corporal punishment has been widely debated on moral, religious, and political grounds (Benjet & Kazdin, 2003; Gershoff, 2002). On the one hand, parents in some cultures and geographical locations see corporal punishment as a typical means of disciplining children. For example, researchers found that in the United States, 94% of parents of toddlers admitted to using corporal punishment for issues of compliance (Straus & Stewart, 1999). Yet, in other areas of the world (e.g., Austria, Finland, Germany, Sweden), corporal punishment is illegal and is banned from use in the home and school (Gershoff, 2002; Kazdin & Benjet, 2003). Opponents of the use of corporal punishment cite countless negative outcomes that have been associated with the use of corporal punishment, including: child aggression, antisocial behavior, and increased tendencies to be victimized (Gershoff, 2002). Other studies have found that children with difficult temperaments (hyperactivity and impulsivity) are particularly at risk for parental use of harsh discipline; however, at the same time, these children are among the most vulnerable to the effects of this form of discipline by demonstrating increased aggressive behavior towards peers (Colder, Lochman, & Wells, 1997).

Global estimates of physical abuse vary widely based on the population sampled and the methods of data collection used. For example, 37% of children surveyed in Egypt claimed to have been beaten or tied up by their parents, while two-thirds of parents in the Republic of Korea admitted to whipping their children; 45% reported that they had hit, kicked, or beaten their children. Almost half of the parents surveyed in Romania admitted to beating their children regularly. The World Studies of Abuse in the Family Environment (WorldSAFE) collected data from mothers on parenting practices in four locations: Chile, Egypt, rural India, and the Philippines. Data are published in the WHO *World Report on Violence and Health* (Krug et al., 2002) and are reported alongside information collected in the United States using the same measure (the Parent–Child Conflict Tactics Scale). Results of the data collection for moderately severe and severe forms of physical punishment are presented in Table 12.2. As is evident in the table, spanking on the buttocks is the most common form of punishment, globally, with the exception of Egypt, where shaking, pinching, or slapping are more common forms of punishment.

Characteristics and outcomes Physical abuse is most likely to occur at the extremes of the age continuum, with 51% of abuse related to children under seven years of age (26% are three years of age or younger) and 20% occurring in adolescence (USDHHS, 2009).

Children who are physically abused can evidence cognitive and behavioral changes, which are apparent in disorganized and disoriented attachment patterns (Lyons-Ruth & Jacobvitz, 1999) or avoidant attachment patterns because the primary caregiver is neither a safe haven nor a source of security. Trauma enactment may take the form of child's play (abusing dolls or stuffed animals) or may show up in children's drawings (Gaensbauer & Siegel, 1995). Cognitively, although not all children demonstrate delays, studies have found deficits in verbal and memory skills, as well as in academic achievement, in children with histories of physical abuse (Friedrich, Einbender, & Luecke, 1983; Hughes & Graham-Bermann, 1998). Prasad, Kramer, and Ewing-Cobbs (2005) found that preschoolers who had been physically abused scored significantly lower than non-abused peers on tests of expressive and receptive language, motor skills, and general cognitive functioning, while Lansford et al. (2002) reported lower grades in language arts and standardized tests for adolescents with a history of abuse.

Munchausen by proxy syndrome

The DSM (APA, 2000) lists Munchausen by proxy syndrome as a fictitious disorder that relates to a parent (usually the mother) inducing illness in a child

Table 12.2　Discipline and punishment by country: incident rates for the past six months

Physical punishment	Chile	Egypt	Rural India	Philippines	United States
Moderately severe forms of punishment					
Spanking on buttocks	51	29	58	75	47
Hit the child on buttocks (with object)	18	28	23	51	21
Slapped the child's face or head	13	41	58	21	4
Shook the child	39	59	12	20	9
Pinched the child	3	45	17	60	5
Pulled the child's hair	24	29	29	23	*
Hit the child with knuckles	12	25	28	8	*
Twisted the child's ear	27	31	16	31	*
Forced the child to kneel or stand in an uncomfortable position	0	6	2	4	*
Put hot pepper in the child's mouth	0	2	3	1	*
Severe forms of punishment					
Hit the child with an object	4	26	36	21	4
Kicked the child	0	2	10	6	0
Burned the child	0	2	1	0	0
Beat the child	0	25	*	3	0
Threatened the child with a knife or gun	0	0	1	1	0
Choked the child	0	1	2	1	0
Verbal or psychological punishment					
Yelled or screamed at the child	84	72	70	82	85
Called the child names	15	44	29	24	17
Cursed at the child	3	51	*	0	24
Refused to speak to the child	17	48	31	15	*
Threatened to kick the child out of the household	5	0	*	26	6
Threatened abandonment	8	10	20	48	*
Threatened evil spirits	12	6	20	24	*
Locked the child out of the Household	2	1	*	12	*
Non-violent disciplinary practices					
Explained why behavior is wrong	91	80	94	90	94
Took privileges away	60	27	43	3	77
Told child to stop	88	69	*	91	*
Gave child something to do	71	43	27	66	75
Made child stay in one place	37	50	5	58	75

Note: *Question was not included in the survey.
Source: Krug et al. (2002).

and subjecting the child to numerous intrusive and painful medical procedures to "cure" a fabricated illness. Children who are victims of Munchausen by proxy suffer extensive physical and emotional abuse.

Children with a history of physical abuse also experience more medical problems, such as failure to thrive, abdominal complaints/injuries, and brain injuries (Bruce, 1992; Ricci, 2000). In addition, these children may show higher pain tolerance (Scannapieco & Connell-Carrick, 2005) and experience delayed physical development. As will be discussed shortly, maltreatment can result in neurodevelopmental outcomes as neural pathways are compromised by living in a chronic state of stress. Children who are physically abused may live in a perpetual state of fear and may produce behaviors consistent with enacting a fight or flight response (Perry, 1997; Perry & Pollard, 1998). Infants may extinguish their crying and dissociate, if the parental response to their cries is physical violence (Perry & Pollard, 1998). Children who live in a physically threatening environment may see the world as a hostile place and in their state of hyperarousal may become the aggressor as a result (Perry, 1997).

Shaken baby syndrome

As was seen in Table 12.2, shaking a child is a common form of punishment. However, when shaking involves an infant, the results can be fatal. Infants have developed intracranial hemorrhages, retinal hemorrhages, and seizures as a result of being shaken repeatedly. It has been estimated that about one-third of shaken babies die as a result of their injuries (Kivlin, Simons, Lazoritz, & Ruttum, 2000).

Early onset of physical maltreatment has been related to increased symptoms of anxiety and depression in adulthood, compared to later onset which is associated with increased behavioral problems (Kaplow & Widom, 2007). If children are emotionally and physically abused prior to the age of five, they are more likely to engage in externalizing and aggressive behaviors, while those who are neglected during this time are more likely to develop internalizing behaviors (Manly, Kim, Rogosch, & Cicchetti, 2001).

Sexual maltreatment

Definition and prevalence rates   The WHO defines sexual abuse as "those acts where a caregiver uses a child for sexual gratification" (Krug et al., 2002, p. 61). According to the WHO, global lifetime prevalence rates for childhood sexual victimization range from 20% of females to 5–10% of males. When peers are considered as perpetrators rates increase by 9%, and when lack of physical contact is included in the definition rates increase by 16% (Krug et al., 2002, p. 64).

Characteristics and outcomes   Middle childhood is the most prevalent age for sexual abuse, with the median age for females being 11 years of age, while the median age for males is eight years of age (USDHHS, 2010). The risk of sexual abuse increases if children live without one of their birth parents for a period of time, or if the mother is not available (Finkelhor & Berliner, 1995). Children who demonstrate inappropriate sexual behavior may be acting out previous abuse, while sexualized behaviors can also place the child at increased risk for future victimization (Friedrich et al., 2001). Other factors which can place a child at risk for sexual abuse include: low self-esteem, depression, external locus of control, introversion, and social isolation (Faust, Runyon, & Kenny, 1995).

A number of studies have found that girls who have been sexually abused obtain lower scores on tests of cognitive abilities and academic achievement than their peers (Sadeh, Hayden, McGuire, Sachs, & Civita, 1993; Trickett, McBride-Chang, & Putnam, 1994). At least one-third of children and youth who have been sexually abused will develop post-traumatic stress disorder, (PTSD) with symptoms of **dissociation** as they try to mentally distance themselves from their thoughts about the abuse (Trickett, Noll, Reiffman, & Putnam, 2001). Their sense of victimization may result in feelings that further victimization is inevitable, leading to revictimization in the future (Boney-McCoy & Finkelhor, 1995). In their discussion of sexual abuse, Finkelhor and Browne (1988) present a four-stage model of the traumatic consequences of abuse, including: traumatic sexualization (age-inappropriate promiscuity and/or avoidance of sexual intimacy), betrayal (sense of manipulation), powerlessness (feelings of victimization), and stigmatization (feeling as if they are damaged goods).

Emotional or psychological maltreatment

Definition and prevalence rates Emotional or psychological abuse is probably the least well defined of all the abusive situations. The WHO defines emotional abuse as:

> the failure of a caregiver to provide an appropriate and supportive environment and includes acts that have an adverse effect on the emotional health and development of a child, such as . . . restricting a child's movements, denigration, ridicule, threats and intimidation, discrimination, rejection and other nonphysical forms of hostile treatment.
>
> (Krug et al., 2002, p. 61)

According to the NIS-4 (2010), approximately one-third of children are subjected to emotional maltreatment. Trickett, Kim, and Prindle (2011) report that youth who are involved with CPS are often multiply maltreated, with emotional maltreatment (54%) or emotional neglect (54%), common factors across other forms of abuse. Some studies have included inter-parental violence (domestic violence) under the rubric of emotional abuse (Ronan, Canoy, & Burke, 2009; Weiss, Waechter, Wekerle, & the MAP Research Team, 2011), while other studies have suggested that emotional abuse be related to an abusive parenting style that predicts a set of acts of omission and commission that do not support development (Glaser, 2011). According to Glaser (2011), the effect of emotional abuse may not be immediately apparent and may not surface until adolescence when identity formation is thwarted as a result. The most common forms of emotional abuse include incidences of verbal abuse, such as "belittling, threatening and terrorizing" (Wekerle, 2011, p. 901). Examples of emotional abuse and prevalence rates for five countries are available in Table 12.2. The table also provides rates for non-violent disciplinary practices for the same countries.

A disturbing statistic from a Canadian study of emotional abuse revealed that the rates for both the categories of emotional-abuse-only and emotional-neglect-only increased threefold between 1998 and 2003 (Chamberland, Fallon, Black, & Trocmé, 2011).

Characteristics and outcomes Children who are emotionally maltreated are significantly more likely to engage in externalizing behaviors such as aggression towards peers and delinquent behaviors (males and females), report more internalizing symptoms, such as depression (in girls) and learned helplessness, have lower levels of self-esteem and self-compassion, and experience more difficulty with emotion regulation than peers (Gabarino, 2011; Herrenkohl, Egolf, & Herrenkohl, 1997; Tanaka, Wekerle, Schmuck, & Paglia-Boak, 2011). While it is important for parents to assist their child in developing ways to limit and regulate their emotions and behaviors through limit setting and the use of appropriate discipline (e.g., temporary removal of privileges, or instituting time outs), emotionally abusive parents exercise control through psychological tactics that undermine the child's sense of emotional security and self-worth through methods such as guilt induction, denigrating remarks, or threats regarding the stability of family relationships, thereby obtaining power through psychologically coercive methods (Bornstein, 2006). These emotionally manipulative practices interfere with the normal development of the child's social, cognitive, and affective responses (Wekerle, Miller, Wolfe, & Spindel, 2006). As a result these children may inhibit emotional responses of distress, such as crying, for fear of retaliation; may become more wary, hypervigilant, and fearful in the future (Klorman et al., 2003); and may misinterpret nonverbal cues in others, such as facial expressions, with an increased tendency to attribute a hostile bias inherent in the expressions of others, by paying more attention to reading expressions of anger and threat than others (Pollak & Tolley-Schell, 2003). Children who are subject to emotionally manipulative tactics report more significant emotional distress and are more likely to develop internalizing disorders, such as anxiety and depression, in the future (Steinberg, 2005).

Neglect

Definition and prevalence rates As with other forms of maltreatment, there are many different definitions of neglect. The NIS-4 (Sedlak et al., 2010) collected data on three forms of neglect (see Table 12.1), namely, physical, emotional, and educational neglect. The overall rate of neglect according to the NIS-4 is 77% using the endangerment standard, and 61% if the harm standard is applied. Physical and emotional neglect are among the highest rates (53% and 52%, respectively, using the endangerment standard). Some researchers consider neglect in two categories, physical and emotional (Gustavsson & Segal, 1994), while other researchers have identified up to five subcategories: physical, emotional, medical, mental health, and educational (Erickson & Egeland, 2002). The WHO reports that manifestations of child neglect can include such situations as:

> non-compliance with health care recommendations, failure to seek appropriate health care, deprivation of food resulting in hunger, failure of a child physically to thrive, exposure to drugs and inadequate protection from environmental dangers, as well as, abandonment, inadequate supervision, poor hygiene and being deprived of an education.
>
> (Krug et al., 2002, p. 61)

The WHO distinguishes between neglect and poverty, stating that neglect can occur "only in cases where reasonable resources are available to the family or caregiver" (Krug et al., 2002, p. 61). In Canada, based on nationally reported cases of neglect to child welfare services, the following breakdown of cases was revealed: 19% physical neglect, 12% abandonment, 11% educational neglect, and 48% lack of supervision resulting in child's physical harm (Trocmé & Wolfe, 2001).

Characteristics and outcomes　In their study of 539 children with a history of neglect, Rogeness, Amrung, Macedo, Harris, and Fisher (1985) found that neglected boys had lower IQ scores than boys with a history of abuse, while girls whose history included both physical abuse and neglect had lower IQ scores than peers. In their study of over 11,000 second-grade students, Fantuzzo, Perlman, and Dobbins (2011) found that substantiated child neglect was associated with poorer outcomes than reported physical abuse.

Compared to all other forms of abuse, neglected children are more likely to encounter school problems in language, reading, and mathematics, and are the most likely to repeat a grade (Veltman & Browne, 2001). Other studies have found that neglect is associated with higher risk for language problems (articulation, comprehension) and school readiness (Strathearn, Gray, O'Callaghan, & Wood, 2001).

Multiple maltreatment

Up to this point, the discussion has focused on different types of abuse, and the prevalence rates and outcomes associated with the various forms of abuse and neglect. However, it has become increasingly evident that maltreated children are often subjected to more than one form of victimization (Finkelhor, Ormrod, & Turner, 2007). As was noted in the initial discussions of maltreatment, our understanding of the different types of abuse has produced at least four different categories of maltreatment (physical, emotional, sexual, and neglect), and while some include domestic violence under the umbrella of emotional abuse (Ronan, Canoy, & Burke, 2009), others prefer to consider it as a distinct category (Edleson, 2001; Herrenkohl & Herrenkohl, 2007).

In their review of the research regarding multiple maltreatment, Herrenkohl and Herrenkohl (2009) found evidence from a number of studies that support the notion that children are often exposed to multiple forms of maltreatment; that is, maltreatment involving more than one of the following: physical abuse, emotional abuse, sexual abuse, neglect, and witnessing domestic violence (Edleson, 2001; Herrenkohl & Herrenkohl, 2007; Higgins & McCabe, 2001). There is a wide range in the estimates of cases of multiple maltreatment depending on the nature of cases studied, and how the data were collected (case reports, versus child and parent interviews). For example, using CPS case records, Herrenkohl and Herrenkohl (1981) found approximately one-third of children were exposed to multiple maltreatment. However, Cicchetti and Rogosch (1997) reported that 73.2% of their sample of 133 maltreated children were subjected to multiple maltreatment, while McGee, Wolfe, and Wilson (1997) found that 94% of 160 maltreated adolescents reported experiencing more than one maltreatment type.

Although more and more researchers are recognizing that multiple forms of maltreatment may coexist for the same victim, research on the cumulative risk that this may pose for child outcomes is lacking (Herrenkohl & Herrenkohl, 2009). However, at least one study has investigated the likelihood of experiencing another form of maltreatment based on exposure to various forms of maltreatment. Lau et al. (2005) report that 94% of children who experience sexual maltreatment also experience another form of abuse, while 78.7% of children who are physically abused also experience another form of maltreatment. In their study of adult female victims of maltreatment, approximately half of those who admitted to being maltreated as children reported two or three different forms of maltreatment (Moeller, Bachman, & Moeller, 1993). Outcomes for children who are exposed to multiple maltreatment, or poly-victimization, will be discussed at greater length in *Chapter 13*.

Child maltreatment: child and family characteristics

Child characteristics: risks and protective factors

Risk factors   Researchers who have investigated age of onset of maltreatment have found differential outcomes based on the nature of the maltreatment and its longevity (Kaplow & Widom, 2007). Children are at the most risk for harm in the first year of life (DfES, 2005). In the United States in 2003, 28% of all child deaths were the result of physical abuse, and of this number almost half (44%) were children under the age of one year (USDHHS, 2005). Globally, infants and very young children are at greatest risk of fatalities, with fatality rates for children under four years of age more than double the rate for those in the five- to 14-year-old category.

In the first two years of life, brain development is rapid, with increased myelination speeding up the efficiency of neural responses, while synaptic pruning provides pathways for future learning. However, in the brains of children exposed to chronic stressful and perhaps even violent conditions, pathways may be wired that set the stage for maladaptive responses to stress in the future. Watts-English, Fortson, Gibler, Hooper, and DeBellis (2006) discuss how the psychobiological pathway, including neurobiological stress response systems and neurodevelopment, can be altered by a child's history of maltreatment. According to Watts-English et al. (2006), brain-related changes can mediate maladaptive "psychiatric, behavioral and neurodevelopmental outcomes experienced by children with histories of maltreatment" (p. 718).

When children are placed in an environment of chronic stress, the **sympathetic nervous system** (**SNS**) responds by repeatedly releasing **catecholamines** (norepinephrine, serotonin, dopamine) into the system, initiating a fight or flight response, which can "influence brain maturation and neurodevelopment" (Watts-English et al., 2006, p. 720). In addition, the **serotonin system** is also affected, since mass production of serotonin eventually depletes reserves and can lead to symptoms of severe depression, suicidal ideation, and PTSD. Finally, the **limbic–hypothalamic–pituitary–adrenal axis** (**LHPA/HPA**) releases cortisol into the bloodstream which may result in greater cortisol production in response to novel stressors in the future. Studies of children exposed to maltreatment have revealed physical differences in the brains of children who had a history of maltreatment (smaller mid area of the corpus callosum; smaller total brain volume in boys) and less volume in the prefrontal cortex and right temporal lobe (De Bellis et al., 2002; Teicher et al., 1997).

Children with disabilities are three to four times more likely to be abused or neglected than peers (Murphy, 2011) and three times more likely to be sexually abused (Sullivan & Knutson, 2000). Within this broad category of disabilities, studies have reported that children with conduct disorders are eight times more likely to be emotionally abused and six to seven times more likely to be sexually abused than children without the disorder (Sullivan & Knutson, 2000). Younger children with behavioral or mental health issues (younger than six years of age) have twice the risk of maltreatment compared to peers.

Protective factors   A young child with an easy temperament is less likely to be a target of maltreatment compared to children with difficult temperaments. Children who have well-developed social skills and positive self-esteem, and are affectionate and cognitively higher functioning, are more likely to be protected from maltreatment (Radke-Yarrow & Sherman, 1990; Wolfe, 1999). Despite being subjected to adversity, such as maltreatment, some children do not develop psychological or social/emotional problems and instead demonstrate resilience. In one study, between 20% and 40% of children who were physically or sexually abused did not suffer negative outcomes as adults; while in another study, half the maltreated children did not develop psychopathology as adults (Collishaw et al., 2007; Finkelhor, 1994).

Family characteristics: risks and protective factors

Risk factors   Parents who have a history of abuse or neglect are at increased risk of abusing their children (Straus, 1994), while the age of the predominant parent has also been found to be a risk factor for maltreatment (a younger age is associated with greater risk) (Cadzow, Armstrong, & Fraser, 1999). Other parental factors that increase the risk for maltreatment include living in poverty, having an income below $15,000, and being a single parent (Chance & Scannapieco, 2002; Sedlak & Broadhurst, 1996). Parents who have a lower level of education and those with an authoritarian or coercive parenting style are at higher risk for abusive behavior (Cadzow et al., 1999). As much as 80% of cases of child maltreatment involve parent substance abuse (Scannapieco & Connell-Carrick, 2004). Parents who are struggling with their own mental health or psychiatric issues (depression, withdrawal, anger, personality disorders) are at significantly higher risk for maltreatment (Berliner & Elliott, 2002; Ferrara, 2002), while other personal problems, such as low self-esteem, lack of self-concept, loneliness, and lack of impulse control under stress, have all been associated with increased risk for maltreatment (Coohey, 1996; Faust, Runyon, & Kenny, 1995).

Protective factors   Protective factors in families that can buffer maltreatment include marital and financial stability, and having at least one supportive adult in an otherwise hostile environment (Dutton, 1998; Wolfe, 1999). Parents who have an understanding of appropriate developmental milestones (e.g., a toddler saying "No" is more likely an assertion of independence rather than willful non-compliance) are less likely to maltreat their children (Cicchetti & Lynch, 1995), while those who manage their home with routines, planning, and consistency are more likely to avoid the stress, conflict, and chaos associated with more abusive environments (Wolfe, 1999). Having a sibling may also be protective for school-age children and serve as an additional buffer from stress in high conflict families and as a source of support throughout adolescence (Caya & Liem, 1998; Campbell, Connidis, & Davies, 1999).

Prevention and intervention for child maltreatment

Prinz, Sanders, Shapiro, Witaker, and Lutzker (2009) suggest two reasons why high rates of child maltreatment and referrals for alleged maltreatment "likely represent only the tip of the iceberg in terms of parenting problems and child adversity," including the fact that many cases are not reported, and many "coercive or inadequate parenting practices" may not meet criteria for abuse, but can still have significant negative outcomes for child development (p. 1). In their discussion of the continuum of emotional sensitivity and expression, Wolfe and McIsaac (2011) suggest an approach to distinguishing between poor/dysfunctional parenting and emotionally abusive/neglectful parenting, by considering the nature, frequency, and intensity of practices and outcomes. For example, *a positive and healthy parenting approach* would be one that entailed positive emotional expressions (joy); interactions that are positive and supportive; consistency across situations; and clear rules and discipline that is moderate with emphasis on behavioral methods, such as time outs, or temporary removal of privileges. *Poor and dysfunctional parenting* would be evident in rigid/inflexible emotional responses; inconsistent patterns that do not balance the need for independence and dependence; and the use of unclear rules, and coercive methods of disciplining that confuse and upset the child. *Emotionally abusive or neglectful parenting* practices would include: placing conditions on parental love; demonstrating ambivalent feelings towards the child; rejecting the child's bids for attention; responding unpredictably to the child and often with high expressed emotion; and the use of coercive, cruel, and harsh controls that threaten and frighten the child (Wolfe & McIsaac, 2011, p. 807). Wolfe and McIsaac (2011) suggest that viewing parenting practices along such a continuum provides the opportunity for the implementation of a public health model for educating parents about healthy and positive parenting practices. In this way, primary or secondary prevention programs can increase parent awareness of such elements as balancing demandingness with support and encouragement in a consistent approach that uses sound behavioral practices to discipline inappropriate and reward appropriate behaviors (e.g., the Incredible Years program; Webster-Stratton, Reid, & Stoolmiller, 2008). For those parents who were identified as emotionally maltreating their children, tertiary prevention programs should focus on programs that have been successful with high-risk populations, such as the Triple P Positive Parenting Program (Prinz et al., 2009) and the Nurse-Home Visiting Program (MacMillan et al., 2009).

A parent's inability to control his or her anger when disciplining a child can contribute to the potential for harsh actions that could result in abuse (Mammen, Kolko, & Pilkonis, 2000). Research has focused on the parent's maladaptive cognitions and negative attributional bias about the child's behaviors and/or inappropriate and unrealistic expectations that can result in increasing anger and aggressive responses (Bugental et al., 2002; Pidgeon & Sanders, 2009).

Dysfunctional or poor parenting practices, including coercive and punitive practices that can be physically or emotionally abusive, place a child at increased risk of abuse, while the promotion of and education in healthy and positive parenting practices may be the most salient feature of programs for preventing abuse (Black, Heyman, & Slep, 2001). Based on social learning theory, several prevention and intervention programs have been developed to increase the use of positive parenting practices. These have achieved positive results whether delivered in the home or community (McNeil, Eyberg, Eisenstadt, & Newcomb, 1991), and have been demonstrated to have long-term benefits (Long, Forehand, Wierson, & Morgan, 1994).

The Triple P Positive Parenting Program   The Triple P program was developed by Sanders (2008) and colleagues at the University of Queensland. The program has been demonstrated to be effective in increasing parent competence and reducing child behavior problems, in different cultures, globally (de Graaf, Speetjens, Smit, de Wolff, & Tavecchio, 2008; Nowak & Heinrichs, 2008).

Sanders and Pidgeon (2011) discuss a derivation of the Triple P program, the PTP, suitable for universal and targeted populations, which has been tailored to meet the needs of parents at risk of abusing their children. The program targets three areas that have been identified in at-risk and abusive parents: (i) parents' anger-intensifying attributional style for their child's negative behaviors; (ii) parents' anger-justifying style for their negative parental behavior; and (iii) parent anger management deficits. Participants attend four two-hour group sessions where they learn and practice strategies for reframing their maladaptive thoughts, with the goal of enhancing their positive attributions about the parent–child relationship and reducing anger-related behaviors.

Prinz et al. (2009) conducted a study of the effectiveness of the Triple P program in 18 counties across the United States. Families were randomly assigned to the Triple P program or to a service-as-usual control. Results revealed that the use of empirically supportive parenting intervention practices resulted in positive prevention for all three populations addressed: substantiated child maltreatment, out of home placements, and child maltreatment injuries.

Self-injurious behaviors

Definition and prevalence rates

Terms such as "deliberate self-harm," "self-mutilation," "non-suicidal self-injury," or "cutting" refer to acts of self-injurious behavior not associated with suicidal intent. Simeon and Favazza (2001) suggest four categories of self-injury: *stereotypic* (repetitive and dissociative type behaviors that may occur in the course of pervasive developmental disorders); *major* (infrequent but significant acts of self-mutilation that may accompany a psychotic episode); *compulsive* (frequent and ritualistic behaviors such as trichotillomania); and *impulsive* (deliberate attempts at self-mutilation often with the intention of relieving tension). Lloyd-Richardson, Perrine, Dierker, and Kelley (2007) suggest the use of the term **non-suicidal self-injury** (**NSSI**) for these behaviors, to distinguish between these behaviors and those involving suicidal intent; that is, **suicidal self-injury** (**SSI**).

Prevalence rates Prevalence rates in England and Australia have been reported as between 6% and 7% (Laukkanen et al., 2009); however, Ross and Heath (2002) report rates as high as 13.9% in a community sample of students, especially girls, admitting to self-mutilation. A meta-analysis of 128 population-based studies found approximately 13% of youth report engaging in acts of self-injurious behaviors, while 20–30% also admitted to having suicidal thoughts (Evans et al., 2005). In a large population-based study of over 4000 Finnish adolescents, Laukkanen et al. (2009) found a lifetime prevalence rate of 11.5% for self-cutting, with both the prevalence rate and frequency of cutting significantly higher in females than males. Jacobson and Gould (2007) report rates for adults engaging in NSSI to be between 1% and 4%, while adolescent rates range from 13% to 23%. Some studies show a significant proportion of those engaging in NSSI are female (Csorba, Dinya, Plener, Nagy, & Páli, 2009;

Laukkanen et al., 2009), while other studies report no gender differences (Hilt, Nock, Lloyd-Richardson, & Prinstein, 2008; Muehlenkamp & Gutierrez, 2004).

Characteristics and populations at risk for self-injury

Although self-cutting is the most common form of self-injury, other forms of NSSI exist, including: scratching, burning, ripping or pulling hair or skin, swallowing toxic substances, bruising, and breaking bones. Although characteristics vary widely, adolescents are the most likely to self-injure and two potential trajectories have been identified: *course persistent*, NSSI which begins in early childhood and continues into adulthood; and *adolescence-limited*, NSSI which begins in early adolescence and then terminates at the end of adolescence (Nixon, Cloutier, & Aggarwal, 2002).

Child maltreatment and self-injury A growing body of research has linked NSSI to child maltreatment, especially childhood sexual abuse (Aglan, Kerfoot, & Pickles, 2008; Briere & Gil, 1998; Yates, Carlson, & Egeland, 2008), and multiple maltreatment (sexual abuse and emotional neglect (Dubo, Zanarini, Lewis, & Williams, 1997); sexual abuse, physical abuse, and witnessing violence (Weiderman, Sansone, & Sansone, 1999)). When viewed within a maltreatment context, NSSI can be seen as a possible compensatory strategy for emotion regulation that has gone awry, becoming a reactive pathway that responds to trauma at a neurobiological level through excitatory and inhibitory processes involved in self-injury (Yates, 2004, 2009). In a healthy environment, secure attachment provides young children with the opportunity of learning how to regulate their emotions effectively. However, in abusive situations, children neither learn how to self-soothe, nor have their feelings validated, and may develop a sense of dissociation or "psychic numbness" as a result (Rodriguez-Srednicki, 2001). Furthermore, maltreatment in childhood has also been related to negative feelings of self-worth, self-blame, and self-criticism that have all been related to increased risk for self-injury (Gratz, 2006).

Childhood maltreatment has been related to self-injury directly and indirectly, with neglect surfacing as either the single most significant predictor of self-injury (van der Kolk, Perry, & Herman, 1991), or predictive of negative feelings of self-worth, self-blame, and self-criticism and increased risk for self-injury (Gratz, 2006). Yates (2009) suggests that chronic stress caused by maltreatment may contribute to alterations in the neurobiological and physiological systems that contribute to self-injury, especially the limbic–hypothalamic–pituitary–adrenal (LHPA) axis responsible for the regulation of chronic, long-term stress responses, and the norepinephrine-sympathetic-adrenal-medullary (NE-SAM) which regulates acute stress responses. Children who are maltreated demonstrate erratic flight or fight responses which result in increased depression, anxiety, suicidal ideation, and tendency to self-injure (Novak, 2003). Childhood maltreatment has also been associated with reduced activity in the frontal cortex, responsible for planning and managing responses (Kaufman & Charney, 2001).

Clinical populations and self-injury Csorba et al. (2009) studied 105 outpatient adolescents (28 males, 77 females) between the ages of 14 and 18, who admitted to engaging in NSSI. In this sample, cutting or scratching was the most common form of NSSI, 60% suffered from a major depressive episode (current or in the past), and two-thirds practiced the impulsive type of NSSI. Csorba et al. (2009) support suggestions made by Favazza (1999) that some individuals (in this case, about one-third of the clinical sample) tend to ruminate or brood about NSSI for some time and engage in rituals surrounding the act.

Nock (2009) proposes a model of NSSI to account for etiology and maintenance based on *intrapersonal factors* (high physiological arousal in response to aversive stimuli and tendencies to avoid or escape aversive stimuli) and *interpersonal factors* (issues in social problem solving and communication). Within this context, NSSI can serve many functions as explained by different theories, including: social learning theory (contagion response), self-punishment, social signaling (communicating one's distress to others in a visual and graphic way), pain analgesia, and implicit identification (emotion regulation becomes associated with NSSI).

Disorders that have been linked to NSSI include: borderline personality disorder, post-traumatic stress disorder (PTSD), depression, eating and substance use/abuse disorders and anxiety (Dyer et al., 2009; Yates, 2004).

Other risk factors   Laukkanen et al. (2009, p. 25) found that adolescents who engaged in self-cutting behaviors were more likely to also engage in more frequent "alcohol consumption, drug abuse, sniffing, cannabis, daily smoking, and use of other illegal drugs." From a psychosocial perspective, having no friends, being aggressive, or experiencing symptoms of depression or somatic complaints were risk factors, while having both parents living together was a protective factor. Negative affective states that motivated adolescent self-injury included: feeling a need to hurt the self, depression, negative feelings towards the self, isolation, and need for distraction (Laye-Gindhu & Schonert-Reichl, 2005).

Whitlock, Powers, and Eckenrode (2006) investigated the role of the internet in adolescent self-injury and found hundreds of message boards devoted to self-injury. Although some of the responses provided a supportive network for those who self-injure, the researchers expressed concern about vulnerable youth's exposure to a culture where self-injury is normalized, and information is available regarding new types of self-injury and purchasing paraphernalia that identify individuals as a member of a "cutting club." The authors conclude that "like other social environments (schools, families or neighbourhoods) the Internet plays a powerful role in shaping opportunities for adaptive and maladaptive social interaction" (Whitlock et al., 2006, p. 416).

Intervention and treatment

Web-based social support networks   Since adolescence is a peak time for self-injurious behaviors, and the majority of youth use the internet for social networking (Whitlock et al., 2006), there has been an increased interest in the possibility of integrating internet social support networks in a therapeutic way for youth with self-injurious behaviors.

In their review of articles about self-injurious behaviors and web-based social networking, Messina and Iwasaki (2011) discuss the pros and cons of using web-based centers for therapeutic purposes. While some report these discussions are beneficial in reducing the incidents of self-harm (Murray & Fox, 2006), other sites can actually trigger episodes of self-harm (Adler & Adler, 2007). Whitlock, Lader, and Conterio (2007) provide guidelines to assist psychotherapists in integrating the internet into their therapy, including the use of questions to determine frequency and nature of usage. Whitlock et al. (2007) also recommend websites affiliated with more quality controlled sources such as WebMD, LifeSIGNS, and SIARI. However, future research is recommended to determine the efficacy of web-based support networks.

Dialectical behavior therapy (DBT) DBT was initially introduced by Linehan, Armstrong, Suarez, Allmon, and Heard (1991) to treat adults with borderline personality disorder (BPD) who engage in high-risk behaviors such as suicide attempts and other self-injurious behaviors. Linehan et al. (1991) use biosocial theory to explain the underlying forces that cause self-injurious behaviors that result from a combination of internal forces (problems in the identification and control of emotions) and external forces such as a history of having one's emotions punished, trivialized, or ignored. The DBT method is an eclectic combination of cognitive-behavioral techniques (CBT), humanistic, and modern psychodynamic approaches. In addition to individual therapeutic sessions focused on the client–therapist relationship supported in an environment fostering empathy and self-affirmation, clients are also instructed in CBT practices that focus on individual homework assignments and in group sessions such as social skills building groups (Comer, 2010).

DBT has used been successful in the treatment of adults and is the treatment of choice for BPD. More recently, DBT was adapted for use with suicidal adolescents (Rathus & Miller, 2002) and has subsequently been successful in reducing self-injurious behavior in youth in a number of investigations (Katz, Gunasekara, Cox, & Miller, 2004; Sunseri, 2004).

Lang and Sharma-Patel (2011) suggest that the success of the DBT approach lies in educating the client that although NSSI behaviors provide temporary relief from immediate tension, this behavior is part of a cycle that comes at a high price of increased long-term dysfunction. Integrating DBT components of *acceptance* (validation of the intensity of distress) and *change* (learning new techniques to reduce stress in a healthy way) provide the necessary balance to address and alleviate the underlying process.

Trauma-focused cognitive behavioral therapy (TF-CBT) Exposure therapies have long been associated with treatment for anxiety disorders where increased tensions are likely to elicit avoidant response patterns (Cohen, Deblinger, Mannarino, & Steer, 2004). Within this context, TF-CBT for self-injury engages individuals in the identification of a hierarchy of stressors associated with self-injury. Future research will determine the efficacy of this treatment method in the reduction of NSSI. There is increasing support for the use of TF-CBT for NSSI (DeRosa et al., as cited in Lang & Sharma-Patel, 2011; Briere & Scott, 2006).

Acceptance and commitment therapy (ACT) The underlying assumptions of ACT are similar to those of DBT and TF-CBT, and focus on acceptance of feelings (rather than avoidance), and positive movement towards healthy alternatives. Using mindfulness as a process, ACT engages youth to focus on the pain (acceptance and tolerance) that accompanies memories rather than avoidance through self-injury. There is some evidence to support the use of ACT for NSSI (Powers, Vording, & Emmelklamp, 2009).

References

Adler, P. A., & Adler, P. (2007). The demedicalization of self-injury: From psychopathology to sociological deviance. *Journal of Contemporary Ethnography, 36*, 537–570.

Aglan, A., Kerfoot, M., & Pickles, A. (2008). Pathways from adolescent deliberate self-poisoning to early adult outcomes: A six-year follow up. *Journal of Child Psychology and Psychiatry, 49*, 508–515.

American Psychological Association (APA). (1996). *Violence and the family (Report of the American Psychological Association Presidential Task Force on Violence and the Family)*. Washington, DC: Author.

American Psychiatric Association (APA). (2000). *Diagnostic and statistical manual of mental disorders* (4th ed., text revision). Washington, DC: Author.

Benjet, C., & Kazdin, A. E. (2003). Spanking children: The controversies, findings and new directions. *Clinical Psychology Review, 23*, 198–224.

Berliner, L., & Elliott, D. (2002). Sexual abuse of children. In J. E. Myers, L. Berliner, J. Briere, C. T. Hendrix, C. Jenny, & T. A. Reid (Eds.), *The APSAC handbook on child maltreatment* (2nd ed.) (pp. 55–78). Thousand Oaks, CA: Sage.

Black, D. A., Heyman, R. E., & Slep, A. M. (2001). Risk factors for child physical abuse. *Aggression and Violent Behaviour, 6*, 121–188.

Boney-McCoy, S., & Finkelhor, D. (1995). Prior victimization: A risk factor for child sexual abuse and for PTSD-related symptomatology among sexually abused youth. *Child Abuse and Neglect, 19*, 1401–1421.

Bornstein, M. H. (2006). Parenting science and practice. In K. A. Renninger, I. E. Sigel, W. Damon, & R. M. Lerner (Eds.), *Handbook of child psychology, Vol. 4., Child psychology in practice* (6th ed.) (pp. 893–949). Hoboken, NJ: John Wiley & Sons, Ltd.

Briere, J., & Gil, E. (1998). Self-mutilation in clinical and general population samples: Prevalence, correlates, and functions. *American Journal of Orthopsychiatry, 68*, 609–620.

Bruce, D. (1992). Neurosurgical aspects of child abuse. In S. Ludwig & A. Kornberg (Eds.), *Child abuse: A medical reference* (2nd ed.) (pp. 117–130). New York: Churchill Livingston.

Bugental, D. B., Ellerson, P. C., Lin, E. K., Rainey, B., Kokotovic, A., & O'Hara, N. (2002). A cognitive approach to child abuse prevention. *Journal of Family Psychology, 16*(3), 243–258.

Cadzow, S. P., Armstrong, K. L., & Fraser, J. A. (1999). Stressed parents with infants: Reassessing physical abuse risk factors. *Child Abuse and Neglect, 23*(9), 845–853.

Campbell, L. D., Connidis, I. A., & Davies, L. (1999). Sibling ties in later life: A social network analysis. *Journal of Family Issues, 20*(1), 114–148.

Cawson, P., Wattam, C., Brooker, S., & Kelly, G. (2000). *Child maltreatment in the United Kingdom: A study of the prevalence of child abuse and neglect.* London: NSPCC.

Caya, M. L., & Liem, J. H. (1998). The role of sibling support in high-conflict families. *American Journal of Orthopsychiatry, 68*(2), 327–333.

Chamberland, C., Fallon, B., Black, T., & Trocmé, N. (2011). Emotional maltreatment in Canada: Prevalence, reporting and child welfare responses. *Child Abuse and Neglect, 35*, 841–854.

Chance, T., & Scannapieco, M. (2002). Ecological correlates of child maltreatment: Similarities and differences between child fatality and nonfatality cases. *Child and Adolescent Social Work Journal, 19*(2), 139–161.

Cicchetti, D., & Lynch, M. (1995). Failures in the expectable environment and their impact on individual development: The case of child maltreatment. In C. Cicchetti & D. J. Cohen (Eds.), *Developmental psychopathology: Vol. 2, Risk, disorder, and adaptation* (pp. 261–279). New York: John Wiley & Sons, Ltd.

Cicchetti, D., & Rogosch, F. (1997). The role of self-organization in the promotion of resilience in maltreated children. *Development and Psychopathology, 9*, 797–815.

Cohen, J. A., Deblinger, E., Mannarino, A. P., & Steer, R. (2004). A multisite randomized controlled trial for multiply traumatized children with sexual abuse-related PTSD. *Journal of the American Academy of Child and Adolescent Psychiatry, 43*, 393–402.

Colder, C. R., Lochman, J. E., & Wells, K. C. (1997). The moderating effects of children's fear and activity level on relations between parenting practices and childhood symptomatology. *Journal of Abnormal Child Psychology, 25*, 251–263.

Collishaw, S., Pickles, A., Messer, J., Rutter, M., Shearer, C., & Maughan, B. (2007). Resilience to adult psychopathology following childhood maltreatment: Evidence from a community sample. *Child Abuse and Neglect, 31*, 211–229.

Comer, R. J. (2010). Eating disorders. In *Abnormal psychology* (7th ed.) (pp. 341–372). New York: Worth Publishers.

Coohey, C. (1996). Child maltreatment: Testing the social isolation hypothesis. *Child Abuse and Neglect, 20*, 241–254.

Csorba, J., Dinya, E., Plener, P., Nagy, E., & Páli, E. (2008). Clinical diagnoses, characteristics of risk behaviour, differences between suicidal and non-suicidal subgroups of Hungarian adolescent outpatients practicing self-injury. *European Child and Adolescent Psychiatry, 18*, 309–320.

De Bellis, M. D., Keshavan, M. S., Shifflett, H., Iyengar, S., Beers, S. R., & Hall, J. (2002). Brain structures in pediatric maltreatment-related PTSD: A sociodemographically matched study. *Biological Psychiatry, 52*, 1066–1078.

de Graaf, I., Speetjens, P., Smit, F., de Wolff, M., & Tavecchio, L. (2008). Effectiveness of the Triple P Positive Parenting Program on parenting: A meta-analysis. *Family Relations, 57*, 553–566.

Department for Education and Skills (DfES). (2005). Departmental report, 2005. Retrieved from http://www.official-documents.gov.uk/document/cm65/6522/6522.pdf

Dubo, E. D., Zanarini, M. C., Lewis, R. E., & Williams, A. A. (1997). Childhood antecedents of self-destructiveness in borderline personality disorder. *Canadian Journal of Psychiatry, 42*, 63–69.

Dutton, D. G. (1998). *The abusive personality: Violence and control in intimate relationships.* New York: Guilford.

Dyer, K. F. W, Dorahy, M. J., Hamilton, G., Corry, M., Shannon, M., MacSherry, A., … McElhill, B. (2009). Anger, aggression, and self-harm in PTSD and complex PTSD. *Journal of Clinical Psychology, 65*, 1099–1114.

Edleson, J. (2001). Studying the co-occurrence of child maltreatment and domestic violence in families. In S. Graham-Bermann & J. Edleson (Eds.), *Domestic violence in the lives of children: The future of research, intervention, and social policy* (pp. 91–110). Washington, DC: APA.

Erickson, M. F., & Egeland, B. (2002). Child neglect. In J. E. Myers, L. Berliner, J. Briere, C. T. Hendrix, C. Jenny, & T. A. Reid (Eds.), *The APSAC handbook on child maltreatment* (2nd ed.) (pp. 3–20). Thousand Oaks, CA: Sage.

Euser, E. M., van IJzendoom, M. H., Prinzie, P., & Bakermans-Kranenburg, M. J. (2010). Prevalence of child maltreatment in the Netherlands. *Child Maltreatment, 15*(1), 5–17.

Evans, E., Hawton, K., Rodman, K., & Deeks, J. (2005). The prevalence of suicidal phenomena in adolescents: A systematic review of population-based studies. *Suicide and Life-Threatening Behavior, 35*, 239–250.

Fantuzzo, J. W., Perlman, S. M., & Dobbins, E. K. (2011). Types and timing of child maltreatment and early school success: A population-based investigation. *Children and Youth Services Review, 33*, 1404–1411.

Faust, J., Runyon, M. K., & Kenny, M. C. (1995). Family variables associated with the onset and impact of intrafamilial childhood sexual abuse. *Clinical Psychology Review, 15*(5), 443–456.

Favazza, A. R. (1999). Self-mutilation. In D. G. Jacobs (Ed.), *The Harvard medical school guide to suicide assessment and intervention* (pp. 125–145). San Francisco: Jossey-Bass.

Feather, J., & Ronan, K. R. (2009). Safeguarding children in the primary care context: Assessment and interventions for child trauma and abuse. In J. Taylor and M. Themessl-Huber (Eds.), *Safeguarding children in primary care: A guide for practitioners working in community settings* (pp. 4–27). London: Kingsley Publishing.

Ferrara, F. F. (2002). *Childhood sexual abuse: Developmental effects across the lifespan.* Pacific-Grove, CA: Brooks/Cole.

Finkelhor, D. (1994). The international epidemiology of child sexual abuse. *Child Abuse and Neglect, 18*(5), 409–417.

Finkelhor, D., & Berliner, L. (1995). Research on the treatment of sexually abused children: Reviewed recommendations. *Journal of the American Academy of Child and Adolescent Psychiatry, 34,* 1–5.

Finkelhor, D., & Browne, A. (1988). Assessing the long-term impact of child sexual abuse: A review and reconceptualization. In L. Walker (Ed.), *Handbook on sexual abuse of children* (pp. 55–71). New York: Springer.

Finkelhor, D., Ormrod, R. K., & Turner, H. A. (2007). Poly-victimization: A neglected component in child victimization. *Child Abuse and Neglect, 31*(1), 7–26.

Friedrich, W. N., Dittner, C., Action, R., Berliner, L., Butler, J., Damon, L. . . . Wright, J. (2001). Child sexual behavior inventory: Normative, psychiatric and sexual abuse comparisons. *Child Maltreatment, 6,* 37–49.

Friedrich, W. N., Einbender, A. J., & Luecke, W. J. (1983). Cognitive and behavioural characteristics of physically abused children. *Journal of Consulting and Clinical Psychology, 51,* 313–314.

Gabarino, J. (2011). Not all bad treatment is psychological maltreatment. *Child Abuse and Neglect, 35,* 797–801.

Gaensbauer, T., & Siegel, C. (1995). Therapeutic approaches to posttraumatic stress disorder in infants and toddlers. *Infant Mental Health, 16*(4), 292–305.

Gershoff, E. T. (2002). Corporal punishment by parents and associated child behaviors and experiences: A meta-analytic and theoretical review. *Psychological Bulletin, 128,* 539–579.

Giovannoni, J. (1989). Definitional issues in child maltreatment. In D. Cicchetti & V. Carlson (Eds.), *Child maltreatment: Theory and research on the consequences and causes of abuse and neglect* (pp. 3–37). Cambridge: Cambridge University Press.

Glaser, D. (2011). How to deal with emotional abuse and neglect? Further development of a conceptual framework (FRAMEA). *Child Abuse and Neglect, 35,* 852–861.

Gratz, K. L. (2006). Risk factors for deliberate self-harm among female college students: The role and interaction of childhood maltreatment, emotional expressivity, and affect intensity/reactivity. *American Journal of Orthopsychiatry, 76,* 238–250.

Gustavsson, N. S., & Segal, E. (1994). *Critical issues in child welfare.* Thousand Oaks, CA: Sage.

Hauser, W., Schmutzer, G., Brahler, E., Glaesmer, H., & Roseveare, D. (2011). Maltreatment in childhood and adolescence. *Deutsches Arzteblatt International, 108*(17), 287–294.

Herrenkohl, R. C., Egolf, B. P., & Herrenkohl, E. C. (1997). Preschool antecedents of adolescent assaultive behavior: A longitudinal study. *American Journal of Orthopsychiatry, 67,* 422–432.

Herrenkohl, R. C., & Herrenkohl, E. C. (1981). Some antecedents and developmental consequences of child maltreatment. *New Directions for Child Development, 11,* 57–76.

Herrenkohl, R. C., & Herrenkohl, T. I. (2009). Assessing a child's experience of multiple maltreatment types: Some unfinished business. *Journal of Family Violence, 24,* 485–496.

Herrenkohl, T. I., & Herrenkohl, R. C. (2007). Examining the overlap and prediction of multiple forms of child maltreatment, stressors, and socioeconomic status: A longitudinal analysis of youth outcomes. *Journey of Family Violence, 22*(7), 553–562.

Higgins, D., & McCabe, M. (2001). Multiple forms of child abuse and neglect: Adult retrospective reports. *Aggression and Violent Behavior, 6*, 547–578.

Hilt, L. M., Nock, M. K., Lloyd-Richardson, E., & Prinstein, M. J. (2008). Longitudinal study of non-suicidal self-injury among young adolescents: Rates, correlates, and preliminary test of an interpersonal model. *Journal of Early Adolescence, 28*, 455–469.

Hobbs, C. (2005). The prevalence of child maltreatment in the United Kingdom. *Child Abuse and Neglect, 29*, 949–951.

Hughes, H. M., & Graham-Bermann, S. A. (1998). Children of battered women: Impact of emotional abuse on adjustment and development. *Journal of Emotional Abuse, 1*, 23–50.

Kaplow, J. B., & Widom, C. S. (2007). Age of onset of child maltreatment predicts long-term mental health outcomes. *Journal of Abnormal Psychology, 116*, 176–187.

Katz, L. Y., Gunasekara, S., Cox, B. J., & Miller, A. L. (2004). Feasibility of dialectical behavior therapy for parasuicidal adolescent inpatients. *Journal of the American Academy of Child and Adolescent Psychiatry, 43*, 276–282.

Kaufman, J., & Charney, D. (2001). Effects of early stress on brain structure and function: Implications for understanding the relationship between child maltreatment and depression. *Development and Psychopathology, Special Issue: Stress and Development: Biological and Psychological Consequences, 13*(3), 451–471.

Kazdin, A. E., & Benjet, C. (2003). Spanking children: Evidence and issues. *Current Directions in Psychological Science, 12*(3), 99–103.

Kempe, C., Silverman, F. N., Steele, B. F., Droegemueller, W., & Silver, H. K. (1962). The battered child syndrome. *Journal of the American Medical Association, 181*, 17–24.

Kivlin, J. D., Simons, K. B., Lazoritz, S., & Ruttum, M. S. (2000). Shaken baby syndrome. *Opthamology, 107*, 1246–1254.

Klorman, R., Cicchetti, D., Thatcher, J. E., & Ison, J. R. (2003). Acoustic startle in maltreated children. *Journal of Abnormal Child Psychology, 31*(4), 359–370.

Krug, E. G., Dahlberg, L. L., Mercy, J. A., Zwi, A. B., & Lozano, R. (2002). *World report on violence and health*. Geneva: WHO.

Lang, C. M., & Sharma-Patel, K. (2011). The relation between childhood maltreatment and self-injury: A review of the literature on conceptualization and intervention. *Trauma, Violence & Abuse, 12*(1), 23–37.

Lansford, J. E., Dodge, K. E., Pettit, G. S., Bates, J. E., Crozier, J., & Kaplow, J. (2002). A 12-year prospective study of the long-term effects of early child physical maltreatment on psychological, behavioral, and academic problems in adolescence. *Archives of Pediatrics and Adolescent Medicine, 156*, 824–830.

Lau, A., Leeb, R., English, D., Graham, J., Briggs, E., & Brody, K. (2005). What's in a name: A comparison of methods for classifying predominant type of maltreatment. *Child Abuse and Neglect, 29*, 533–551.

Laukkanen, E., Rissanen, M., Honkalampi, K., Kylmä, J., Tolmunen, T., & Hintikka, J. (2009). The prevalence of self-cutting and other self-harm among 13- to 18-year old Finnish adolescents. *Social Psychiatry and Psychiatric Epidemiology, 44*, 23–28.

Laye-Gindhu, A., & Schonert-Reichl, K. A. (2005). Nonsuicidal self-harm among community adolescents: Understanding the "whats" and "whys" of self-harm. *Journal of Youth and Adolescence, 34*(5), 447–457.

Linehan, M. M., Armstrong, H. E., Suarez, A., Allmon, D., & Heard, H. L. (1991). Cognitive-behavioural treatment of chronically parasuicidal borderline patients. *Archives of General Psychiatry, 48*, 1060–1064.

Lloyd-Richardson, E. E., Perrine, N., Dierker, L., & Kelley, M. L. (2007). Characteristic and functions on non-suicidal self-injury in a community sample of adolescents. *Psychological Medicine, 37*(8), 1183–1192.

Long, P., Forehand, R., Wierson, M., & Morgan, A. (1994). Does parent training with young noncompliant children have long-term effects? *Behaviour Research and Therapy, 32,* 101–107.

Lyons-Ruth, K., & Jacobvitz, D. (1999). Attachment disorganization: Unresolved loss, relational violence, and lapses in behavioural and attentional strategies. In J. Cassidy & P. R. Shaver (Eds.), *Handbook of attachment* (pp. 520–554). New York: Guilford.

MacMillan, H. L., Wathen, C. N., Barlow, J., Fergusson, D. M., Leventhal, J. M. & Taussig, H. (2009). Interventions to prevent child maltreatment and associated impairment. *The Lancet, 373*(9659), 250–266.

Mammen, O. K., Kolko, D. J., & Pilkonis, P. A. (2002). Negative affect and parental aggression in child physical abuse. *Child Abuse and Neglect, 26*(4), 407–424.

Manly, J. T., Kim, J. E., Rogosch, F. A., & Cicchetti, D. (2001). Dimensions of child maltreatment and children's adjustment: Contributions of developmental timing and subtype. *Development and Psychopathology, 13,* 759–782.

McNeil, C. B., Eyberg, S., Eisenstadt, T. H., & Newcomb, K. (1991). Parent–child interaction therapy with behaviour problem children: Generalization of treatment effects to the school setting. *Journal of Clinical Child Psychology, 20,* 140–151.

McGee, R., Wolfe, D., & Wilson, S. (1997). Multiple maltreatment experiences and adolescent behavior problems: Adolescents' perspectives. *Development and Psychopathology, 9,* 131–149.

Messina, E. S., & Iwasaki, Y. (2011). Internet use and self-injurious behaviors among adolescents and young adults: An interdisciplinary literature review and implications for health professionals. *Cyberpsychology, Behavior and Social Networking, 14*(3), 161–168.

Moeller, T., Bachman, G., & Moeller, J. (1993). The combined effects of physical, sexual and emotional abuse during childhood: Long term health consequences. *Child Abuse and Neglect, 17,* 623–640.

Muehlenkamp, J. J., & Gutierrez, P. M. (2004). An investigation of differences between self-injurious behavior and suicide attempts in a sample of adolescents. *Suicide & Life-Threatening Behavior, 34,* 12–24.

Murphy, N. (2011). Maltreatment of children with disabilities: The breaking point. *Journal of Child Neurology, 26*(8), 1054–1056.

Murray, C. D., & Fox, J. (2006). Do internet self-harm discussion groups alleviate or exacerbate self-harming behavior? *Australian e-Journal for the Advancement of Mental Health, 5,* 1–9.

Nixon, M. K., Cloutier, P. F., & Aggrawal, S. (2002). Affect regulation and addictive aspects of repetitive self-injury in hospitalized adolescents. *Journal of the American Academy of Child and Adolescent Psychiatry, 41*(11), 1333–1341.

Nock, M. K. (2009). Why do people hurt themselves? New insights into the nature and functions of self-injury. *Current Directions in Psychological Science, 18,* 78–83.

Novak, M. A. (2003). Self-injurious behavior in rhesus monkeys: New insights into its etiology, physiology, and treatment. *American Journal of Primatology, 1,* 3–19.

Nowak, C., & Heinrichs, N. (2008). A comprehensive meta-analysis of Triple P – Positive Parenting Program using hierarchical linear modeling: Effectiveness and moderating Variables. *Clinical Child and Family Psychology Review, 11,* 114–144.

Perry, B. (1997). Incubated in terror: Neurodevelopmental factors in the "cycle of violence." In J. Osofsky (Ed.), *Children, youth and violence: A search for solutions* (pp. 124–148). New York: Guilford.

Perry, B., & Pollard, R. (1998). Homeostasis, trauma, and adaptations: A neurodevelopmental view of childhood trauma. *Child and Adolescent Psychiatric Clinics of North America, 7*(1), 33–51.

Pidgeon, A. M., & Sanders, M. R. (2009). Attributions, parental anger and risk of maltreatment. *International Journal of Child Health and Human Development, 2*(1), 57–69.

Pollak, S. D., & Tolley-Schell, S. A. (2003). Selective attention to facial emotion in physically abused children. *Journal of Abnormal Psychology, 112*(3), 323–338.

Powers, M. B., Vording, M. B., & Emmelkamp, P. M. G (2009). Acceptance and commitment therapy: a meta-analytic review. *Psychotherapy and Psychosomatics, 78*, 73–80.

Prasad, M. R., Kramer, L. A., & Ewing-Cobbs, L. (2005). Cognitive and neuroimaging findings in physically abused preschoolers. *Archives of Disease in Childhood, 90*, 82–85.

Prinz, J. P., Sanders, R. S., Shapiro, C. J., Witaker, D. J., & Lutzker, J. R. (2009). Population-based prevention of child maltreatment: The US Triple P system population trial. *Prevention Science, 10*(1), 1–12.

Radke-Yarrow, M., & Sherman, T. (1990). Hard growing: Children who survive. In J. Rolf, A. S. Masten, D. Cicchetti, K. H. Nüchterlein, & S. Weintraub (Eds.), *Risk and protective factors in the development of psychopathology* (pp. 97–119). New York: Cambridge University Press.

Rathus, J. H., & Miller, A. L. (2002). Dialectical behavior therapy adapted for suicidal adolescents. *Suicide and Life-Threatening Behavior, 32*, 146–157.

Ricci, L. (2000). Initial medical treatment of the physically abused child. In R. Reece (Ed.), *Treatment of child abuse: Common ground for mental health, medical, and legal practitioners* (pp. 81–94). Baltimore, MD: John Hopkins University Press.

Rodriguez-Srednicki, O. (2001). Childhood sexual abuse, dissociation and adult self-destructive behavior. *Journal of Child Sexual Abuse, 10*, 75–90.

Rogeness, G. A., Amrung, S., Macedo, C., Harris, W., & Fisher, C. (1985). Psychopathology in abused or neglected children. *Journal of the American Academy of Child Psychiatry, 25*, 659–665.

Ronan, K. R., Canoy, D. F., & Burke, K. J. (2009). Child maltreatment: Prevalence, risk, solutions, obstacles. *Australian Psychologist, 44*(3), 195–213.

Ross, S., & Health, N. (2002). A study of the frequency of self mutilation in a community sample of adolescents. *Journal of Youth and Adolescence, 31*, 61–77.

Sadeh, A., Hayden, R., McGuire, J., Sachs, H., & Civita, R. (1993). Somatic, cognitive and emotional characteristics of abused children in a psychiatric hospital. *Child Psychiatry and Human Development, 24*, 191–200.

Sanders, M. R. (2008). The Triple P – Positive Parenting Program as a public health approach to strengthening parenting. *Journal of Family Psychology, 22*(4), 506–517.

Sanders, M., & Pidgeon, A. (2011). The role of parenting programs in the prevention of child maltreatment. *Australian Psychologist, 46*, 199–209.

Scannapieco, M., & Connell-Carrick, K. (2004). Families in poverty: Those who maltreat their infants and those who do not. *Journal of Family Social Work, 7*(3), 49–70.

Scannapieco, M., & Connell-Carrick, K. (2005). *Understanding child maltreatment: An ecological and developmental perspective.* New York: Oxford University Press.

Schwartz, D. (2000). Failure to thrive: An old nemesis in the new millennium. *Pediatrics in Review, 21*(8), 257–264.

Sedlak, A. J., & Broadhurst, D. D. (1996). *Executive summary of the Third National Incidence Study of Child Abuse and Neglect.* Washington, DC: National Clearing House on Child Abuse and Neglect.

Sedlak, A. J., Mettenburg, J., Basena, M., Petta, J., McPherson, K., Greene, A., & Spencer, L. (2010). *Fourth National Incidence Study of Child Abuse and Neglect (NIS–4): Report to Congress.* Washington, DC: US Department of Health and Human Services, Administration for Children and Families.

Simeon, D., & Favazza, A. R. (2001). Self-injurious behaviors: Phenomenology and assessment. In D. Simeon & E. Hollander (Eds.), *Self-injurious behaviors: Assessment and treatment* (pp. 1–28). Washington, DC: American Psychiatric Publishing.

Spitz, A. (1946). Anaclitic depression. *Psychoanalytic Study of the Child, 2*, 313–342.

Steinberg, L. (2005). Psychological control: Style or substance? *New Directions for Child and Adolescent Development, 108,* 71–78.

Strathearn, L., Gray, P. H., O'Callaghan, M., & Wood, D. (2001). Childhood neglect and cognitive development in extremely low birth weight infants: A prospective study. *Pediatrics, 108,* 142–151.

Straus, M. (1994). *Beating the devil out of them: Corporal punishment in American families.* Durham, NH: New Hampshire University, Family Research Lab.

Straus, M. A., & Stewart, J. H. (1999). Corporal punishment by American parents: National data on prevalence, chronicity, severity, and duration in relation to child and family characteristics. *Clinical Child and Family Psychology Review, 2,* 55–70.

Sullivan, P. M., & Knutson, J. F. (2000). Maltreatment and disabilities: A population-based epidemiological study. *Child Abuse and Neglect, 24,* 1257–1273.

Sunseri, P. A. (2004). Preliminary outcomes on the use of dialectical behavior therapy to reduce hospitalization among adolescents in residential care. *Residential Treatment for Children & Youth, 21,* 59–76.

Tanaka, M., Wekerle, C., Schmuck, M., & Paglia-Boak, A. (2011). The linkages among childhood maltreatment, adolescent mental health, and self-compassion in child welfare adolescents. *Child Abuse and Neglect, 35,* 873–884.

Teicher, M. H., Ito, Y., Glod, C. A., Andersen, S. L., Dumont, N., & Ackerman, E. (1997). Preliminary evidence for abnormal cortical development in physically and sexually abused children using EEG coherence and MRI. *Annals of the New York Academy of Sciences, 821,* 160–175.

Trickett, P., Kim, K., & Prindle, J. (2011). Variations in emotional abuse experiences among multiply maltreated young adolescents and relations with developmental outcomes. *Child Abuse and Neglect, 35,* 862–872.

Trickett, P., McBride-Chang, C., & Putnam, F. (1994). The classroom performance and behavior of sexually abused females. *Development and Psychopathology, 6,* 183–194.

Trickett, P., Noll, J. G., Reiffman, A., & Putnam, F. W. (2001). Variants of intrafamilial sexual abuse experience: Implications for short- and long-term development. *Development and Psychopathology, 13,* 1001–1019.

Trocmé, N. H., & Wolfe, D. (2001). *Child maltreatment in Canada: Selected results from the Canadian Incidence Study of Reported Child Abuse and Neglect.* Ottawa: Minister of Public Works and Government Services Canada. Retrieved from http://dsp-psd.pwgsc.gc.ca/collections/collection_2010/sc-hc/H49-152-2000-eng.pdf

United States Department of Health and Human Services (USDHHS). (2005). *Child maltreatment 2005.* Retrieved from http://www.acf.hhs.gov/programs/cb/pubs/cm05/cm05.pdf

United States Department of Health and Human Services (USDHHS). (2009). *Child maltreatment 2007.* Retrieved from http://www.acf.hhs.gov/programs/cb/pubs/cm07/cm07.pdf

United States Department of Health and Human Services (USDHHS). (2010). *Child maltreatment 2010.* Retrieved from http://www.acf.hhs.gov/programs/cb/pubs/cm10/cm10.pdf

van der Kolk, B. A., Perry, C. J., & Herman, J. L. (1991). Childhood origins of self-destructive behavior. *American Journal of Psychiatry, 12,* 1665–1671.

Veltman, M., & Browne, K. (2001). Three decades of child maltreatment research. *Trauma, Violence and Abuse, 2,* 215–239.

Watts-English, T., Fortson, B. L., Gibler, N., Hooper, S. R., & DeBellis, M. D. (2006). The psychobiology of maltreatment in childhood. *Journal of Social Issues, 62,* 717–736.

Webster-Stratton, C., Reid, M. J., & Stoolmiller, M. (2008). Preventing conduct problems and improving school readiness: Evaluation of the Incredible Years Teacher and Child Training Programs in high-risk schools. *Journal of Child Psychology and Psychiatry, 49,* 471–488.

Weiderman, M. W., Sansone, R. A., & Sansone, L. A. (1999). Bodily self harm and its relationship to childhood abuse among women in a primary care setting. *Violence Against Women, 5,* 155–163.

Weiss, J. A., Waechter, R., Wekerle, C., & the MAP Research Team (2011). The impact of emotional abuse on psychological distress among Child Protective Services-involved adolescents with borderline-to-mild intellectual disability. *Journal of Child and Adolescent Trauma, 4,* 142–159.

Wekerle, C. (2011). Emotionally maltreated: The under-current of impairment? *Child Abuse and Neglect, 35,* 899–903.

Wekerle, C., Miller, A., Wolfe, D. A., & Spindel, C. B. (2006). *Childhood maltreatment, advances in psychotherapy: Evidence-based practice* (series Ed. D. Wedding). Cambridge, MA: Hogrefe and Huber.

Whitlock, J., Lader, W., & Conterio, K. (2007). The Internet and self-injury: What psychotherapists should know. *Journal of Clinical Psychology, 63,* 1135–1143.

Whitlock, J. L., Powers, J. L., & Eckenrode, J. (2006). The virtual cutting edge: The internet and adolescent self-injury. *Developmental Psychology, 42,* 407–417.

Wolfe, D. A. (1999). *Child abuse: Implications for child development and psychopathology.* Thousand Oaks, CAL Sage.

Wolfe, D., & McIsaac, C. (2011). Distinguishing between poor/dysfunctional parenting and child emotional maltreatment. *Child Abuse and Neglect, 35,* 802–813.

Yates, T. M. (2004). The developmental psychopathology of self-injurious behavior: Compensatory regulation in posttraumatic adaptation. *Clinical Psychological Review, 24,* 35–74.

Yates, T. M. (2009). Developmental pathways from child maltreatment to nonsuicidal self-injury. In M. K. Nock (Ed.), *Understanding nonsuicidal self-injury: Origins, assessment, and treatment* (pp. 117–137). Washington, DC: APA.

Yates, T. M., Carlson, E. A., & Egeland, B. (2008). A prospective study of child maltreatment and self-injurious behavior in a community sample. *Development and Psychopathology, 20,* 651–671.

13

Trauma and Trauma Disorders

Chapter preview and learning objectives

The discussion of childhood disorders in *Chapter 6* introduced the *adjustment disorders* which the DSM describes as a psychological response to an identifiable stressor (or stressors) that results in significantly distressing, emotional, and behavioral reactions (APA, 2000). The response can be distressing, is often more intense than would be expected, and can result in significant impairment in functioning. However, the response is a temporary one, occurring within three months of the stressful situation, but lasting no longer than six months after the stressor is removed.

Clinical and Educational Child Psychology, First Edition. Linda Wilmshurst.
© 2013 John Wiley & Sons, Ltd. Published 2013 by John Wiley & Sons, Ltd.

Distress

When capacity to cope with existing demands, exceeds our ability to cope, then Stress becomes Distress.

Children who experience distress resulting from chronic interpersonal trauma often do so within the context of an environment where exposure to adverse early life experiences includes caregivers who do not provide security and a safe haven from harm. In this chapter, severe forms of stress-related disorders are introduced that are triggered by traumatic situations or events that result in symptoms of re-experiencing the event, attempts to avoid potential triggers of the event, and heightened agitation and arousal. These symptoms can be acute, lasting for less than one month, as in acute stress disorder, or more pervasive, lasting for more than a month and potentially for years, as can be the case with post-traumatic stress disorder (PTSD). Prior to discussing the traumatic stress disorders, the focus will be on reactive attachment disorder, a severe disorder with onset prior to age five which can develop in response to various forms of maltreatment and results in disturbances in the child–parent attachment relationship.

Child and adolescent trauma disorders: an introduction

Costello, Erkanli, Fairbank, and Angold (2002) conducted a longitudinal survey of 1420 children and adolescents from middle childhood through adolescence who were living in western North Carolina regarding exposure to traumatic events. In this sample, one in four children reported that they had been exposed to a "high magnitude" traumatic event (an extreme stressor, such as witnessing or hearing about the death of a loved one, a serious illness, a serious accident, a natural disaster, a fire, or being a victim of violence, rape, or sexual abuse) by 16 years of age, while one-third had been exposed to a "low magnitude event" (such as a new child in the home, pregnancy, parental separation/divorce/new parental figure, or parent arrest) in the previous three months.

It has long been suspected and more recently confirmed that childhood maltreatment can have a profound impact on development, extending into the adult years. In *Chapter 12*, the focus was on different types of maltreatment, as well as the potential outcomes, risks, and protective factors. In this chapter there will be more discussion about the nature and outcomes of multiple maltreatment, as well as the nature of the maltreatment in terms of Type I and Type II trauma.

Type I and Type II trauma

Terr (1991) suggested that childhood trauma could be best conceptualized as two distinct forms of trauma: **Type I traumas** which consist of single event incidences; and **Type II traumas** which refer to chronic and long-term victimization where the child is exposed to a repeated traumatic event, such as repeated physical, sexual, or emotional abuse, or prolonged neglect. Within this framework, Terr (1991) proposed that symptoms and outcomes would be more severe (including dissociation and emotional numbing) for children who experienced Type II trauma, and may ultimately result in the development of personality disorders in the future. Subsequently, researchers have provided support for Terr's theory, demonstrating that children exposed to chronic physical or sexual abuse were at greater risk for depression and schizophrenia, relative to peers who experienced Type I trauma (Kiser, Heston, Millsap, & Pruitt, 1991), as well as for the development of borderline personality disorder as adults (Sansone, Sansone, & Gaither, 2004).

More recently Allen and Lauterbach (2007) found that adults who experienced Type I or Type II trauma as children rated significantly higher on the *neuroticism* (symptoms of anxiety and depression) and *openness to new experiences* subscales of the brief Big Five Personality Measure (Goldberg, 1992) relative to controls, while those who experienced Type II trauma also scored significantly higher on the neuroticism scale than those who experienced Type I trauma. The authors suggest that while endorsement of the neuroticism scale was not unexpected, scoring high on the openness to new experiences scale may increase the chances of individuals engaging in risky behaviors, which would make them more vulnerable to revictimization in the future.

Poly-victimization   In addition to looking at outcomes related to experiencing single versus repeated trauma, studies have also investigated the impact of exposure to multiple different types of abuse. Finkelhor, Ormrod, and Turner (2007) surveyed 2000 children (aged two to 17 years) through random digit dialing, and found that 70% of respondents (children, or parents of younger children) reported at least one adverse and stressful incident of victimization, while 64% also admitted experiencing a different type of victimization. The mean number of victimizations in this sample was 2.8 episodes. Continued data collection with a national sample of 4549 children (aged 0 to 17 years) yielded the following prevalence rates for poly-victimization: close to 66% reported more than one type of victimization; 30% experienced five or more different types; and 10% admitted to 11 or more different forms of victimization (Turner, Finkelhor, & Ormrod, 2010). The authors conclude that poly-victimization is more significantly related to trauma symptoms than Type II trauma (repeated victimization of a single type) and emphasize the need to recognize the impact of experiencing multiple victimizations and the role that cumulative trauma can have on development in all areas.

Determining the number of episodes of victimization is important, since research has shown that adult outcomes for multiple victimization in childhood are associated with more severe and negative consequences (Marx, Heidt, & Gold, 2005). Researchers have also investigated the likelihood of certain types of maltreatment increasing the risk for other forms of maltreatment. Exposure to domestic violence has been linked to general child maltreatment in 30–60% of cases, and to child physical abuse in 45–70% of cases (Edleson, 1999; Margolin, 1998).

In their development of *Practice Parameters for the Assessment and Treatment of Children and Adolescents with Posttraumatic Stress Disorder,* the American Academy of Child and Adolescent Psychiatry (AACAP, 2010) has cautioned that although children may present with behavioral problems or may be referred due to their exposure to a single traumatic event, practitioners should be cognizant that other traumatic events may be at the core of the problem, even if these are not immediately discernible.

In their study of poly-traumatic victims, Kira, Lewandowski, Somers, Yoon, and Chiodo (2012) found that for individuals who experienced Type I trauma, numbness/dissociation provided a protective effect against hyperarousal and re-experiencing which can damage IQ performance. However, for youth who experienced cumulative traumas, negative effects on information processing were evident in all areas of IQ functioning (memory, perceptual reasoning, verbal comprehension, and processing speed).

Developmental trauma disorder   Recognizing the impact of interpersonal trauma on young children and the implications this has for psychological well-being, van der Kolk and Pynoos (2009) have advocated for the establishment of a new classification for children, **developmental trauma disorder** (**DTD**), which they proposed should be added to the DSM-V. In their proposal, DTD is conceptualized as encompassing facets of post-traumatic stress disorder (PTSD), but providing a more appropriate and comprehensive description of symptoms that children experience resulting from interpersonal trauma (often involving multiple victimizations) and the disruption of caregiver support systems. The current diagnostic system does not recognize symptoms unique to children, nor post-traumatic sequelae, such as disturbances in affect regulation, attention and concentration, impulse control, aggression, and risk taking that are not part of the criteria or characteristics associated with PTSD. As a consequence, deficiencies in the current diagnostic system often result in a lack of diagnosis, inaccurate diagnosis, or inadequate diagnosis for traumatic disorders in children.

There is research support for the proposal put forth by van der Kolk and Pynoos (2009). Cloitre et al. (2009) studied cumulative trauma in children and adults and concluded that "exposure to multiple or repeated forms of maltreatment and trauma in childhood can lead to outcomes that are not simply more severe than the sequelae of a single incident trauma, but are qualitatively different in their tendency to affect multiple affective and interpersonal domains" (p. 405). As a result of their findings, Cloitre et al. (2009) suggest that DTD may provide a new way of classifying the complex profiles produced by these traumatized children.

Traumatic stress disorders: a developmental perspective   As it currently stands, there are a number of options for classifying trauma disorders in children: traumatic attachment disorders (reactive attachment disorder; inhibited and disinhibited types) and the traumatic stress disorders (acute and post-traumatic disorder). The current classification system is in transition and there are many conceptual issues that are in the process of being resolved that will likely impact how we classify stress disorders in the future. There is consensus between the DSM and ICD that traumatic attachment disorders can manifest in two different symptoms clusters: an inhibited type and a disinhibited type. However, whether these two types represent two different disorders, or subtypes of one disorder, is a point of contention.

As for the stress disorders, as has already been discussed, there is much controversy as to whether symptoms for post-traumatic stress disorder are broad enough to encompass situations of multiple, poly-traumatic, and chronic stress conditions, and whether the unique symptom constellations should be recognized with a more appropriate classification, such as DTD (which was previously discussed) or disorders of extreme stress not otherwise specified (DESNOS, to be discussed shortly) (Blaz-Kapusta, 2008; Ford, 1999; Herman, 1997; van der Kolk & Pynoos, 2009).

Reactive attachment disorder (RAD)/disinhibited social engagement disorder

Definition   Historically, RAD first appeared in the third revision of the DSM (APA, 1980), and criteria were modified over the course of the next two editions. In the current edition of the DSM (APA, 2000) reactive attachment disorder is described as a marked disturbance in social relatedness with onset prior to five years of age, and causing one of two predominant behavioral patterns, indicating one of two types of RAD:

1. *inhibited type:* an excessively inhibited response to social interaction which might be characterized by hypervigilant, ambivalent, or contradictory responses (e.g., approach/avoidance, resistance to being soothed, or frozen watchfulness);
2. *disinhibited type:* indiscriminate and diffuse social responses accompanied by an inability to display selective and appropriate social affiliations (e.g., lack of selectivity in attachment figures, or excessive familiarity with individuals who have minimal contact).

The disorder is not due to an intellectual disability or autism spectrum disorder, and is manifested in response to "pathogenic care" which may be evident in persistent neglect and disregard for the child's basic, emotional needs, or basic physical needs; or frequent and repeated changes in primary caregiver, resulting in poor formation of normal and stable attachments. The two forms of RAD have been identified in populations of maltreated, and institutionalized or formerly institutionalized, children (Rutter et al., 2007; Smyke, Dumitrescu, & Zeanah, 2002; Zeanah et al., 2005).

A controversial question is whether the two forms represent variants of one disorder or if they are best represented as two distinct disorders. While the current DSM considers these responses as two subtypes of the same disorder, the ICD conceptualizes the variants as two distinct disorders: reactive attachment disorder (RAD), which aligns with the inhibited pattern in the DSM, and disinhibited attachment disorder (DAD) which aligns more with the indiscriminately social disinhibited type of RAD.

In the proposed DSM-V, it has been recommended that the two be recognized as separate disorders, which is in keeping with the current ICD classification: namely, reactive attachment disorder of infancy or early childhood (RAD), and disinhibited social engagement disorder (DSED). In addition to conceptually altering the way that RAD is perceived, the proposed changes also suggest a more comprehensive list of symptoms that match findings from empirical research. With these changes in mind the following suggestions for criteria have evolved.

Reactive attachment disorder of infancy or early childhood (RAD)   This disorder has onset between nine months and five years of age and describes children who in times of distress manifest a marked disturbance in attachment, rarely seeking out the caregiver as a source of comfort and instead demonstrating a consistent pattern of inhibited and emotionally withdrawn behavior, displaying *two* of the following characteristics: lack of emotional responsiveness to others; low positive affect; or episodic and random responses to caregivers that demonstrate sad, irritable, or fearful behaviors. Exclusionary criteria require that the above characteristics are not the result of autism spectrum disorder.

Precipitating conditions A diagnosis of RAD requires one of the following cardinal precipitating conditions: neglect of care and disregard for basic emotional needs; neglect of basic physical needs; or adverse living conditions, including frequent changes of primary caregivers (different caregivers, different foster placements), or care provided in an institution or setting with a large child-to-caregiver ratio.

Disinhibited social engagement disorder (DSEG) Children in this category demonstrate an indiscriminate and active effort to engage with unfamiliar adults, involving *two* of the following four conditions: a lack of shyness or inhibition in approaching unfamiliar adults; a lack of social referencing or checking back with the caregiver after wandering off; a lack of hesitation in venturing off with a stranger; or engaging in social solicitation that demonstrates a disregard for social boundaries (overly familiar, verbally or physically). An exclusionary criterion for DSEG is that the above characteristics are not better accounted for by ADHD.

Precipitation conditions: The child's early history would be seen as responsible for the development of the disorder by including *one* of the three precipitating conditions, as noted for RAD, above. Gleason et al. (2011) provide data from their longitudinal studies of children adopted from institutions (e.g., the Bucharest Early Intervention Project) that support conceptualizing two separate forms of RAD. The researchers found that 17.6% exhibited the socially disinhibited version of RAD/DSEG at 54 months post-institutionalization, while 4.1% exhibited the emotionally withdrawn/ inhibited version of RAD. The authors suggest support for two different versions of RAD, in keeping with the proposed revision.

Differential diagnosis: RAD and disorganized/disoriented attachment: Main and Solomon (1990) describe a disorganized/disoriented attachment pattern that infants display in the strange situation experiments (Ainsworth, Blehar, Waters, & Wall, 1978) which has been associated with child maltreatment and/or parent psychopathology (Lyons-Ruth & Jacobvitz, 1999). In this pattern, children demonstrate a number of odd behaviors when the caregiver leaves or returns to the laboratory setting. However, in this case, the impairment is in the attachment relationship itself and may not be evident in other areas, unlike RAD which influences the child's ability to establish normal social relationships. While children with disorganized/disoriented patterns are at higher risk for aggression towards peers and externalizing behaviors beginning in preschool (Troy & Sroufe, 1989) and persisting into elementary school (Renken, Egeland, Marvinney, Mangelsdorf, & Sroufe, 1989), children with reactive attachment disorders may also demonstrate significant internalizing problems, and withdraw from contact with others.

Nature and course Given that attachment disorders derive from situations of "pathogenic care" involving emotional or physical maltreatment or some form of institutionalized care, it is not surprising to see that many children meet criteria for both an attachment disorder and PTSD (Hinshaw-Fuselier, Boris, & Zeanah, 1999). As will be discussed at greater length later in the chapter, symptoms of PTSD can manifest in different ways during the course of development; however, one common symptom of PTSD in young children is "emotional numbing" (Carrion, Weems, Ray, & Reiss, 2002) which can be attributed to chronic fatigue or exhaustion due to pervasive and on-going experiencing of high levels of arousal (Weems, Saltzman, Reiss, &

Carrion, 2003). Children are also more likely to be exposed to Type II trauma, which involves the repeated exposure to abuse over time, than Type I trauma, like a natural disaster or traumatic event which occurs once (Terr, 1991). Given that the attachment disorders represent exposure to Type II trauma, symptoms of PTSD such as emotional numbing can be seen in children with the inhibited form of the attachment disorder.

The inhibited type of attachment disorder represents an extreme form of withdrawal and inhibition that has developed in the absence of an attachment to a caregiver and is related to severe forms of maltreatment and neglect. Other characteristics of the disorder that have been found in the literature include: a failure to seek out or respond to comfort when distressed, flat affect, unpredictable bouts of irritability or fearfulness, low levels of social or emotional reciprocity, and poor emotion regulation (Smyke, Dumitrescu, & Zeanah, 2002; Tizard & Rees, 1975; Zeanah et al., 2005). While those with the inhibited type have been found to be very responsive to enhanced caregiving, those who are socially disinhibited may develop attachments when caregiving becomes more positive and stable but nevertheless still tend to exhibit socially inappropriate and disinhibited responses to other unfamiliar adults (Zeanah & Smyke, 2008).

Research has provided several documented cases of attachment disorders that conform to descriptions of the socially disinhibited form of attachment disorder, including: tendencies to approach strangers and unfamiliar adults without reservation; a lack of hesitation in venturing off with strangers; and tendencies to ignore appropriate social boundaries in their interactions with adults, while soliciting social contact by seeking close proximity to unfamiliar adults and being intrusive, verbally or physically (O'Connor, 2002; O'Connor & Zeanah, 2003; Zeanah, Smyke, & Dumitrescu, 2002).

Etiology and prevalence

Etiology Researchers have investigated the relationship between early maltreatment/deprivation and attachment theory and have suggested several possible causes for negative outcomes, including: perinatal exposure to toxins; lack of goodness of fit between child and parent temperament; and poor or dysfunctional parenting practices (Kemph & Voeller, 2008). For example, Lyons-Ruth, Bureau, Riley, and Atlas-Corbett (2009) found that the indiscriminate and uninhibited form of attachment disorder was exhibited by high-risk infants only if they also experienced maltreatment or if their mother was hospitalized for psychiatric problems. Lyons-Ruth et al. (2009) suggest that the attachment disorder and subsequent indiscriminant behaviors resulted from the disruption in emotional caregiving. According to Hardy (2007, p. 28), an inability to develop a consistent internal working model (IWM) based on secure affective interactions can result in altering "neurological development and lead to the creation of neural networks (particularly in the right hemisphere) that will influence the infant's personality and relationships with others throughout life."

Hariri (2002) suggests that early maternal deprivation may also alter brain development, by causing overactivity of the hypothalamic–pituitary–adrenal (HPA) system resulting in the production of elevated levels of the stress hormone cortisol. Support for HPA activation is found in reports of increased levels of cortisol in traumatized infants when they are reunited with their caregivers (Nachmias, Gunnar, Mangelsdorf, Parritz, & Buss, 1996). In addition, Barr et al. (2003) suggest that some children may be more vulnerable to dysfunctional parenting practices due to their biological make-up, such as possessing the 5-HTT short allele of the serotonin transporter polymorphism associated with heightened activity and arousal of the amygdale and cortisol systems.

Prevalence   In their follow-up studies of Romanian children, O'Connor (2002) and Zeanah (2000) found that the disinhibited type was most prevalent among those who were adopted out of the institutional setting, while Smyke, Dumitrescu, and Zeanah (2002) reported that the inhibited type was most prevalent among those children who remained at the orphanage. In addition, the disinhibited/indiscriminate behaviors associated with the socially disinhibited attachment disorder persisted for years, even if the children eventually established a secure attachment with their adopted parent (Chisholm, 2009; O'Connor, Marvin, Rutter, Orlick, & Britner, 2003).

Gleason et al. (2011) report the following prevalence rates for the two forms of attachment disorders found in their longitudinal sample of previously institutionalized children: *social/disinhibited children* at baseline (31.8%), 30 months (17.9%), 42 months (18%), and 54 months (17.6%); and withdrawn/inhibited children at baseline (4.6%), 30 months (3.3%), 42 months (1.6%), and 54 months (4.1%).

Assessment and treatment

Assessment   Diagnosis of RAD has been problematic in the past because of the high degree of overlap in symptoms of RAD with other childhood disorders, such as ADHD, anxiety disorders, and PTSD (Balbernie, 1997; Kemph & Voeller, 2008) or in situations of less severe symptom presentations (O'Connor, Rutter, Beckett, Keaveney, & Kreppner, 2000).

In the absence of a suggested protocol for assessing RAD, Sheperis et al. (2003) suggest a test battery, including evaluation of intelligence, obtaining a developmental and medical history, conducting interviews and observations, and completion of a number of behavioral rating scales, such as the Child Behavior Checklist (Achenbach & Rescorla, 2001).

More recently, Thrall, Hall, Golden, and Sheafer (2010) evaluated two screening measures designed to aid in diagnosing RAD: the Reactive Attachment Disorder-Checklist (RAD-C; Hall, 2007) and the Relationship Problems Questionnaire (RPQ; Minnis, Rabe-Hesketh, & Wolkind, 2002) which has been used in Great Britain to aid in the diagnosis of RAD. Results revealed that scores on the RPQ and RAD-C discriminated significantly between children with RAD and the control groups, both statistically and clinically.

The American Association of Child and Adolescent Psychiatry (AACAP, 2005, p. 1214) has made several suggestions for the assessment of children with RAD, including: direct observations of the child with primary caregivers and unfamiliar adults; obtaining a complete history of the child and caregivers; reporting of maltreatment to the appropriate authorities; accessing the safety of the current placement; and appropriate referrals for assessments of developmental delays, language delays, or medical concerns.

Treatment   The AACAP (2005) recommends that treatments be based on the individual needs of the child, including caregiver education when needed, and recognizing that "the building blocks of secure attachment are interactive moments" where the caregiver needs to be attuned to the child's needs, in order for the child to develop "an internal sense of security" (AACAP, 2005, p. 1215). The AACAP (2005) suggests that service delivery can occur at three levels: working through the caregiver; working with the child and caregiver dyad; or working individually, with the child; and that adjunct therapeutic interventions should be used if aggression or opposition/defiance are issues. The AACAP (2005) cautions strongly against the use of "non-contingent physical restraints or coercion (Therapeutic Holding) or reworking the trauma (Rebirthing Therapy) since these practices have no empirical support and have in fact resulted in serious harm, including death" (p. 1216).

Failure to develop a sense of "affective sharing" could negatively influence the development of self-awareness and other awareness which usually develops at about 18 months of age; however, an absence of shared emotional communication might be the precursor to "shunning of sharing" or avoidance of a caregiver who causes distress (Lyons-Ruth, 2008). In these cases, intervention would be directed towards rebuilding emotional and affective channels of communication and sharing. Securely attached children are better able to regulate their emotions and manage physiological stress responses than those with insecure attachments, while those with disorganized attachment have even greater dysregulation (Gunnar & Quevedo, 2007). Children who are maltreated are over five times more likely to have insecure attachments (Carlson, Cicchetti, Barnett, & Braunwald, 1989), while traumatic stress responses are more often associated with traumatized children who have insecure attachments, likely due to their inability to seek comfort from the caregiver (Lynch & Cicchetti, 1998).

According to Kemph and Voeller (2008, p. 174), repairing the damage resulting from RAD requires an acknowledgement that some of these children may be "attachment resistant," and enhancing their ability to develop social relationships may pose a challenge that requires patience and practice and "many repetitions of appropriate thoughts and behaviors over a prolonged period of time" in order to form "new neuronal patterns" which may ultimately enable the child or adolescent to develop socially meaningful relationships.

Hardy (2007) suggests that treatment focus on enhancing existing or creating new attachment relationships and reducing problematic behaviors, while Corbin (2007) stresses the need to foster secure attachments in the development of self-confidence. Cornell and Hamrin (2008) suggest the need to provide psycho-educational and psychotherapeutic supports that target primary attachment relationships and limit exposure to multiple caregivers.

Chaffin et al. (2006) summarize the Task Force position of the American Professional Society on the Abuse of Children (APSAC) on attachment therapy, RAD, and attachment disorder problems. In their document, similar to AACAP, they also take a strong stand against the use of coercive "holding techniques" which have no empirical basis and have even resulted in fatalities. Chaffin et al. (2006) suggest that in addition to potential physical harm, the technique can also be psychologically damaging to the child who is already feeling victimized, and would be subjected to even further harsh and controlling tactics that would likely increase feelings of victimization and helplessness. As an alternative, empirically based behavioral training programs have had an excellent success rate with child behavior problems, similar to those demonstrated by children with attachment disorders. Examples of empirically supported programs for behavior problems, some of which were discussed in *Chapter 12*, and in previous chapters, include: behavioral management training (BMT; Barkley, 1997); the Incredible Years (Webster-Stratton & Reid, 2003); the Triple P Program (Prinz, Sanders, Shapiro, Witaker, & Lutzker, 2009; Sanders & Pidgeon, 2011), and parent–child interactive therapy (PCIT; Eyberg & Boggs, 1998), a program which targets preschool children.

Buckner, Lopez, Dunkel, and Joiner (2008) selected BMT for their case study of a seven-year-old girl with RAD. Results of their case study revealed that BMT was successful in reducing problematic behaviors, and increasing compliance with caregiver and teacher requests, as well as improving age-appropriate play with peers.

What is behavioral management training (BMT)?

BMT (Barkley, 1997) is a manualized 10-session program for caregivers of school-age children. The program targets behavioral problems (compliance, defiance, attention/concentration), and provides parents/caregivers with psycho-educational information about precipitating and maintaining causes of behaviors, opportunities for practice sessions to enhance parenting skills/effectiveness, and techniques to assist in developing a home-based reward system.

Based on their investigation of neurological explanations of problems in self-regulation experienced by children with traumatic attachment histories, Huang-Storms, Bodenhamer-Davis, Davis, and Dunn (2007) used EEG biofeedback to instruct children in self-regulation to enhance attention, control impulses, and help better manage their physiological and emotional arousal states. Initial results showed a reduction in the majority of behavioral categories evaluated by the Child Behavior Checklist (CBCL; Achenbach & Rescorla, 2001). Future research will provide more insight into the efficacy of this neuro-feedback approach.

Interventions for children with RAD in the school system   Children with a history of disrupted attachment have not met key attachment goals (proximity, security, safety, and self-regulation) and the school psychologist can assist in educating school personnel on ways to enhance the child's sense of security. Schwartz and Davis (2006) suggest furthermore that the school psychologist can help teachers understand the importance of the student–teacher relationship in "providing a sense of safety and security and enhancing self-regulation" that may "enable children to explore the environment, regulate behaviors and emotions and join others in the process of learning" (p. 477). Within the context of the school environment, Lieberman and Zeneah (1999) also emphasize the need to use interventions that are child-specific and developmentally appropriate, and minimize emotional pressure and negative practices (scolding, condemning).

Post-traumatic stress disorder

Post-traumatic stress disorder (PTSD) is also triggered by a stressor, the nature of which is extreme, traumatic, and often life-altering. Examples of the types of trauma include: natural disasters (floods, hurricanes, earthquakes), accidents (car wreck, being struck by a car), wars, victimization, and witnessing or experiencing a life-threatening event. However, what constitutes a trauma for a child may be difficult to determine since some events, although not violent or life-threatening, may still have traumatic outcomes for children (such as inappropriate sexual touching). In addition, what is traumatic may also differ by developmental level. Children who suffer from PTSD can experience flashbacks, numbing, avoidance, heightened physiological arousal, and a sense of a foreshortened future.

Definition: PTSD in children and adolescents   The DSM currently defines PTSD as a cluster of symptoms which develop in the aftermath of exposure to an extremely traumatic episode or event. There are six criteria, the first of which contains two parts:

A1. the relationship between the individual and the event such that the person is either directly exposed to an event, or has witnessed an event that is either life-threatening, or results in serious injury to the person or others;
A2. the individual experiences a response of "fear, helplessness or horror" as a result.

Both criteria (A1 and A2) are required for a diagnosis of PTSD. However, for children, the response (A2) may be one of "disorganized or agitated behavior" (APA, 2000, p. 467).

The DSM groups the symptoms into three broad criterion clusters:

B. re-experiencing of intrusive thoughts and images;
C. avoidance and numbing; and
D. hyperarousal.

Symptoms from these clusters must be evident for more than a month and cause significantly impaired functioning.

Re-experiencing   Re-experiencing of the trauma can be invasive and intrusive, unpredictable, and uncontrollable, and can result in significant anxiety and distress. The diagnosis of PTSD requires *one symptom* from this cluster. This category includes five symptoms, namely: recurring thoughts about the trauma; recurrent dreams; flashbacks; intense psychological distress; and intense physiological responses to triggers or cues about the trauma.

Symptoms of re-experiencing in children

In children recurrent thoughts or images may appear as repetitive play, and while they may experience nightmares, they may not be aware of how these are related to the trauma. Dreams can have themes of monsters or rescue. Flashbacks may appear as re-enacting parts of the trauma, while distress may manifest in complaints of headaches and stomachaches. Research suggests that re-experiencing might be one of the most prevalent symptoms of PTSD in children of school age (Carrion et al., 2002; La Greca, Silverman, Vernberg, & Prinstein, 1996).

Avoidance and numbing   Individuals with PTSD will attempt to avoid people, events, or situations that might trigger thoughts or images of the traumatic situation. This is often accomplished by physical distancing and emotional numbing. There is usually a loss of interest in normal activities and a stunted perspective on the future. The DSM requires *three symptoms* from a list of seven potential symptoms, namely: avoidance of conversations about the trauma; inability to recall details about the trauma; avoidance of activities associated with the trauma; loss of interest in normal activities; restricted range of affect; detachment; and a sense of a foreshortened future.

Symptoms of avoidance and numbing in children

Children may avoid talking about the event or engaging in activities associated with the event, or develop a sense of **time skew** which results in their inability to recall trauma-related events in the correct sequence. Parents and teachers may report diminished interest in activities and restricted range of affect. Although emotional numbing is not typically one of the most prevalent symptoms in children (Carrion et al., 2002), it has been observed at all developmental levels.

Increased agitation and arousal   There may be evidence of interrupted sleep/ nightmares, difficulties concentrating/distractibility, and irritability or anger. There are two symptoms required from a list of five problem areas: difficulty in falling or staying asleep; problems with concentration/task completion; hypervigilance; exaggerated startle response; and angry or irritable outbursts. If symptoms subside within a month, then a diagnosis of **acute stress disorder** is made instead of PTSD.

Symptoms of increased agitation and arousal in children

In addition to exhibiting symptoms of heightened arousal, disorganization, and agitated behaviors, children may also exhibit **omen formation**, a belief that they can detect warning signs about the traumatic event, and become hypervigilant in their attempt to detect clues or early warning signs about an impending trauma.

Other associated features of the disorder that may incur in children and adolescents who are survivors of physical or sexual abuse or have witnessed violence may involve:

* impulsive and destructive behaviors;
* social withdrawal;
* dissociative symptoms;
* impaired social relationships;
* somatic complaints;
* difficulties with affect regulation;
* change in personality;

- feeling threatened, on guard;
- feelings of shame. (APA, 2000)

Definition: PTSD in preschool children   Although it has been widely recognized that very young children can experience trauma, it has only been within the past two decades that researchers have advocated for different DSM criteria for very young children. Scheeringa, Zeanah, Drell, and Larrieu (1995) reported that almost half (eight out of 18) of the necessary criteria for PTSD are only accessible through verbal descriptions of experiences and internal status, placing children at a disadvantage for diagnosis, due to their limited verbal skills. Scheeringa, Zeanah, Myers, and Putnam (2003) evaluated 62 traumatized preschoolers and 63 healthy controls (aged 20 months to six years) who had experienced various forms of trauma, including abuse, accidental injuries, vehicle collisions, and witnessing violence. In their sample, no cases met DSM criteria for PTSD. They reported the percentage of responses that met criteria for each of the symptoms clusters. Cluster B (re-experiencing) was endorsed by 67.9%. However, Cluster C (avoidance/numbing) was only endorsed by 2% for the required three symptoms, 11% when reduced to two symptoms, and 73% when one symptom was required. Cluster D (agitation/arousal) met criteria for 45% when two symptoms were required and 73% when one symptom was required. Based on their results, they suggest that for the preschool population, the best fit was one that required one symptom from cluster B, one from cluster C, and two from cluster D, which would derive a rate of diagnosis of PTSD for this population of 26%.

Based on findings from several studies, Sheeringa (2008) has questioned whether DSM-IV criteria are developmentally sensitive enough to diagnose the disorder in preschoolers. In their study of young child survivors of motor vehicle accidents, Meiser-Stedman, Smith, Glucksman, Yule, and Dalgleish (2008) found that using the DSM resulted in 1.7% of the children being diagnosed with PTSD compared to 10% when using alternative (proposed) criteria, even though, on the average, children demonstrated 10 traumatic symptoms. Furthermore, the symptoms remained stable six months later, suggesting that PTSD in children may be more stable and unremitting than in adults; a finding that was supported by results of child survivors of Hurricane Andrew whose symptoms were still evident when they were re-evaluated almost two years later (Shaw, Applegate, & Schorr, 1996). As a result, a proposed set of criteria has been suggested for children under six years of age.

Proposed DSM criteria for PTSD in preschool children   The proposed criteria contain three possible ways of identifying the event (experiencing, witnessing, or learning about the event in relation to close relatives or friends) while feelings of "fear, helplessness and horror" have been excluded from the event criteria for preschoolers (De Young, Kenardy, & Cobham, 2011). It has been recommended that symptom requirements be altered, such that: Cluster B (re-experiencing) requires only one symptom (distressing memories, dreams, distress at exposure, re-experiencing, and physiological response to triggers); Cluster C (avoidance) requires one symptom (avoiding activities, avoiding talking about the event); and Cluster E (increased arousal) requires at least two symptoms (irritability/aggressive behaviors, reckless/self-destructive behavior, hypervigilance, exaggerated startle response, sleep disturbance, and problems concentrating). An additional symptom cluster has been recommended which describes negative moods and thoughts, and this cluster (Cluster D) would require one symptom (frequent negative moods and states/fears, withdrawn, diminished interest, loss of positive emotion). Symptom duration for PTSD would be more than one month.

Nature and course   There has been significant research activity surrounding how symptom presentations might differ between adults and children, and what symptoms might look like across the developmental spectrum. Although there are common symptoms shared by PTSD victims at all ages, it should not be surprising that children would also have some symptoms that differ from adults, due to the impact of "divergent stressors, developmental themes, family issues and collateral symptoms" (Amaya-Jackson & March, 1995b, p. 294).

   McDermott and Palmer (2002) studied responses of 2379 students (Grades 4 to 12) to an Australian bush firebush disaster six months after the event and found responses differed based on developmental level: younger children (Grades 4 to 6) were more likely to respond with *depressive symptoms*; middle school children reported the most symptoms of *emotional distress* (peaking in the eighth grade); while the oldest children (Grades 11 to 12) were most likely to demonstrate symptoms of *depression*.

Characteristics evident in preschool children   Studies have investigated early memory to determine how early trauma can register in infants, and suggest that although infantile amnesia precludes the ability to recall information prior to 18 months of age (Howe, Toth, & Cicchetti, 2006), children who were traumatized between seven and 13 months of age spontaneously re-enacted or verbally described events seven years later (Gaensbauer, 2002), while children between 30 and 36 months of age are able to recall distressing events accurately several years later (Scheeringa, 2009). Furthermore, children 18 months of age would likely be able to recall the gist of a traumatic event, in the absence of more specific details (Howe, Toth, & Cicchetti, 2006). However, due to cognitive limitations, very young children are not likely to express coherent memories, which places the burden of assessment on caregivers or professionals to look for behavioral manifestations of PTSD (Coates & Gaensbauer, 2009).

   Trauma that is experienced during the early years will by necessity involve the child–caregiver relationship at some level. Scheeringa and Zeanah (2001) discuss possible ramifications of the parent–child relationship in what they refer to as *relational PTSD*, where symptomatology in the parent can exacerbate symptoms in the child. Within this framework, although parent and child may not be exposed to the same trauma, a parent's unresolved history of trauma may negatively influence child outcomes. Examples include the parent who is emotionally unavailable (the parent responds to the child's symptoms by avoidance and numbing); the parent who re-experiences the event, intrusively (an overprotective and constricting pattern due to guilt for not having protected the child from harm); or parent preoccupation with the trauma (the parent floods the child with questions, causing the child to relive the event).

   While traumatic responses vary depending on the nature and severity of the trauma, Scheeringa and Zeanah (1995) found that one of the most consistent predictors of PTSD in very young children was witnessing a threat to the caregiver which resulted in hyperarousal, increased aggressive and fear responses, and a decrease in numbing symptoms. Some of the most common symptoms at this age include: separation anxiety, increases in irritability, tantrums, sleep problems, and nightmares (Graham-Bermann et al., 2008; Klein, DeVoe, Miranda-Julian, & Linas, 2009; Zerk, Mertin, & Proeve, 2009).

Characteristics evident in school-age children   In school-age children, sleep problems are common, with episodes of sleep walking or bed wetting, while dreams and nightmares may result in night terrors (Amaya-Jackson & March, 1995b). Repetitive play often replaces "flashbacks" in children (Scheeringa & Zeanah, 2001), while trauma play may contain themes of happy endings to achieve mastery over an otherwise helpless situation (Amaya-Jackson & March, 1995b). Attention and concentration problems may interfere with school achievement (Amaya-Jackson & March, 1995a), and hyperarousal may result in an exaggerated startle response to unsuspected school drills or fire alarms (March, Amaya-Jackson, & Pynoos, 1994). Play may be subdued and restricted, while anxiety may take the form of vague somatic complaints of headaches or stomachaches. It has also been noted that for some children, numbing and avoidance may take the form of restlessness, poor concentration, hypervigilance, and behavioral problems (Malmquist, 1986). Problems may be more evident at bedtime, with new or renewed fears of the dark, fears of sleeping alone, and worry about possible nightmares.

Younger children may engage in post-traumatic play (repeating some aspect of the trauma, which does not serve to relieve anxiety; e.g., repeatedly smashing two cars together after being in a car accident) or reenactment play (behavioral response to the traumatic event, such as securely fastening a belt around the doll so she will not be injured in the crash).

Variations in response to trauma

In addition to developmental factors, responses can vary based on the degree of exposure, the proximity to the event, and the nature of the personal impact. The closer the child is to the actual trauma, the greater the impact of PTSD (Pynoos, 1994).

Characteristics evident in adolescence   PTSD in adolescence has more in common with adult forms of the disorder; however, there are some features unique to adolescence, such as engaging in increased risk-taking behaviors and re-enacting the trauma through these behaviors. Pynoos and Nader (1993) suggest that because youth are at a stage where the focus is on identity formation, the impact of a trauma at this time could be particularly devastating and alter the course of the youth's future (Pynoos, 1990; Pynoos & Nader, 1993). Given their physical make-up and hormonal changes that take place during this period of development, males may be more likely to respond with impulsive or aggressive impulses, while females may be more prone to depression and withdrawal.

If the trauma involves the death of a family member or friend, then the situation becomes even more complex (Pynoos & Nader, 1993). In this case, interactions

between trauma and grief responses can cause increased focus on the traumatic circumstances surrounding the death and interfere with the grieving process and subsequent
adaptation. Trauma victims may also experience significant **survivor guilt**, especially
if the teen was responsible for the accident which caused the trauma (e.g., by being
the driver of a car in a fatal crash).

Etiology and prevalence

Etiology   As has been discussed, there is a growing body of research linking traumatic
and stressful events to physical changes that take place in several areas, including:
activation of the hypothalamic–pituitary–adrenal (HPA) pathway and sympathetic
nervous system pathway (see *Chapter 2* for a review); the amygdale; prefrontal cortex;
hippocampus, and corpus callosum; as well as the serotonin and dopamine systems,
all of which evidence dysregulation. There is evidence that early maltreatment and
duration of maltreatment result in greater symptom presentations of PTSD (DeBellis,
Hooper, & Sapia, 2005). Abnormal activity of the neurotransmitter *norepinephrine*
and elevated levels of the hormone *cortisol* have both been implicated in the process
(Baker et al., 2010).

The fight or flight response pattern

When we encounter a stressful/traumatic situation, the hypothalamus causes
activation of two pathways: the autonomic nervous system (ANS) and sympathetic **nervous system pathway** initiating a fight or flight response pattern. The
hypothalamus also activates the hypothalamic–pituitary–adrenal (HPA) pathway which causes the pituitary gland to release adrenocorticotropic hormone
(ACTH) and prompts the adrenal cortex to release corticosteroids.

There is also evidence that enduring heightened arousal over time may actually
damage key brain areas (Carlson, 2008), including the hippocampus and amygdale.
The *hippocampus* (the portion of the brain that regulates stress hormones and memory)
may malfunction, resulting in reduced ability to manage future stressful situations, and
may be instrumental in the repetition of intrusive memories (Bremner, 1999; Bremner,
Vythilingan, Vermetten, Vaccarino, & Charney, 2004). Furthermore, the amygdale
may be involved in intensifying the emotional responses that accompany the traumatic
memories (Shin et al., 2005).

There is also evidence of genetic and environmental interactions in the trauma
research. For example, women who were pregnant during the September 11, 2001
terrorist attack in the United States, and who developed PTSD, actually gave birth
to infants who registered higher levels of cortisol than the norm (Yehuda & Bierer,
2007). One study of nature/nurture interactions in physically abused children found
that children with the lowest genetic risk showed an increased probability of conduct
disorder of 2%, while those with the highest genetic risk demonstrated an increased
probability of 24% (Jaffee et al., 2005). Furthermore, Brewin et al. (1996) suggest
that traumatic memories may become activated as "situationally accessible memories"

(SAMs) that are distinct from other memories because they are not readily accessed by conscious effort, but rather are triggered by environmental cues.

In addition to biological explanations for the development of PTSD, cognitive-behavioral models suggest the possibility that *re-experiencing* a traumatic event can be equated to a conditioned fear response. Although the trauma is not likely to be repeated, extinction does not occur, because the fear is continually re-energizing through stimulus generalization and increased connections. Emotional processing can alter how future threat is appraised, turning relatively innocuous events into signals of potential threat (Foa & Kozak, 1986). Other cognitive theorists stress the maladaptive cognitive assumptions and appraisals resulting in dysfunctional beliefs about the future (Ehlers & Clark, 2000).

Prevalence   The difficulty in obtaining accurate prevalence rates for PTSD relates to the wide variability of populations from which these rates are drawn, variability in the nature of the trauma, cumulative versus single event situations, and the question-able sensitivity of current DSM criteria for the preschool population. According to community-based studies, the lifetime prevalence rate for adult PTSD is approximately 8%; while the prevalence rate for adolescent PTSD (mean age 17 years) is reported to be 6.3% (Giaconia et al., 1994). A more recent national sample of adolescents (aged 12 to 17 years) found that 3.7% of males and 6.3% of female adolescents met the full criteria for PTSD (Kilpatrick et al., 2003). The rates for young children are less clear due to the additional problem of methods of data collection and criteria used to determine whether a diagnosis of PTSD is warranted. Using modified criteria, prevalence rates for single event trauma were reported to be between 6.5% and 29% (Meiser-Stedman et al., 2008) and for mass trauma reported to be between 17% and 50% (De Voe, Bannon, & Klein, 2006; Scheeringa & Zeanah, 2008).

Where data collection involves clinical populations, and samples of urban popu-lations, substantially higher rates have been reported. Horowitz, Weine, and Jekel (1995) interviewed 79 girls (12 to 21 years of age) attending an urban adolescent health clinic and found that 67% met criteria for a diagnosis of PTSD; while Berton and Stabb (1996) report that 27% of their sample (97 juniors attending five high schools in a major metropolitan area) endorsed PTSD symptoms at a clinical level. Berton and Stabb (1996) suggest that "community violence" was the variable most highly asso-ciated with PTSD in their sample. McLeer, Deblinger, Henry, and Orvaschel (1992) found that 43.9% of 92 sexually abused children (three to 16 years of age) met criteria for PTSD.

Gender and PTSD

Studies of adult populations have found that women are at least twice as likely to develop PTSD, with 20% of women developing the disorder post-trauma, compared to only 8% of men (Koch & Haring, 2008; Russo & Tartaro, 2008).

Young girls who have been abused sexually are two to three times more likely to experience repeated victimization in adulthood and to be victims of family violence (Cloitre, Tardiff, Marzuk, Leon, & Portera, 1996). Furthermore, Deblinger, McLeer,

Atkins, Ralphe, and Foa (1989) suggest that the PTSD symptom profile of sexually abused children may differ from other forms of abuse, with more symptoms of re-experiencing and inappropriate sexual behaviors.

Assessment and treatment/intervention

Assessment The difficulty in appropriately assessing PTSD symptoms in children, especially young children, has been addressed throughout this chapter. Loeb, Stettler, Gavila, Stein, and Chinitz (2011) investigated the sensitivity of several scales and criteria in screening PTSD symptoms in a clinic sample of 51 preschool-aged children with high exposure to trauma and found wide variations in the diagnosis of PTSD. Researchers compared several identification procedures and instruments, including the PTSD scale of the CBCL (Achenbach & Recorla, 2001), DSM-IV criteria (APA, 2000), and the Zero to Three (2005) diagnostic criteria. In this sample, 24% were diagnosed with PTSD using the Zero to Three criteria, while only 4% were diagnosed using the DSM criteria. Results revealed that although the CBCL PTSD subscale had previously been found to screen for PTSD in preschool children (Dehon & Sheeringa, 2006), positive results were not replicated in this study.

There are several screening instruments available for children and adolescents with suspected PTSD. The *Juvenile Victimization Questionnaire* (Finkelhor, Hamby, Ormrod, & Turner, 2005) is suitable for children aged two to 17 years, and has been validated on diverse ethnic samples. Informants complete the questionnaire for children under seven years of age. The *Trauma Symptom Checklist for Children* (Briere, 1996) is a self-report measure for children aged eight to 16 years, which provides measures of avoidance/symptom denial (under-response) and heightened responding (hyper-response), in addition to the clinical scales (anxiety, depression, anger, PTSD, and dissociation). The *Trauma Symptom Checklist for Young Children* (Briere et al., 2001) is a caretaker response report available for children aged three to 12 years. Measures of generalized anxiety, depression, and mental status can be obtained using the more general child behavior rating scales discussed earlier, while the *Personality Inventory for Youth* (PIY; Lachar & Gruber, 1995) contains a number of scales assessing emotional and behavioral adjustment in the home and school environments that would be helpful, including a somatic scale to evaluate vegetative symptoms.

Treatment The AACAP (2010) makes several recommendations for the treatment of children with PTSD, including the need for a comprehensive approach that includes consultation with school personnel and primary care physicians and includes trauma-focused therapy. Because avoidance of talking about trauma topics is a common symptom of PTSD, trauma-focused treatment has been proven superior to other non-directive treatment models (Cohen, Deblinger, Mannarino, & Steer, 2004), while including the parent in the treatment has also been found to reduce trauma-related symptoms (Deblinger, Lippmann, & Steer, 1996). The AACAP (2010) recommends the use of trauma-focused cognitive behavioral therapy (TF-CBT) and psychodynamic trauma-focused therapy. Although AACAP (2010, p. 424) recognizes that selective serotonin reuptake inhibitor (SSRI) treatment may benefit children with comorbid symptoms of depression, generalized anxiety disorder, or obsessive compulsive disorder, and that combined SSRI treatment and TF-CBT might benefit some children, research results suggest beginning with TF-CBT alone.

Cognitive behavioral therapy (CBT)   Recently, Cohen et al. (2004) evaluated a multisite, randomized controlled trial of TF-CBT for 224 children (aged eight to 14 years) with PTSD resulting from sexual abuse. The cognitive behavioral program TF-CBT and a therapeutic treatment alternative (child-centered therapy (CCT)) were manualized and delivered in 12 weekly sessions to parent–child dyads. The TF-CBT program emphasized skills in feeling expression, emotional management, and cognitive abuse processing. The CCT program was an ego-supportive alternative that focused on trust-building and empowerment of the parent–child dyad in processing the abuse. Children who participated in the TF-CBT program demonstrated significantly greater improvement of PTSD abuse associated areas (behavior problems, social problems, shame, depression, and abuse attributions) compared to children in the CCT program. Furthermore, parents also reported less depression and more support of their child as a result of their involvement in the TF-CBT program. The authors conclude that TF-CBT is an effective treatment intervention for children who have experienced sexual abuse. Cohen, Mannarino, and Deblinger (2006) summarize the essential components of their TF-CBT program using the acronym PRACTICE: *psycho-education, parenting skills, relaxation skills, affective modulation skills, cognitive coping and processing skills, trauma narrative* (correcting cognitive distortions and time skew), *in vivo mastery of trauma reminders, conjoint child–parent sessions*, and *enhancing future safety and development*. Preschool-specific CBT has been successfully used to treat preschoolers exposed to traumatic events (Gleason et al., 2007).

Stein et al. (2003) developed Cognitive Behavior Intervention for Trauma in Schools (CBITS) as a group program for use in schools. The program is very similar to TF-CBT, substituting a teacher component for the parent component, and has been demonstrated to be efficacious through the use of several randomized controlled trials.

Eye Movement Desensitization and Reprocessing (EMDR)   The *Eye Movement Desensitization and Reprocessing* (EMDR) technique (Shapiro, 1995) involves evoking a traumatic memory while engaging in a rapid eye tracking task (following the therapist's finger as it moves back and forth). Results from at least two studies, one with Swedish children and one with Japanese children, report positive results in symptom reduction of PTSD in children (Ahmad, Larsson, & Sundelin-Wahlsten, 2007; Chemtob, Nakashima, & Carlson, 2002).

Psychodynamic trauma-focused psychotherapies   Child–parent psychotherapy (CPP; Lieberman & Van Horn, 2005, 2008) is a therapeutic relationship-based intervention that targets children under seven years of age. CPP is based on psychoanalytic, attachment, and trauma theory and attempts to restore trust in the attachment relationship and to modulate stress associated with the trauma. The program has been demonstrated to be successful in randomized clinical trials and with diverse populations.

References

Achenbach, T. M., & Rescorla, L. A. (2001). *Manual for the ASEBA school-age forms and profiles.* Burlington, VT: University of Vermont, Research Center for Children, Youth and Families.

Ahmad, A., Larsson, B., & Sundelin-Wahlsten, V. (2007). EMDR treatment for children with PTSD: Results of a randomized controlled trail. *Nordic Journal of Psychiatry, 61*(5), 349–354.

Ainsworth, M. D., Blehar, M. S., Waters, E., & Wall, S. (1978). *Patterns of attachment: A psychological study of the Strange Situation*. Hillsdale, NJ: Erlbaum.

Allen, B., & Lauterbach, D. (2007). Personality characteristics of adult survivors of childhood trauma. *Journal of Traumatic Stress*, 20(4), 587–595.

Amaya-Jackson, L., & March, J. (1995a). Posttraumatic stress disorder in adolescents: Risk factors, diagnosis and intervention. *Adolescent Medicine*, 6, 251–269.

Amaya-Jackson, L., & March, J. (1995b). Posttraumatic stress disorder. In J. S. March (Ed.), *Anxiety disorders in children and adolescents* (pp. 276–300). New York: Guilford.

American Academy of Child and Adolescent Psychiatry (AACAP). (2005). Practice parameter for the assessment and treatment of children and adolescents with reactive attachment disorder in infancy and early childhood. *Journal of the American Academy of Child and Adolescent Psychiatry*, 44, 1206–1219.

American Academy of Child and Adolescent Psychiatry (AACAP). (2010). Practice parameter for the assessment and treatment of children and adolescent with posttraumatic stress disorder. *Journal of the American Academy of Child and Adolescent Psychiatry*, 49, 414–430.

American Psychiatric Association (APA). (1980). *Diagnostic and statistical manual of mental disorders* (3rd ed.). Washington, DC: Author.

American Psychiatric Association (APA). (2000). *Diagnostic and statistical manual of mental disorders* (4th ed., text revision). Washington, DC: Author.

Baker, D. G., West, S. A., Nicholson, W. E., Ekhator, N., Kasckow, J., Hill, K. K., . . . Geracioti, T. D. (1999). Serial CSF corticotropin-releasing hormone levels and adrenocortical activity in combat veterans with posttraumatic stress disorder. *American Journal of Psychiatry*, 156, 585–588.

Balbernie, R. (2010). Reactive attachment disorder as an evolutionary adaptation. *Attachment and Human Development*, 12, 265–281.

Barkley, R. A. (1997). *Defiant children: A clinician's manual for assessment and parent training* (2nd ed.). New York: Guilford.

Barr, C. S., Newman, T. K., Shannon, C., Parker, C., Dvoskin, R. L., & Becket, M. L. (2003). Rearing condition and the rh5-HTTLPR interact to influence limbic-hypothalamic-pituitary-adrenal axis response to stress in infant macaques. *Biological Psychiatry*, 455, 733–738.

Berton, M. W., & Stabb, D. D. (1996). Exposure to violence and post-traumatic stress disorder in urban adolescents. *Adolescence*, 31, 489–498.

Blaz-Kapusta, B. (2008). Disorders of extreme stress not otherwise specified (DESNOS)–a case study. *Archives of Psychiatry and Psychotherapy*, 2, 5–11.

Bremner, J. D. (1999). Does stress damage the brain? *Biological Psychiatry*, 45, 797–805.

Bremner, J. D., Vythilingan, M., Vermetten, E., Vaccarino, V., & Charney, D. S. (2004). Deficits in hippocampal and anterior cingulate functioning during verbal declarative memory encoding in midlife major depression. *American Journal of Psychiatry*, 161(4), 637–645.

Brewin, C. R. (1996). Cognitive processing of adverse experiences. *International Review of Psychiatry*, 8(4), 333–339.

Briere, J. (1996). *Trauma Symptom Checklist for Children (TSCC)*. Odessa, FL: Psychological Assessment Resources.

Briere, J., Johnson, K., Bissada, A., Damon, L., Crouch, J., Gil, E., . . . Ernst, V. (2001). The Trauma Symptom Checklist for Young Children (TSCYC): Reliability and association with abuse exposure in a multi-site study. *Child Abuse and Neglect*, 25, 1001–1014.

Buckner, J. D., Lopez, C., Dunkel, S., & Joiner, Jr., T. E. (2008). Behavior management training for the treatment of reactive attachment disorder. *Child Maltreatment*, 13, 289–297.

Carlson, N. R. (2008). *Foundations of physiological psychology* (7th ed.). Boston: Pearson.

Carlson, V., Cicchetti, D., Barnett, D., & Braunwald, K. (1989). Disorganized/disoriented attachment relationships in maltreated infants. *Developmental Psychology*, 25, 525–531.

Carrion, V. G., Weems, C. F., Ray, R., & Reiss, A. L. (2002). Towards an empirical definition of pediatric PTSD: The phenomenology of PTSD symptoms in youth. *Journal of the American Academy of Child and Adolescent Psychiatry*, 41, 166–173.

Chaffin, M., Hanson, R., Saunders, B. E., Nichols, T., Barnett, D., Zeanah, C., ... Miller-Perrin, C. (2006). Report on the APSAC Task Force on attachment therapy, reactive attachment disorder, and attachment problems. *Child Maltreatment*, 11(1), 76–89.

Chemtob, C. M., Nakashima, J., & Carlson, J. (2002). Brief treatment for elementary school children with disaster-related posttraumatic stress disorder: A field study. *Journal of Clinical Psychology*, 58(1), 99–112.

Chisholm, K. (1998). A three year follow-up of attachment and indiscriminate friend liness in children adopted from Romanian orphanages. *Child Development*, 69, 1092–1106.

Cloitre, M., Stolbach, B. C., Herman, J. L., van der Kolk, B., Pynoos, R., Wang, J., & Petkova, E. (2009). A developmental approach to complex PTSD: childhood and adult cumulative trauma as predictors of symptom complexity. *Journal of Traumatic Stress*, 22(5), 399–408.

Cloitre, M., Tardiff, K., Marzuk, P. M., Leon, A. V., & Portera, L. (1996). Childhood abuse and subsequent sexual assault among female inpatients. *Journal of Traumatic Stress*, 9, 473–482.

Coates, S., & Gaensbauer, T. J. (2009). Event trauma in early childhood: Symptoms, assessment, intervention. *Child and Adolescent Psychiatric Clinics of North America*, 18(3), 611–626.

Cohen, J. A., Deblinger, E., Mannarino, A. P., & Steer, A. (2004). A multisite, randomized controlled trial for children with sexual abuse-related PTSD symptoms. *Journal of the American Academy of child and Adolescent Psychiatry*, 43(4), 393–402.

Cohen, J. A., Mannarino, A. P., & Deblinger, E. (2006). *Treating trauma and traumatic grief in children and adolescents*. New York: Guilford Press.

Corbin, J. R. (2007). Reactive attachment disorder: A biopsychosocial disturbance of attachment. *Child and Adolescent Social Work Journal*, 24(6), 539–552.

Cornell, T., & Hamrin, V. (2008). Clinical interventions for children with attachment problems. *Journal of Child and Adolescent Psychiatric Nursing*, 21(1), 35–47.

Costello, E. J., Erkanli, A., Fairbank, J. A., & Angold, A. (2002). The prevalence of potentially traumatic events in childhood and adolescence. *Journal of Traumatic Stress*, 15, 99–112.

DeBellis, M. D., Hooper, S. R., & Sapia, J. L. (2005). Early trauma exposure and the brain. In J. J. Vasterling & C. R. Brewin (Eds.), *Neuropsychology of PTSD – biological, cognitive and clinical perspectives* (pp. 153–177). New York: Guilford.

Deblinger, E., Lippmann, J., & Steer, R. (1996). Sexually abused children suffering posttraumatic stress symptoms: Initial treatment outcome findings. *Child Maltreatment*, 1(4), 310–321.

Deblinger, E., McLeer, S. V., Atkins, M. S., Ralphe, D., & Foa, E. (1989). Posttraumatic stress in sexually abused, physically abused and nonabused children. *Child Abuse and Neglect*, 13, 403–408.

Dehon, C., & Sheeringa, M. (2006). Screening for preschool posttraumatic stress disorder with the child behavior checklist. *Journal of Pediatric Psychology*, 31, 431–435.

DeVoe, E. R., Bannon, W. M., & Klein, T. P. (2006). Post-9/11 helpseeking by New York City parents on behalf of highly exposed young children. *American Journal of Orthopsychiatry*, 76(2), 167–175.

DeYoung, A. C., Kenardy, J. A., & Cobham, V. E. (2011). Trauma in early childhood: A neglected population. *Clinical Child and Family Psychology Review*, 14, 231–250.

Edleson, J. L. (1999). The overlap between child maltreatment and woman battering. *Violence Against Women*, 5, 134–154.

Ehlers, A., & Clark, D. M. (2000). A cognitive model of posttraumatic stress disorder. *Behavior Research and Therapy*, 38, 319–345.

Eyberg, S. M., & Boggs, S. R. (1998). Parent–child interaction therapy: A psychosocial intervention for the treatment of young conduct-disordered children. In J. M. Briesmeister & C. S. Schaefer (Eds.), *Handbook of parent training: Parents as co-therapists for children's behavior* (2nd ed.) (pp. 61–97). New York: John Wiley & Sons, Ltd.

Finkelhor, D., Hamby, S. L., Ormrod, R., & Turner, H. (2005). The Juvenile Victimization Questionnaire: Reliability, validity and national norms. *Child Abuse and Neglect*, 29(4), 383–412.

Finkelhor, D., Ormrod, R. K., & Turner, H. A. (2007). Polyvictimization and trauma in a national longitudinal cohort. *Development and Psychopathology*, 19, 149–166.

Foa, E. B., & Kozak, M. J. (1986). Emotional processing of fear: Exposure to corrective information. *Psychological Bulletin*, 99, 220–235.

Ford, J. D. (1999). Disorders of extreme stress following war-zone military trauma: Associated features of posttraumatic stress disorder or comorbid but distinct syndromes? *Journal of Consulting and Clinical Psychology*, 67, 3–12.

Gaensbauer, T. J. (2002). Representations of trauma in infancy: Clinical and theoretical implications for the understanding of early memory. *Infant Mental Health Journal*, 23(3), 259–277.

Giaconia, R. M., Reinherz, H. Z., Silverman, A. B., Pakiz, B., Frost, A. K., & Cohen, E. (1994). Ages of onset of psychiatric disorders in a community population of older adolescents. *Journal of the American Academy of Child and Adolescent Psychiatry*, 33, 706–717.

Gleason, M. M., Egger, J. L., Emslie, G. H., Greenhill, L. L., Kowatch, R. A., Lieberman, J., ... Scheeringa, M. (2007). Psychopharmacological treatment for very young children: Contexts and guidelines. *Journal of the American Academy of Child and Adolescent Psychiatry*, 46, 1532–1572.

Gleason, M. M., Fox, N. A., Drury, S., Smyke, A., Egger, H., Nelson, C. Gregas, M. C., & Zeanah, C. H. (2011). Validity of evidence-derived criteria for reactive attachment disorder: Indiscriminately social/disinhibited and emotionally withdrawn/inhibited types. *Journal of the American Academy of Child and Adolescent Psychiatry*, 50(3), 216–231.

Goldberg, L. R. (1992). The development of markers for the Big-Five factor structure. *Psychological Assessment*, 4, 26–42.

Graham-Bermann, S. A., Howell, K., Habarath, J., Krishnan, S., Loree, A., & Bermann, E. A. (2008). Toward assessing traumatic events and stress symptoms in preschool children from low-income families. *American Journal of Orthopsychiatry*, 78(2), 220–228.

Gunnar, M. R., & Quevedo, K. (2007). The neurobiology of stress and development. *Annual Review of Psychology*, 58, 145–173.

Hall, C. (2007). *Reactive Attachment Disorder Checklist – RAD-C*. Greenville, NC: Department of Psychology, East Carolina University.

Hardy, L. T. (2007). Attachment theory and reactive attachment disorder: Theoretical perspectives and treatment implications. *Journal of Child and Adolescent Psychiatric Nursing*, 20(1), 27–39.

Hariri, A. (2002). Serotonin transporter genetic variation and the response of the human amygdale. *Science*, 297, 400–403.

Herman, J. (1997). *Trauma and recovery: The aftermath of violence from domestic abuse to political terror*. New York: Basic Books.

Hinshaw-Fuselier, S., Boris, N. W., & Zeanah, C. H. (1999). Reactive attachment disorder in maltreated twins. *Infant Mental Health Journal*, 20, 42–59.

Horowitz, K., Weine, S., & Jekel, J. (1995). PTSD symptoms in urban adolescent girls: Compounded community trauma. *Journal of the American Academy of Child and Adolescent Psychiatry*, 34, 1353–1361.

Howe, M. L., Toth, S. L., & Cicchetti, D. (2006). Memory and developmental psychopathology. In D. Cicchetti & D. H. Cohen (Eds.), *Developmental psychopathology, Vol. 2: Developmental neuroscience* (2nd ed.) (pp. 629–655). Hoboken, NJ: John Wiley & Sons, Ltd.

Huang-Storms, L., Bodenhamer-Davis, E., Davis, R., & Dunn, J. (2007). QEEG-guided neurofeedback for children with histories of abuse and neglect: Neurodevelopmental rationale and pilot study. *Journal of Neurotherapy*, 10(4), 3–19.

Jaffee, S. R., Caspi, A., Moffitt, T. E., Dodge, K. A., Rutter, M., & Taylor, A. (2005). Nature x nurture: Genetic vulnerabilities interact with physical maltreatment to promote conduct problems. *Developmental Psychopathology*, 17, 67–84.

Kemph, J., & Voeller, K. (2008). Reactive attachment disorder in adolescence. In L. Flaherty (Ed.), *Adolescent psychiatry*, vol. 30 (pp. 159–178). New York: Analytic Press/Taylor and Francis Group.

Kilpatrick, D. G., Ruggiero, K. J., Acierno, R., Saunders, B. E., Resnick, H. S., & Best, C. L. (2003). Violence and risk of PTSD, major depression, substance abuse/dependence, and comorbidity: Results from the National Survey of Adolescents. *Journal of Consulting and Clinical Psychology*, 71(4). 692–700.

Kira, I., Lewandowski, L., Somers, C. L., Yoon, J. S., & Chiodo, L. (2012). The effects of trauma types, cumulative trauma and PTSD on IQ in two highly traumatized adolescent groups. *Psychological Trauma, Theory, Research, Practice and Policy*, 4, 128–139.

Kiser, L. J., Heston, J., Millsap, P. A., & Pruitt, D. B. (1991). Physical and sexual abuse in childhood: Relationship with post-traumatic stress disorder. *Journal of the American Academy of Child and Adolescent Psychiatry*, 30, 776–783.

Klein, T. P., DeVoe, E. R., Miranda-Julian, C., & Linas, K. (2009). Young children's responses to September 11th: The New York City experience. *Infant Mental Health Journal*, 30(1), 1–22.

Koch, W. J., & Haring, M. (2008). Posttraumatic stress disorder. In M. Hersen & J. Rosqvist (Eds.), *Handbook of psychological assessment, case conceptualization and treatment, Vol.1: Adults* (pp. 263–290). Hoboken, NJ: John Wiley & Sons, Ltd.

Lachar, D., & Gruber, C. P. (1995). *Personality Inventory for Youth (PIY). Manual.* Los Angeles: Western Psychological Services.

La Greca, A. M., Silverman, W. K., Vernberg, E. M., & Prinstein, M. (1996). Symptoms of posttraumatic stress in children after Hurricane Andrew: A prospective study. *Journal of Consulting and Clinical Psychology*, 64, 712–723.

Lieberman, A. F., & Van Horn, P. (2005). *"Don't hit my mommy!" A manual for child–parent psychotherapy with young witnesses of family violence.* Washington, DC: Zero to Three Press.

Lieberman, A. F., & Van Horn, P. (2008). *Psychotherapy with infants and young children: Repairing the effects of stress and trauma on early attachment.* New York: Guilford.

Lieberman, A. F., & Zeanah, C. H. (1999). Contributions of attachment theory to infant parent psychotherapy and other interventions with infants and young children. In P. R. Shaver & J. Cassidy (Eds.), *Handbook of attachment: Theory, research, and clinical applications* (pp. 555–574). New York: Guilford.

Loeb, J., Stettler, E. M., Gavila, T., Stein, A., & Chinitz, S. (2011). The child behavior checklist PTSD scale: Screening for TPSD in young children with high exposure to trauma. *Journal of Traumatic Stress*, 24(4), 430–434.

Lynch, M., & Cicchetti, D. (1998). An ecological-transactional analysis of children and contexts: The longitudinal interplay among child maltreatment, community violence and children's symptomatology. *Development and Psychopathology*, 10, 235–257.

Lyons-Ruth, K. (2008). Contributions of the mother–infant relationship to dissociative, borderline and conduct symptoms in young adulthood. *Infant Mental Health Journal*, 29, 203–218.

Lyons-Ruth, K., Bureau, J., Riley, C. D., & Atlas-Corbett, A. F. (2009). Socially indiscriminate attachment behavior in the strange situation: Convergent and discriminant validity in relation to caregiving risk, later behavior problems, and attachment insecurity. *Development and Psychopathology*, 21(2), 355–372.

Lyons-Ruth, K., & Jacobvitz, D. (1999). Attachment disorganization: Unresolved loss, relational violence and lapses in behavioral and attentional strategies. In P. R. Shaver & J. Cassidy (Eds.), *Handbook of attachment: Theory, research, and clinical applications* (pp. 520–554). New York: Guilford.

Main, M., & Solomon, J. (1990). Parents' unresolved traumatic experiences are related to infant disorganized attachment status: Is frightening and/or frightened parental behavior the linking mechanism? In M. T. Greenburg, D. Cicchetti, & E. M. Cummings (Eds.), *Attachment in the preschool years* (pp. 161–182). Chicago: University of Chicago Press.

Malmquist, C. P. (1986). Children who witness parental murder: Posttraumatic aspects. *Journal of the American Academy of Child and Adolescent Psychiatry*, 25, 320–325.

March, J., Amaya-Jackson, L., & Pynoos, R. S. (1994). Pediatric posttraumatic stress disorder. In J. W. Weiner (Ed.), *Textbook of child and adolescent psychiatry* (pp. 507–527). Washington, DC: APA.

Margolin, G. (1998). Effects of witnessing violence on children. In P. K. Trickett & C. J. Schellenbach (Eds.), *Violence against children in the family and the community* (pp. 57–101). Washington, DC: APA.

Marx, B. P., Heidt, J. M., & Gold, S. D. (2005). Perceived uncontrollability and unpredictability, self-regulation and sexual revictimizations. *Review of General Psychology*, 9, 67–90.

McDermott, B. M., & Palmer, L. J. (2002). Postdisaster emotional distress, depression and event-related variables: Findings across child and adolescent developmental stages. *Australian and New Zealand Journal of Psychiatry*, 36, 754–761.

McLeer, S., Deblinger, E., Henry, D., & Orvaschel, H. (1992). Sexually abused children at high risk for post-traumatic stress disorder. *Journal of the American Academy of Child and Adolescent Psychiatry*, 32, 875–879.

Meiser-Stedman, R., Smith, P., Glucksman, E., Yule, W., & Dalgleish, T. (2008). The posttraumatic stress disorder diagnosis in preschool and elementary school-age children exposed to motor vehicle accidents. *American Journal of Psychiatry*, 165, 1326–1337.

Minnis, H., Rabe-Hesketh, S., & Wolkind, S. (2002). Development of a brief, clinically relevant, scale for measuring attachment disorders. *International Journal of Methods in Psychiatric Research*, 11(2), 90–98.

Nachmias, M., Gunnar, M., Mangelsdorf, S., Parritz, R., & Buss, K. (1996). Behavioral inhibition and stress reactivity: The moderating role of attachment security. *Child Development*, 67, 508–522.

O'Connor, T. G. (2002). Attachment disorders in infancy and childhood. In M. Rutter & E. Taylor (Eds.), *Child and adolescent psychiatry: Modern approaches* (4th ed.) (pp. 776–792). Oxford: Blackwell.

O'Connor, T. G., Marvin, R. S., Rutter, M., Orlick, J. T., & Britner, P. A. (2003). Child–parent attachment following early institutional deprivation. *Development and Psychopathology*, 15, 19–38.

O'Connor, T., Rutter, M., Beckett, C., Keaveney, L., & Kreppner, J. (2000). English and Romanian adoptee teams. The effects of global severe privation on cognitive competence: Extension and longitudinal follow-up. *Child Development*, 71, 376–390.

O'Connor, T. G., & Zeanah, C. H. (2003). Attachment disorders: Assessment strategies and treatment approaches. *Attachment and Human Development*, 15(3), 223–244.

Prinz, J. P., Sanders, R. S., Shapiro, C. J., Witaker, D. J., & Lutzker, J. R. (2009). Population-based prevention of child maltreatment: The US Triple P system population trial. *Prevention Science*, 10(1), 1–12.

Pynoos, R. S. (1990). Post-traumatic stress disorder in children and adolescence. In B. Garfinkel, G. Carlson, & E. Weller (Eds.), *Psychiatric disorders in children and adolescents* (pp. 48–63). Philadelphia, PA: W.B. Saunders Company.

Pynoos, R. S. (1994). Traumatic stress and developmental psychopathology in children and adolescents. In R. S. Pynoos (Ed.), *Posttraumatic stress disorder: A clinical review* (pp. 64–98). Lutherville, MD: Sidran Press.

Pynoos, R. S., & Nader, K. (1993). Issues in the treatment of posttraumatic stress in children and adolescents. In J. P. Wilson & B. Raphael (Eds.), *International handbook of traumatic stress syndromes* (pp. 535–549). New York: Plenum Press.

Renken, B., Egeland, B., Marvinney, D., Mangelsdorf, S., & Sroufe, L. A. (1989). Early childhood antecedents of aggression and passive-withdrawal in early elementary school. *Journal of Personality*, 57, 257–281.

Russo, N. F., & Tartaro, J. (2008). Women and mental health. In F. L. Denmark and M. A. Paludi (Eds.), *Psychology of women: A handbook of issues and theories* (2nd ed.) (pp. 440–483). Westport, CT: Praeger.

Rutter, M., Beckett, C., Castle, J., Colvert, E., Kreppner, J., Mehta, M., ... Sonuga-Barke, E. (2007). Effects of profound early institutional deprivation: An overview of findings from a UK longitudinal study of Romanian adoptees. *European Journal of Developmental Psychology*, 4(3), 332–350.

Sanders, M., & Pidgeon, A. (2011). The role of parenting programs in the prevention of child maltreatment. *Australian Psychologist*, 46, 199–209.

Sansone, R. A., Sansone, L. A., & Gaither, G. A. (2004). Multiple types of childhood trauma and borderline personality symptomatology among a sample of diabetic patients. *Traumatology*, 10, 257–266.

Scheeringa, M. S. (2008). Developmental considerations for diagnosing PTSD and acute stress disorder in preschool and school-age children. *American Journal of Psychiatry*, 165, 1237–1239.

Scheeringa, M. S. (2009). Posttraumatic stress disorder. In C. H. Zeanah, Jr. (Ed.), *Handbook of infant mental health* (3rd ed.) (pp. 345–361). New York: Guilford.

Scheeringa, M. S., & Zeanah, C. H. (1995). Symptom expression and trauma variables in children under 48 months of age. *Infant Mental Health Journal*, 16(4), 259–270.

Scheeringa, M. S., & Zeanah, C. H. (2001). A relational perspective on PTSD in early childhood. *Journal of Traumatic Stress*, 14(4), 799–815.

Scheeringa, M. S., & Zeanah, C. H. (2008). Reconsideration of harm's way: Onsets and comorbidity patterns of disorders in preschool children and their caregivers following Hurricane Katrina. *Journal of Clinical Child and Adolescent Psychology*, 37(3), 508–518.

Scheeringa, M. S., Zeanah, C. H., Drell, M. J., & Larrieu, J. A. (1995). Two approaches to the diagnosis of posttraumatic stress disorder in infancy and early childhood. *Journal of the American Academy of Child and Adolescent Psychiatry*, 34, 191–200.

Scheeringa, M. S., Zeanah, C. H., Myers, L., & Putnam, F. W. (2003). Predictive validity in a prospective follow-up of PTSD in preschool children. *Journal of the American Academy of Child and Adolescent Psychiatry*, 44(9), 561–570.

Schwartz, E., & Davis, A. S. (2006). Reactive attachment disorder: Implications for school readiness and school functioning. *Psychology in the Schools*, 43(4), 471–479.

Shapiro, F. (1995). *Eye movement desensitization and reprocessing: Basic principles, protocols and procedures*. New York: Guilford.

Shaw, J., Applegate, B., & Schorr, C. (1996). Twenty-one-month follow-up study of school-age children exposed to Hurricane Andrew. *Journal of the American Academy of Child and Adolescent Psychiatry*, 35, 359–364.

Sheperis, C. J., Doggett, R. A., Hoda, N. E., Blanchard, T., Renfro-Michel, E. L., Holdiness, S. & Schlagheck, R. (2003). The development of an assessment protocol for reactive attachment disorder. *Journal of Mental Health Counseling*, 25(4), 291–310.

Shin, L. M., Wright, C. L., Cannistraro, P. A., Wedig, M. M., McMullin, K., & Martis, B. (2005). A functional magnetic resonance imaging study of amygdale and medial prefrontal cortex responses to overtly presented fearful faces in posttraumatic stress disorder. *Archives of General Psychiatry*, 62(3), 273–281.

Smyke, A. T., Dumitrescu, A., & Zeanah, C. H. (2002). Disturbances of attachment in young children: 1. The continuum of caretaking casualty. *Journal of the American Academy of Child and Adolescent Psychiatry*, 41, 972–982.

Stein, B. D., Jaycox, L., Kataoka, S. H., Wong, M., Tu, W., Elliott, M., & Fink, A. (2003). A mental health intervention for school children exposed to violence: A randomized controlled trial. *Journal of the American Medical Association*, 290(5), 603–611.

Terr, L. C. (1991). Childhood traumas: An outline and overview. *American Journal of Psychiatry*, 148, 10–20.

Thrall, E. E., Hall, C. W., Golden, J. A., & Sheafer, B. L. (2009). Screening measures for children and adolescents with reactive attachment disorder. *Behavioral Development Bulletin*, 15, 4–10.

Tizard, B., & Rees, J. (1975). The effect of early institutional rearing on the behaviour problems and affectional relationships of four-year-old children. *Journal of Child Psychology and Psychiatry*, 16(1), 61–73.

Troy, M., & Sroufe, L. A. (1989). Victimization among preschoolers: Role of attachment relationship history. *Journal of the American Academy of Child and Adolescent Psychiatry*, 26, 166–172.

Turner, H. A., Finkelhor, D., & Ormrod, R. (2010). Poly-victimization in a national sample of children and youth. *American Journal of Preventive Medicine*, 38, 323–330.

van der Kolk, B. A., & Pynoos, R. S. (2009). Proposal to include developmental trauma disorder diagnosis for children in the DSM-V. Retrieved from http://www.cathymalchiodi .com/dtd_nctsn.pdf

Webster-Stratton, C., & Reid, M. J. (2003). The Incredible Years Parents, Teachers, and Children Training Series: A multifaceted treatment approach for young children with conduct problems. In A. E. Kazdin & J. R. Weisz (Eds.), *Evidence-based psychotherapies for children and adolescents* (pp. 224–240). New York: Guilford.

Weems, C., Saltzman, K. M., Reiss, A. L., & Carrion, V. G. (2003). A prospective test of the association between hyperarousal and emotional numbing in youth with a history of traumatic stress. *Journal of Clinical Child and Abnormal Psychology*, 32, 166–171.

Yehuda, R., & Bierer, L. K. (2007). Transgenerational transmission of cortisol and PTSD risk. *Progress in Brain Research*, 167, 121–135.

Zeanah, C. H. (2000). Disturbances of attachment in young children adopted from institutions. *Journal of Developmental and Behavioral Pediatrics*, 21, 230–236.

Zeanah, C. H., & Smyke, A. T. (2008). Attachment disorders in family and social context. *Infant Mental Health Journal*, 29(3), 219–233.

Zeanah, C. H., Smyke, A. T., & Dumitrescu, A. (2002). Attachment disturbances in young children. II: Indiscriminate behavior and institutional care. *Journal of the American Academy of Child and Adolescent Psychiatry*, 41, 983–989.

Zeanah, C. H., Smyke, A. T., Koga, S., Carlson, E., & The BEIP Core Group (2005). Attachment in institutionalized and community children in Romania. *Child Development*, 76, 1015–1028.

Zerk, D. M., Mertin, P. G., & Proeve, M. (2009). Domestic violence and maternal reports of young children's functioning. *Journal of Family Violence*, 24(7), 423–432.

Zero to Three. (2005). Diagnostic classification of mental health and developmental disorders of infancy and early childhood (revised ed.). Washington, DC: Author.

Index

Printed and bound by CPI Group (UK) Ltd, Croydon, CR0 4YY

17/04/2025

14658912-0001